Solutions Manual

to Accompany

PHYSICAL CHEMISTRY

Second Edition

Not For Resale
THIS IS A FREE BOOK
www.bookthing.org
THIS BOOK THING OF BALTIMORE, INC.

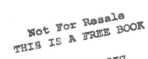

Solutions Manual

to Accompany

PHYSICAL CHEMISTRY

Second Edition

Joseph H. Noggle
University of Delaware

John M. Pope

Juliana G. Serafin

Scott, Foresman and Company
Glenview, Illinois   London, England

ISBN 0-673-39818-8

Printed in the United States of America.

123456-EBI-949392919089

Contents

1 Properties of Matter 1

2 The First Law of Thermodynamics 28

3 The Second Law of Thermodynamics 56

4 Equilibrium in Pure Substances 86

5 Statistical Thermodynamics 106

6 Chemical Reactions 143

7 Solutions 186

8 Ionic Solutions 209

9 Transport Properties 249

10 Chemical Kinetics 268

11 Quantum Theory 311

12 Atoms 342

13 Diatomic Molecules 374

14 Polyatomic Molecules 407

15 Statistical Mechanics 439

16 Structure of Condensed Phases 450

1

Properties of Matter

1.1 Dry air is roughly 79% N_2 and 21% O_2 by volume. Calculate its average molecular weight and density at STP using the ideal gas law.

$$\overline{M}_{air} = \text{average molecular weight} = 0.79M_{N_2} + 0.21M_{O_2}$$

$$\overline{M}_{air} = 0.79(28.013\ g) + 0.21(31.999\ g) = 28.85\ g\ .$$

The density is given by Eq. (1.1c)

$$\rho = \frac{P\overline{M}}{RT} = \frac{(101325\ Pa)(28.85\ g)}{(8.3145\ J\ K^{-1})(273.15\ K)} = 1287\ g\ m^{-3}$$

$$\rho = 0.001287\ g\ cm^{-3}\ .$$

1.2 Use the van der Waals equation to calculate the pressure exerted by SO_2 at 500 K if the density is 100 g/dm^3.

From Eqs. (1.1b) and (1.1c),

$$V_m = \frac{M}{\rho} = \frac{64.06\ g}{100\ g\ dm^{-3}} = 0.6406\ dm^3\ .$$

The van der Waals Eq. (1.3) is:

$$P = \frac{RT}{V_m - b} - \frac{a}{V_m^2}$$

$$P = \frac{(0.08206\ dm^3\ atm\ K^{-1})(500K)}{(0.6406\ dm^3 - 0.0564\ dm^3)} - \frac{(6.71\ dm^6\ atm)}{(0.6406\ dm^3)^2} = 53.9\ atm\ .$$

1.3 Calculate the molecular diameter (σ) of CO_2 from its van der Waals constant.

From Eq. (1.4), $\sigma = \left(\frac{3b}{2\pi L}\right)^{1/3}$. Using data from Table 1.1,

$$\sigma = \left(\frac{3(0.0427\ \text{dm}^3)}{2\pi(6.02214 \times 10^{23})}\right)^{1/3} = 3.23 \times 10^{-9}\ \text{dm} .$$

1.4 Calculate the pressure exerted by 3.00 moles of CO_2 in a 2.00-dm^3 container at 400 K using (a) ideal gas, (b) van der Waals, (c) Redlich-Kwong equations.

a) From the ideal gas law, $P = \frac{nRT}{V}$ so that

$$P = \frac{(3.00\ \text{mol})(0.08206\ \text{dm}^3\ \text{atm mol}^{-1}\ \text{K}^{-1})(400\text{K})}{(2.00\ \text{dm}^3)} = 49.24\ \text{atm} .$$

b) The van der Waals equation is: $P = \frac{nRT}{V - nb} - \frac{n^2a}{V^2}$.

For CO_2, $a = 3.59\ \text{dm}^6\ \text{atm mol}^{-2}$ and $b = 0.0427\ \text{dm}^3\ \text{mol}^{-1}$,

so that

$$P = \frac{(3.00\ \text{mol})(0.08206\ \text{dm}^3\ \text{atm mol}^{-1}\ \text{K}^{-1})(400\ \text{K})}{(2.00\ \text{dm}^3) - (3.00\ \text{mol})(0.0427\ \text{dm}^3\ \text{mol}^{-1})} - \frac{(3.00\ \text{mol})^2(3.59\ \text{dm}^6\ \text{atm mol}^{-2})}{(2.0\ \text{dm}^3)^2}$$

$$P = 44.53\ \text{atm} .$$

c) The Redlich - Kwong equation is:

$$P = \frac{nRT}{V - nb} - \frac{n^2a}{T^{1/2}V(V + nb)} .$$

For CO_2 , $a = 63.64\ \text{dm}^6\ \text{atm K}^{1/2}\ \text{mol}^{-2}$ and $b = 0.02963\ \text{dm}^3\ \text{mol}^{-1}$,

so that

$$P = \frac{(3.00\ \text{mol})(0.08206\ \text{dm}^3\ \text{atm mol}^{-1}\ \text{K}^{-1})(400\ \text{K})}{(2.00\ \text{dm}^3) - (3.00\ \text{mol})(0.02963\ \text{dm}^3\ \text{mol}^{-1})} -$$

$$\frac{(3.00\ \text{mol})^2(63.64\ \text{dm}^6\ \text{atm K}^{1/2}\ \text{mol}^{-2})}{(400\ \text{K})^{1/2}(2.00\ \text{dm}^3)(2.00\ \text{dm}^3 + (3.00\ \text{mol})(0.02963\ \text{dm}^3\ \text{mol}^{-1}))}$$

$$P = 51.53 - 6.85 = 44.68\ \text{atm} .$$

1.5 Calculate the density of CCl_2F_2 at 300°C, 50 atm, using the Redlich-Kwong equation.

The Redlich - Kwong equation may be written as:

$$P = \frac{RT}{V_m - b} - \frac{a}{T^{1/2}\ V_m(V_m + b)} .$$

This may be rearranged to:

$$V_m = \frac{RT}{P + \dfrac{a}{T^{1/2}\ V_m(V_m + b)}} + b .$$

For CCl_2F_2 , $a = 206.4\ \text{dm}^6\ \text{atm K}^{1/2}\ \text{mol}^{-2}$ and $b = 0.06744\ \text{dm}^3\ \text{mol}^{-1}$. Estimate $V_m^{(1)}$ from the ideal gas law:

$$V_m^{(1)} = \frac{RT}{P} = \frac{(0.08206\ \text{dm}^3\ \text{atm mol}^{-1}\ \text{K}^{-1})(573.15\ \text{K})(1\ \text{mol})}{(50\ \text{atm})}$$

$$V_m^{(1)} = 0.941\ \text{dm}^3 .$$

Now use this value in the right-hand side of the Redlich - Kwong equation to find: $V_m^{(2)} = 0.863\ \text{dm}^3$. Similarly, $V_m^{(3)} = 0.842\ \text{dm}^3$, $V_m^{(4)} = 0.835\ \text{dm}^3$, and $V_m^{(5)} = 0.833\ \text{dm}^3$. The density is the reciprocal of the molar volume times the molecular weight:

$$\rho = \frac{M}{V_m} = (1.201\ \text{mol/dm}^3)(1\ \text{dm}/10\ \text{cm})^3(120.91\ \text{g/mol}).$$

$$\rho = 0.145\ \text{g/cm}^3 .$$

1.6 Calculate the molar volume of CH_4 at 298 K and 10.0 atm using (a) ideal gas, (b) van der Waals equation, (c) Redlich-Kwong equation.

a) From Eq. (1.1b),

$$V_m = \frac{RT}{P} = \frac{(0.08206\ dm^3\ atm\ mol^{-1}\ K^{-1})(298\ K)(1\ mol)}{(10\ atm)} = 2.445\ dm^3.$$

b) Start with Eq. (1.9), $V_m = \dfrac{RT}{P + \left(\dfrac{a}{V_m^2}\right)} + b$. Use the ideal gas solution from part a) to find the right-hand side and continue iterating: $V_m^{(1)} = 2.445\ dm^3$, $V_m^{(2)} = 2.399\ dm^3$, $V_m^{(3)} = 2.396\ dm^3$, $V_m^{(4)} = 2.396\ dm^3$.

c) The Redlich - Kwong equation may be written as:

$$V_m = \frac{RT}{P + \dfrac{a}{T^{1/2}\ V_m(V_m + b)}} + b\ .$$

For CH_4, $a = 31.52\ dm^3\ atm\ K^{1/2}\ mol^{-2}$ and $b = 0.02959\ dm^3\ mol^{-1}$.

Use $V_m^{(1)} = 2.445\ dm^3$.

$$V_m^{(2)} = (0.08206\ dm^3\ atm\ mol^{-1}\ K^{-1})(298\ K)(1\ mol) \times \left[10\ atm + \frac{31.52\ dm^3\ atm\ K^{1/2}\ mol^{-2}}{(298\ K)^{1/2}(2.445\ dm^3\ mol^{-1})[(2.445 + 0.02959)\ dm^3\ mol^{-1}]}\right]^{-1}$$

$$+ (0.02959\ dm^3\ mol^{-1})(1\ mol)$$

$V_m^{(2)} = 2.403\ dm^3$.

Similarly, $V_m(3) = 2.402\ dm^3$, and the iteration has converged.

1.7 Use the van der Waals equation to calculate the volume occupied by 100 grams of NH_3 at 300 K, 7.00 atm.

With a molecular weight of 17.03, 100 g of NH_3 = 5.87 mol .

From the van der Waals equation, we find:

$$V = \frac{nRT}{P + \left(\frac{n^2a}{V^2}\right)} + nb \ .$$

Use the ideal gas law to estimate:

$$V^{(1)} = \frac{nRT}{P} = \frac{(5.87\ \text{mol})(0.08206\ \text{dm}^3\ \text{atm mol}^{-1}\ \text{K}^{-1})(300\ \text{K})}{(7.0\ \text{atm})}$$

$$V^{(1)} = 20.65\ \text{dm}^3 \ .$$

Use this value with $a = 4.17\ \text{dm}^6\ \text{atm mol}^{-2}$ and $b = 0.0371\ \text{dm}^3\ \text{mol}^{-1}$ in the van der Waals equation to find:

$$V^{(2)} = 19.91\ \text{dm}^3 \ .$$

Similarly, $V^{(3)} = 19.85\ \text{dm}^3$, $V^{(4)} = 19.84\ \text{dm}^3$ and the iteration has converged.

1.8 Show that the Dieterici equation is mathematically similar to the van der Waals equation at high temperatures or low densities (i.e., when $a/RTV_m \ll 1$).

The Dieterici equation is: $P = \frac{RT}{V_m - b} \exp\left(-\frac{a}{RTV_m}\right)$. The exponential term may be expanded in a Taylor series (Appendix A1.2) so that: $P = \frac{RT}{V_m - b}\left[1 - \frac{a}{RTV_m} + \frac{1}{2}\left(\frac{a}{RTV_m}\right)^2 \cdots\right]$. If $\frac{a}{RTV_m} \ll 1$, then: $P \cong \frac{RT}{V_m - b}\left(1 - \frac{a}{RTV_m}\right) = \frac{RT}{V_m - b} - \frac{a}{V_m(V_m - b)}$.

This is similar to the van der Waals equation:

$$P = \frac{RT}{V_m - b} - \frac{a}{V_m^2} \ .$$

1.9 The data below for acetylene at 25°C give the PV product divided by P_0V_0 (at 0°C and 1 atm). Use a graphical or least-squares method to determine P_0V_0 and the second virial coefficient at this temperature.

P/atm	(PV/P_0V_0)	P/atm	(PV/P_0V_0)
0.5	1.0989	6	1.0531
1	1.0937	8	1.0385
2	1.0841	10	1.0255
4	1.0684	12	1.0139

From Eq. (1.13), $PV \cong RT + BP$. Dividing by P_0V_0 gives:

$\frac{PV}{P_0V_0} = \frac{RT}{P_0V_0} + P\left(\frac{B}{P_0V_0}\right)$. Regressing $\frac{PV}{P_0V_0}$ vs. P yields

slope $= \frac{B}{P_0V_0} = -7.4227 \times 10^{-3} \pm 2.0258 \times 10^{-4}$ and

intercept $= \frac{RT}{P_0V_0} = 1.0999 \pm 0.0014$. Then

$P_0V_0 = 22.243$ dm^3 atm mol^{-1} and $B = -0.165$ dm^3 mol^{-1}.

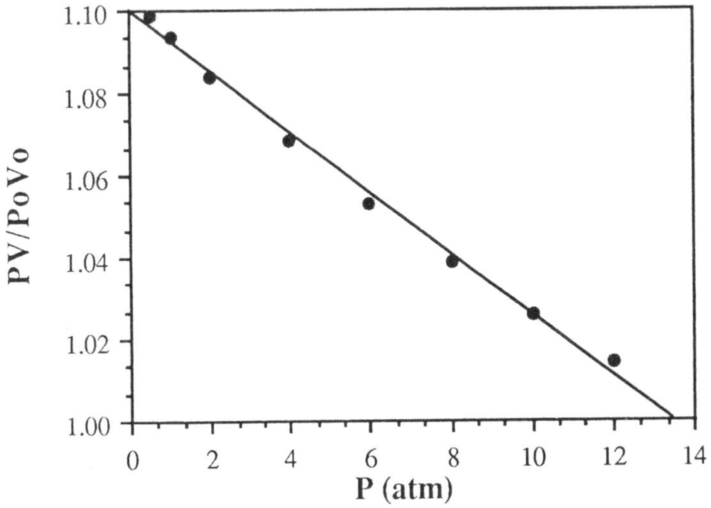

1.10 Use the measured compressibility factors given below for methane at 203 K to calculate the second virial coefficient. You could also get an estimate of the third virial coefficient (C) from these data.

P/atm	z
1	0.9940
10	0.9370
20	0.8683
30	0.7928

From Eqs. (1.10) and (1.11), $V_m(z - 1) = B + \frac{C}{V_m}$ with $V_m = \frac{zRT}{P}$. A plot of $V_m(z - 1)$ vs. $\frac{1}{V_m}$ gives slope = C = 0.0038 dm^6 and intercept = B = -0.100 $dm^3\ mol^{-1}$.

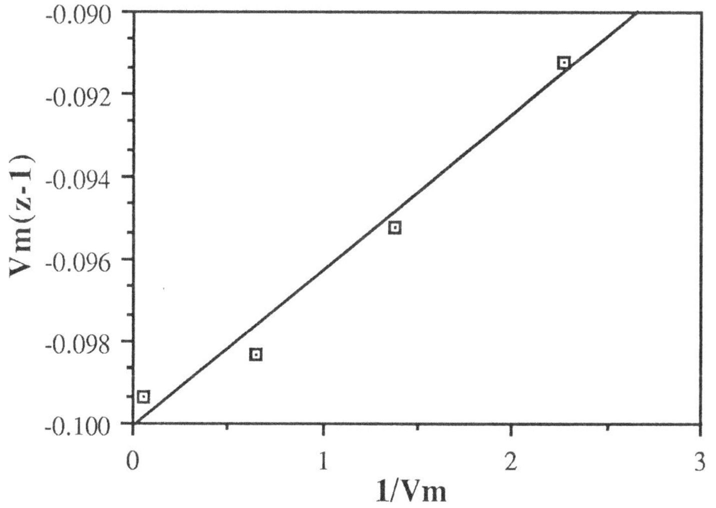

1.11 The virial coefficients [for Eq. (1.13)] of hydrogen at 223 K are given below (PV in dm^3 atm); use them to calculate the compressibility of this gas at 50 atm.

$B = 1.2027 \times 10^{-2}$ $\delta = -1.741 \times 10^{-8}$

$\gamma = 1.164 \times 10^{-5}$ $\varepsilon = 1.022 \times 10^{-11}$

Rearrange Eq. (1.13) to $z = 1 + \frac{BP}{RT} + \frac{\gamma P^2}{RT} + \frac{\delta P^3}{RT} + \frac{\xi P^4}{RT}$. Plugging in the data, z = 1.0343 .

1.12   Calculate the second virial coefficient of N_2 at 473.15 K using (a) van der Waals, (b) Beattie-Bridgeman, (c) Berthelot equations. The observed value is 14.76 cm³.

a)   From Eq. (1.18), $B = b - \frac{a}{RT}$.   Using the data of

Table 1.1, $B = 3.3$ cm³ mol⁻¹ for N_2 .

b)   From Eq. (1.16), $B = B_0 - \frac{A_0}{RT} - \frac{C}{T^3}$. Using the data of

Table 1.2, $B = 15.4$ cm³ mol⁻¹ .

c)   For the Redlich - Kwong equation: $B(T) = b - \frac{a}{RT^{3/2}}$. With

$a = 15.31$ dm⁶ atm K$^{1/2}$ mol⁻¹ and $b = 0.02674$ dm³ mol⁻¹ we find

$B(T) = 8.612$ cm³ mol⁻¹.

1.13   Calculate the Boyle temperature of argon using (a) van der Waals and (b) Berthelot forms of the second virial coefficient. (c) Use the Beattie-Bridgeman form of the second virial coefficient to calculate the Boyle temperature of argon. The actual value is 410 K.

a)   From Eq. (1.18), $T_B = \frac{a}{bR}$.   Using the data of Table 1.1,

$$T_B = 509 \text{ K} .$$

b)   From Eq. (1.17), $T_B = \sqrt{6}\, T_C$.   Thus $T_B = 370$ K .

c)   Setting $B(T_B) = 0$, $B(T_B) = B_0 - \frac{A_0}{RT_B} - \frac{C}{T_B^3} = 0$ and

$T_B^3 - \left(\frac{A_0}{RB_0} \right) T_B^2 - \frac{C}{B_0} = 0$.   Using Table 1.2,

$T_B^3 - 400.12\, T_B^2 - 1.5238 \times 10^6$ K³ $= 0$.   The solution is (see

Appendix I of text) $T_B = 409$ K .

1.14 Calculate the Boyle temperature of He using the (a) van der Waals, (b) Berthelot, (c) Beattie-Bridgeman forms for $B(T)$.

a) Same method as 1.13a, $T_B = 17\ \text{K}$.

b) Same method as 1.13a, $T_B = 13\ \text{K}$.

c) Same method as 1.13a, $T_B = 24\ \text{K}$.

1.15 Derive an expression for the second virial coefficient of a gas in terms of the Dieterici constants from Eq. (1.6).

Multiply Eq. (1.6) by $\frac{V_m}{RT}$ to get $z \equiv \frac{PV_m}{RT} = \frac{V_m}{V_m - b}\exp\left(\frac{-a}{RTV_m}\right)$.

Expanding the exponential in a Taylor series,

$z = \frac{V_m}{V_m - b}\left(1 - \frac{a}{RTV_m} + \frac{1}{2}\left(\frac{a}{RTV_m}\right)^2 + \ldots\right)$. Also

$\frac{V_m}{V_m - b} = \frac{1}{1 - \frac{b}{V_m}} = \left(1 + \frac{b}{V_m} + \left(\frac{b}{V_m}\right)^2 + \ldots\right)$. Thus

$$z = \left(1 + \frac{b}{V_m} + \ldots\right)\left(1 - \frac{a}{RTV_m} + \ldots\right)$$

$$z = 1 + \left(b - \frac{a}{RT}\right)\frac{1}{V_m} - \left(\frac{ab}{RT}\right)\frac{1}{V_m^2} + \ldots$$

Comparison to Eq. (1.11) shows $B = b - \frac{a}{RT}$.

1.16 Use the data below to determine the critical constants of Cl_2.

t/°C	Liquid density (g/cm^3)	Vapor density (g/cm^3)
98.9	1.115	0.124
104.4	1.087	0.139
110.0	1.057	0.156
115.6	1.025	0.179
121.1	0.989	0.203
126.7	0.949	0.231
132.2	0.894	0.268
137.8	0.814	0.321
143.3	0.599	0.523

Use the method illustrated in Figure 1.4. Calculate

$\rho_{avg} = \frac{1}{2}(\rho_{liq} + \rho_{vap})$ and make the following plot:

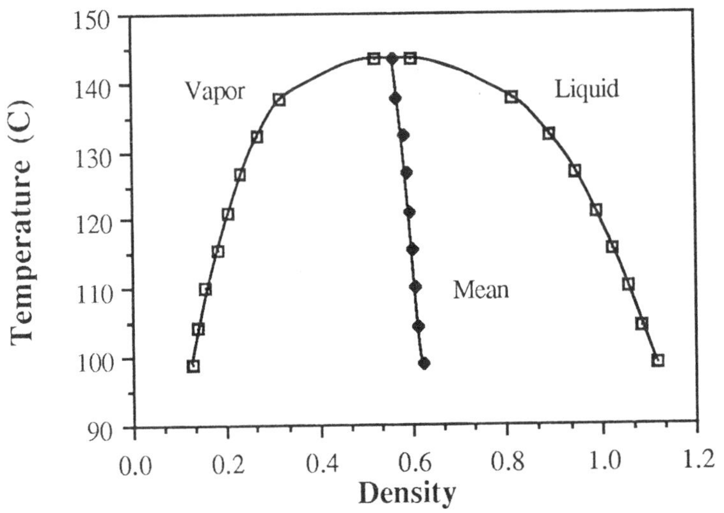

From the plot, the critical point is at $t_c = 144°C$ and

$\rho_c = 0.57\ g/cm^3$. For Cl_2, M = 70.906 g and

$$V_c = \frac{M}{\rho_c} = 124\ cm^3\ mol^{-1}.$$

1.17 Use the Berthelot equation (1.5) at the critical point to derive relationships between the critical constants and the constants a and b.

For Eq. (1.5) at the critical point, $P = \frac{RT_c}{V_c - b} - \frac{a}{T_cV_c^2}$.

$\frac{\partial P_c}{\partial V_c} = \frac{-RT_c}{(V_c - b)^2} + \frac{2a}{T_cV_c^3} = 0$, $\frac{\partial^2 P_c}{\partial^2 V_c} = \frac{2RT_c}{(V_c - b)^3} - \frac{6a}{T_cV_c^4} = 0$. We combine the last two equations to find $V_c = 3b$. Substitute this into $\frac{\partial P_c}{\partial V_c}$ to find $T_c = \sqrt{\frac{8a}{27Rb}}$. Substitute this and $V_c = 3b$ into the expression for P_c, $P_c = \sqrt{\frac{Ra}{216b^3}}$.

1.18 Use the law of corresponding states (Fig. 1.10) to calculate the molar volume of NO at 165 K and 19.5 atm.

From Table 1.1, we have for NO: $T_r = \frac{T}{T_c} = \frac{165}{183} = 0.902$, $P_r = \frac{P}{P_c} = \frac{19.5}{65} = 0.300$. From the "low pressure region" part of Figure 1.10 we find $z = \frac{PV_m}{RT} = 0.83$ so $V_m = \frac{0.83RT}{P} = 0.58\ dm^3$.

1.19 Silicon tetrafluoride (SiF_4) has a critical temperature 259.1 K and critical pressure 36.7 atm. Calculate the van der Waals constants; then use the van der Waals equation to calculate the vapor density of this gas at STP.

From Table 1.4, the van der Waals constants are

$$a = \frac{27R^2T_c^{\,2}}{64P_c} = \frac{27(0.08206\ \text{dm}^3\ \text{atm K}^{-1})^2(259.1\ \text{K})^2}{64(36.7\ \text{atm})} = 5.197\ \text{dm}^6\ \text{atm}$$

$$b = \frac{RT_c}{8P_c} = \frac{(0.08206\ \text{dm}^3\ \text{atm K}^{-1})(259.1\ \text{K})}{8(36.7\ \text{atm})} = 0.0724\ \text{dm}^3\ .$$

Calculating the molar volume with Eq. (1.19) as in problem 1.6 b) with the first $V_m = \frac{RT}{P}$, $V_m^{(1)} = 22.415\ \text{dm}^3$, $V_m^{(2)} = 22.258\ \text{dm}^3$, $V_m^{(3)} = 22.254\ \text{dm}^3$, and $V_m^{(4)} = 22.254\ \text{dm}^3$.

The density is $\rho = \frac{M}{V} = \frac{104.079\ \text{g}}{22.254\ \text{dm}^3} = 4.679\ \text{g/dm}^3$.

1.20 (a) Calculate the Dieterici constants of methane from the critical constants.
(b) Use these constants to calculate the pressure of methane when $T = 270$ K, $V_m = 0.1$ dm^3.
(c) Use successive approximations and the Dieterici equation to calculate V_m when $P =$ 10 atm and $T = 270$ K.

a) From Table 1.4, the Dieterici constants are

$$a = \frac{4R^2T_c^{\,2}}{e^2P_c} = \frac{4(0.08206\ \text{dm}^3\ \text{atm K}^{-1})^2(190.6\ \text{K})^2}{e^2(45.8\ \text{atm})} = 2.891\ \text{dm}^6\ \text{atm}$$

$$b = \frac{RT_c}{e^2P_c} = \frac{(0.08206\ \text{dm}^3\ \text{atm K}^{-1})(190.6\ \text{K})}{e^2(45.8\ \text{atm})} = 0.04622\ \text{dm}^3\ .$$

b) From Eq. (1.6), $P = \frac{RT}{V_m - b}\exp\left(\frac{-a}{RTV_m}\right) = 111.7$ atm .

c) Rewriting Eq. (1.6) as $V_m = \frac{RT}{P}\exp\left(\frac{-a}{RTV_m}\right) + b$, we solve this as we did in problem 1.6 b), with $V_m^{(1)} = \frac{RT}{P} = 2.216\ \text{dm}^3$

as a first approximation. Then $V_m^{(2)} = 2.135\ dm^3$,

$V_m^{(3)} = 2.130\ dm^3$, $V_m^{(4)} = 2.130\ dm^3$.

1.21 Calculate the number density n^* of an ideal gas at 298 K and 1 atm.

From Eq. (1.22b), the number density is

$$n^* = \frac{PL}{RT} = \frac{(1\ atm)(6.02214 \times 10^{23})}{(0.08206\ dm^3\ atm\ K^{-1})(298\ K)} = 2.463 \times 10^{19}\ cm^{-3} .$$

1.22 Calculate the number of collisions which hydrogen molecules would make with 1 cm^2 of a wall in one second at 150 K and a pressure of (a) 1 torr, (b) 1 atm.

a) From Eq. (1.22b),

$$n^* = \frac{PL}{RT} = \frac{\left(\frac{1}{760}\ atm\right)(6.02214 \times 10^{23})}{(0.08206\ dm^3\ atm\ K^{-1})(150\ K)} = 6.437 \times 10^{16}\ cm^{-3} .$$

From Eq. (1.33),

$$z_{wall} = n^*\left(\frac{RT}{2\pi M}\right)^{1/2}$$

$$z_{wall} = (6.437 \times 10^{16}\ cm^{-3})\left(\frac{8.3145 \times 10^7\ erg\ K^{-1}(150\ K)}{2\pi(2.016\ g)}\right)^{1/2}$$

$$z_{wall} = 2.02 \times 10^{21}\ cm^{-2}\ s^{-1} .$$

b) At P = 1 atm , $n^* = 4.892 \times 10^{19}\ cm^{-3}$,

$$z_{wall} = 1.54 \times 10^{24}\ cm^{-2}\ s^{-1} .$$

1.23 In a Knudsen experiment, a substance with a molecular weight of 0.210 kg is placed in a cell with a hole of area 3×10^{-5} m^2. At 500 K, the weight lost in 10 minutes is 30 mg. Calculate the vapor pressure of this substance.

$$\mu = \frac{\Delta W}{A\Delta t} = \frac{(3 \times 10^{-5}\ \text{kg})}{(3 \times 10^{-5}\ \text{m}^2)(600\ \text{s})} = 1.67 \times 10^{-3}\ \text{kg m}^{-2}\ \text{s}^{-1}.$$

From Eq. (1.34), the vapor pressure is

$$P = \mu\left(\frac{2\pi RT}{M}\right)^{1/2}$$

$$= 1.67 \times 10^{-3}\ \text{kg m}^{-2}\ \text{s}^{-1}\left(\frac{2\pi(8.3145\ \text{J K}^{-1})(500\ \text{K})}{0.210\ \text{kg}}\right)^{1/2}$$

$$P = 0.589\ \text{kg m}^{-1}\ \text{s}^{-2} = 5.80 \times 10^{-6}\ \text{atm}.$$

1.24 Derive a formula for the speed distribution of a two-dimensional gas. This has application in the study of adsorbed species which may have freedom of motion about the surface of the adsorbent.

Proceed as in 3 dimensions, $f(v_x, v_y) = a^2 e^{-bv_x^2} e^{-bv_y^2} = a^2 e^{-bv^2}$

where $a = \sqrt{\frac{m}{2\pi kT}}$, $b = \frac{m}{2kT}$. Points in velocity space with speeds between v and v + dv will lie within a ring of area $A = 2\pi v dv$, thus

$$f(v)dv = a^2 e^{-bv^2} 2\pi v dv = \frac{mv}{kT} \exp\left(\frac{-mv^2}{2kT}\right)dv \quad \text{in 2-D space.}$$

1.25 Calculate the average and rms speeds of N_2 at 500°C.

From Eq. (1.38), the average speed is

$$\bar{v} = \sqrt{\frac{8RT}{\pi M}} = \sqrt{\frac{8(8.3145\ \text{J K}^{-1})(773.15\ \text{K})}{\pi(0.0280\ \text{kg})}} = 765\ \text{m/s}.$$

From Eq. (1.28),

$$u = \sqrt{\frac{3RT}{M}} = \sqrt{\frac{3(8.3145\ \text{J K}^{-1})(773.15\ \text{K})}{(0.0280\ \text{kg})}} = 830\ \text{m/s}.$$

1.26 Calculate the average, rms, and most probable speeds for CO_2 at 300 K.

From Eq. (1.38),

$$\bar{v} = \sqrt{\frac{8RT}{\pi M}} = \sqrt{\frac{8(8.3145\ \text{J K}^{-1})(300\ \text{K})}{\pi(0.04401\ \text{kg})}} = 380\ \text{m/s}\ .$$

From Eqn (1.28),

$$u = \sqrt{\frac{3RT}{M}} = \sqrt{\frac{3(8.3145\ \text{J K}^{-1})(300\ \text{K})}{(0.04401\ \text{kg})}} = 412\ \text{m/s}\ .$$

$$v_p = \sqrt{\frac{2RT}{M}} = \sqrt{\frac{2(8.3145\ \text{J K}^{-1})(300\ \text{K})}{(0.04401\ \text{kg})}} = 337\ \text{m/s}\ .$$

1.27 Calculate the fraction of molecules in a gas with velocities greater than $3v_p$. The required integral can be done numerically (Appendix I).

The fraction of molecules with speeds in a given interval is $P(v_1 \text{ to } v_2) = \frac{4}{\sqrt{\pi}}\int_{w_1}^{w_2} e^{-w^2} w^2 dw$, Eq. (1.40b), where $w = \frac{v}{v_p}$. For the interval from $w_1 = 3v_p$ to $w_2 = \infty$: $P = \frac{4}{\sqrt{\pi}}\int_{3}^{\infty} e^{-w^2} w^2 dw$. A numerical solution (Appendix I, Simpson's Rule) gives

$$P = 440\ \text{ppm}\ .$$

1.28 Calculate the fraction of molecules in a gas with kinetic energy greater than $10kT$.

A molecule with kinetic energy $E = 10\ kT = \frac{1}{2}mv_0^2$ has

$v_0 = \sqrt{\frac{20kT}{m}}$. The fraction of molecules with $v > v_0$ is given by

Eq. (1.40b), $P(v > v_0) = \frac{4}{\sqrt{\pi}}\int_{w_0}^{\infty} e^{-w^2} w^2 dw$ where

$w_0 = \frac{v}{v_p} = \frac{\sqrt{\frac{20kT}{m}}}{\sqrt{\frac{2kT}{m}}} = \sqrt{10}$. Thus from numerical integration

(Appendix I, Simpson's Rule) $P(v > v_0) = 1.7 \times 10^{-4}$.

1.29 Find the distance r/σ at which the Lennard-Jones potential $U(r)$ is a minimum. Show that the value of $U(r)$ at the minimum is $-\varepsilon$.

$U(r)$ is a minimum when $\frac{dU(r)}{dr} = 0$. From Eq. (1.43),

$U(r) = 4\epsilon\left(\left[\frac{\sigma}{r}\right]^{12} - \left[\frac{\sigma}{r}\right]^{6}\right)$; $\frac{dU(r)}{dr} = 4\epsilon\left(\frac{-12\sigma^{12}}{r_m^{13}} + \frac{6\sigma^6}{r_m^7}\right) = 0$. Thus

$r_{min} = 2^{1/6}\sigma$. It is easily verified that $\frac{d^2U}{dr^2} > 0$, so r is a

minimum . Then $U(r_m) = 4\epsilon\left[\frac{1}{4} - \frac{1}{2}\right] = -\epsilon$.

1.30 Calculate the third virial coefficient (C) of CO at 300 K from its Lennard-Jones constants (Table 1.7).

From Eq. (1.45) and Table 1.7, $T^* = \frac{T}{(\xi/k)} = \frac{300\ K}{100.2\ K} = 2.994$.

From Figure 1.22, we read $C^* = 0.35$. From Eq. (1.48),

$$C = b_0^2 C^* = 1.6 \times 10^{-3}\ dm^6 .$$

1.31 Derive a formula for the second virial coefficient from the Sutherland potential with $n = 6$. Assume $\varepsilon/kT < 1$ so that the exponential can be expanded with $e^x = 1 + x + x^2/2 + x^3/6 + \cdots$ (keep exactly that number of terms).

The Sutherland potential is $\begin{cases} U = \infty & 0 < r < \sigma \\ U = -\epsilon\left(\frac{\sigma}{r}\right)^6 & \sigma < r < \infty \end{cases}$

Using Eq. (1.41) over 2 regions of integration

$$B(T) = 2\pi L\left[\int_0^\sigma r^2\,dr + \int_\sigma^\infty \left(1 - e^{-U/kT}\right)r^2\,dr\right].$$

The first integral is $2\pi L\int_0^\sigma r^2\,dr = \frac{2}{3}\pi L\sigma^3 = b_0$. Expanding the exponential of the second integral

$$2\pi L\int_\sigma^\infty \left(1 - e^{-U/kT}\right)r^2\,dr = -2\pi L\int_\sigma^\infty \left(\frac{\epsilon\sigma^6}{r^4 kT} + \frac{1}{2}\frac{\epsilon^2\sigma^{12}}{r^{10}(kT)^2} + \frac{1}{6}\frac{\epsilon^3\sigma^{18}}{r^{16}(kT)^3} + \ldots\right)dr$$

$$2\pi L\int_\sigma^\infty \left(1 - e^{-u/kT}\right)r^2\,dr = -b_0\left(\frac{\epsilon}{kT} + \frac{1}{6}\left(\frac{\epsilon}{kT}\right)^2 + \frac{1}{30}\left(\frac{\epsilon}{kT}\right)^3 + \ldots\right)$$

thus $B(T) = b_0\left(1 - \frac{\epsilon}{kT} - \frac{1}{6}\left(\frac{\epsilon}{kT}\right)^2 - \frac{1}{30}\left(\frac{\epsilon}{kT}\right)^3 + \ldots\right).$

1.32 Derive Eq. (1.49) for the second virial coefficient of a gas with a square-well potential.

The square well potential is $\begin{cases} U = \infty & 0 < r < \sigma \\ U = -\epsilon & \sigma < r < R\sigma \\ U = 0 & R\sigma < r < \infty \end{cases}$

Proceeding as in problem 1.31, Eq. (1.41) gives

$$B(T) = 2\pi L\left[\int_0^\sigma r^2 dr + \int_\sigma^{R\sigma}\left(1 - e^{-U/kT}\right)r^2 dr\right].$$ Integration gives

$B(T) = b_0\left[1 - (R^3 - 1)\left(e^{\epsilon/kT} - 1\right)\right]$ where $b_0 = \frac{2\pi L\sigma^3}{3}$.

1.33 Name, with examples, four types of molecules or atoms whose interactions would *not* be accurately approximated by the Lennard-Jones potential.

The Lennard - Jones Potential is characterized by the parameters σ (molecular diameter) and ϵ (energy well depth). The equation will work well for approximately spherical, non polar species. Four types of species which would not conform to a Lennard - Jones potential are:

1. Charged atoms or molecules, such as He^+
2. Polar molecules, such as HF
3. Long chain molecules, such as $CH_3(CH_2)_nCH_3$
4. Open-shell species, such as Cl , CH_2 , etc.

1.34 (a) For the square-well potential, find a relationship between the well depth (ε) and the Boyle temperature.
(b) Calculate the Boyle temperature of argon using the potential constants of Table 1.7. Compare this to the value predicted by the Lennard-Jones potential.

a) At the Boyle temperature, for a square well potential

$B(T_B) = b_0[1 - (R^3 - 1)(e^{\epsilon/kT} - 1)] = 0$, or solving for T_B

$$T_B = \frac{\epsilon}{k}\left[\ln\left(1 + \frac{1}{(R^3 - 1)}\right)\right]^{-1}.$$

b) Using data for Ar from Table 1.7,

$$T_B = (69.4\ \text{K})\left[\ln\left(1 + \frac{1}{((1.85)^3 - 1)}\right)\right]^{-1} = 404\ \text{K}.$$ From

Eq. (1.47), for a Lennard - Jones gas

$$T_B = 3.42\ \frac{\epsilon}{k} = 3.42(119.8\ \text{K}) = 410\ \text{K}.$$

1.35 (a) Use the square-well potential constants for nitrogen (Table 1.7) to calculate its second virial coefficients at 223.15 and 473.15 K. These may be compared to the results in Table 1.3.
(b) With the same constants, estimate the Boyle temperature of nitrogen.

a) From Eq. (1.49), $B(T) = b_0[1 - (R^3 - 1)(e^{\epsilon/kT} - 1)]$ or at

T = 223.15 ,

$$B(T) = (45.29 \text{ cm}^3)[1 - ((1.87)^3 - 1)(e^{53.7/223.15} - 1)]$$

$$B(T) = -22.96 \text{ cm}^3 .$$

At T = 473.15 K , $B(T) = 15.14 \text{ cm}^3$.

b) Using the result of problem 1.34,

$$T_B = \frac{\epsilon}{k}\left[\ln\left(1 + \frac{1}{(R^3 - 1)}\right)\right]^{-1} = 53.7 \text{ K}\left[\ln\left(1 + \frac{1}{((1.87)^3 - 1)}\right)\right]^{-1}$$

$T_B = 323.6$ K .

1.36 A mixture of hydrogen and ammonia has a volume at STP of 153.2 cm^3. The mixture is chilled with liquid nitrogen, the remaining gas drawn off; the volume then (again at STP) is 98.7 cm^3. Calculate the mole fraction of ammonia in the original mixture using Amagat's law.

Amagat's law: $V = \sum V_i = V_{NH_3} + V_{H_2}$. Given $V_{H_2} = 98.7 \text{ cm}^3$ and $V_{NH_3} = 153.2 - 98.7 = 54.5 \text{ cm}^3$ and that the mole fraction of NH_3 is $\frac{V_{NH_3}}{V}$, then $X_{NH_3} = \frac{V_{NH_3}}{V} = \frac{54.5}{153.2} = 0.356$.

1.37 Calculate the partial pressure of oxygen and nitrogen in air that has been compressed to 32 atm. Neglect other components.

In air, $X_{O_2} = 0.2095$ and $X_{N_2} = 0.7808$. From Dalton's Law,

$P_i = X_iP$, so that $P_{O_2} = (0.2095)(32\text{ atm}) = 6.704\text{ atm}$ and

$$P_{N_2} = (0.7808)(32\text{ atm}) = 24.99\text{ atm} .$$

1.38 Use Dalton's law to calculate the pressure exerted by a mixture of 7.0 moles of H_2, 3.0 moles of CO_2, and 2.00 moles of NH_3 at $T = 300$ K if the total volume is 0.84 dm^3. (Use the van der Waals equation for the pure gases.)

From Eq. (1.50), $P = \Sigma P_i$. Use the van der Waals eq. to find P_i, $P = \dfrac{nRT}{V - nb} - \dfrac{n^2a}{V^2}$. Using the data from Table 1.1:

Species	a	b	n	P_i
H_2	0.244	0.0266	7.0	246.6
CO_2	3.59	0.0427	3.0	57.9
NH_3	4.17	0.0371	2.0	40.6

Thus $P = P_{H_2} + P_{CO_2} + P_{NH_3} = 345\text{ atm}$.

1.39 Calculate the volume occupied by 7.00 moles of CO and 5.00 moles of H_2O at 700 K and 1000 atm using Amagat's law (use the van der Waals equation for the pure gases).

Amagat's law states $V = \Sigma V_i$. The pure component volumes may be found from Eq. (1.9), using the method illustrated in problem 1.6b. We have $V = \dfrac{nRT}{P + \dfrac{n^2a}{V^2}} + nb$. As a first approximation for the r.h.s. we use $V^{(1)} = \dfrac{nRT}{P} = 0.402\text{ dm}^3$.

Using parameters from Table 1.1 for CO,

$V^{(2)} = 0.556\ dm^3$, . . . , $V^{(5)} = 0.616\ dm^3$. For H_2O,

$V^{(2)} = 0.308\ dm^3$, . . . , $V^{(7)} = 0.238\ dm^3$. Thus

$$V = V_{CO} + V_{H_2O} = 0.854\ dm^3 .$$

1.40 Use the square-well potential constants:

CCl_3F: $b_0 = 117.6\ cm^3$, $\varepsilon/k = 339\ K$, $R = 1.545$

CCl_2F_2: $b_0 = 140.6\ cm^3$, $\varepsilon/k = 345\ K$, $R = 1.394$

to estimate the second virial coefficient of a 50/50 mixture of these gases at 273.15 K and, from that, the compressibility factor of this mixture at STP.

Designate CCl_3F species 1 and CCl_2F_2 species 2 . Using Eq. (1.57),

$$b_{012} = \left(b_{01}{}^{1/3} + b_{02}{}^{1/3}\right)^3/8 = \left((117.6)^{1/3} + (140.6)^{1/3}\right)^3/8$$

$$b_{012} = 128.8\ cm^3 .$$

Also, $\frac{\epsilon_{12}}{k} = \sqrt{\frac{\epsilon_1\epsilon_2}{k^2}} = \sqrt{(339\ K)(345\ K)} = 342\ K$ and

$R_{12} = \frac{(R_1 + R_2)}{2} = \frac{(1.545 + 1.392)}{2} = 1.470$. From Eq. (1.49)

$B(T) = b_0\left[1 - (R^3 - 1)(e^{\epsilon/kT} - 1)\right]$, thus, $B_{12} = -571.4\ cm^3$,

$B_1 = -659.8\ cm^3$, $B_2 = -468.8\ cm^3$. From Eq. (1.54),

$$B = X_1{}^2B_1 + X_2{}^2B_2 + 2X_1X_2B_{12} = (0.5)^2(-659.8) + (0.5)^2\ (-468.8) +$$
$$2(0.5)^2(-571.4)$$

$$B = -567.8\ cm^3 = -0.568\ dm^3 .$$

Since $z \cong 1 + \frac{BP}{RT}$, $z(STP) = 0.9747$.

1.41 Use the Lennard-Jones potential to calculate the second virial coefficient of air at 25°C.

Designate N_2 species 1 and O_2 species 2 . Using Eq. (1.55) and Table 1.7, $\frac{\epsilon_{12}}{k} = \sqrt{\frac{\epsilon_1\epsilon_2}{k^2}} = \sqrt{(95\ K)(117.5\ K)} = 105.7\ K$. From Eq. (1.45), $T_{12}^* = \frac{T}{\left(\frac{\epsilon_{12}}{k}\right)} = 2.82$. B_{12}^* may be read from Figure 1.20, $B_{12}^* = -0.20$. Similarly for N_2 and O_2 $T_1^* = 3.138$, $B_1^* = -0.10$, $T_2^* = 2.537$, $B_2^* = -0.30$. From Eq. (1.45) $B = b_0B^*$. With $b_{012} = \left(b_{01}^{1/3} + b_{02}^{1/3}\right)^3/8 = 60.79\ cm^3$, $B_{12} = -12.16\ cm^3$. Also $B_1 = -6.38$ and $B_2 = -17.37$. With $X_1 = 0.79$ and $X_2 = 0.21$, $B = X_1^2B_1 + X_2^2B_2 + 2X_1X_2B_{12} = -8.8\ cm^3$.

1.42 Use the van der Waals equation for mixed gases to calculate the pressure when 6 moles of CO and 4 moles of H_2 are together in a 5-dm^3 container at 500 K.

Designate CO species 1 and H_2 species 2 . Using Eq. (1.56) and Table 1.1, the van der Waals constants are

$a = a_1^{1/2}X_1 + a_2^{1/2}X_2 = 0.865\ dm^6\ atm\ mol^{-2}$ and

$b = b_1X_1^2 + b_2X_2^2 + 2b_1b_2X_1X_2$, where $b_{12} = \left(b_1^{1/3} + b_2^{1/3}\right)^3/8$.

Then $b_{12} = 0.0328\ dm^3\ mol^{-1}$, $b = 0.0344\ dm^3\ mol^{-1}$. From Eq. (1.3), $P = \frac{nRT}{V - nb} - \frac{n^2a}{V^2} = 84.66\ atm$.

1.43 (a) Use the van der Waals equation for mixed gases to calculate the volume occupied by 3 moles of H_2 and 5 moles of N_2 at 398 K, 10 atm.
(b) What is the partial pressure of H_2?

a) Designate H_2 as species 1 and N_2 as species 2 , so that

$X_1 = 0.375$, $a_1 = 0.244\ dm^6\ atm^{-1}\ mol^{-2}$ and $b_1 = 0.0266\ dm^3\ mol^{-1}$;

$X_2 = 0.625$, $a_2 = 1.39\ dm^6\ atm^{-1}\ mol^{-2}$ and $b_2 = 0.0391\ dm^3\ mol^{-1}$.

For the mixture: $a = (a_1^{1/2}X_1 + a_2^{1/2}X_2)^2$,

$b = (b_1X_1^2 + b_2X_2^2 + 2b_{12}X_1X_2)$ and $b_{12} = (b_1^{1/3} + b_2^{1/3})^3/8$.

The van der Waals equation may be written as:

$V = \dfrac{nRT}{P + \left(\dfrac{n^2a}{V^2}\right)} + nb$. As a first approximation, we find from

the ideal gas law:

$$V^{(1)} = \frac{nRT}{P} = \frac{8(0.08206\ dm^3\ atm\ mol^{-1}\ K^{-1})(398\ K)}{10\ atm} = 26.13\ dm^3 .$$

Using the van der Waals equation, we now find by successive

approximations $V^{(2)} = 26.20\ dm^3$, $V^{(3)} = 26.20\ dm^3$.

b) $P_{H_2} = X_{H_2}P = 0.375(10\ atm) = 3.75\ atm$.

1.44 The specific volume of H_2O (liq.) is given by the following empirical formula:

$$\ln v = -6.70781 + 1.012566 \ln T + \frac{280.663}{T}$$

Derive from this a formula for the coefficient of thermal expansion of water.

From Eq. (1.59), $\alpha \equiv \frac{1}{V}\left(\frac{\partial V}{\partial T}\right)_P = \left(\frac{d(\ln V)}{dT}\right)_P$. Since

$\ln V = -6.70781 + 1.012566(\ln T) + \dfrac{280.663}{T}$, then

$$\alpha = \frac{1.012566}{T} - \frac{280.663}{T^2} .$$

1.45 Derive an expression for the coefficient of thermal expansion of a van der Waals gas.

The van der Waals eq. may be written $T = \left(P + \frac{a}{V_m^2}\right)\left(\frac{V_m - b}{R}\right)$

Then $\left(\frac{\partial T}{\partial V_m}\right)_P = \frac{P}{R} - \frac{a}{RV_m^2} + \frac{2ba}{RV_m^3}$ or $V_m\left(\frac{\partial T}{\partial V_m}\right)_P = \frac{PV_m^3 - aV_m + 2ba}{RV_m^2}$.

Since $\alpha = \frac{1}{V}\left(\frac{\partial V}{\partial T}\right)_P = \left[V_m\left(\frac{\partial T}{\partial V_m}\right)_P\right]^{-1} = \frac{RV_m^2}{PV_m^3 - aV_m + 2ba}$,

substituting into $P = \frac{RT}{V_m - b} - \frac{a}{V_m^2}$ and rearranging gives

$$\alpha = \frac{R(V_m - b)}{RTV_m - 2a\left(\frac{(V_m - b)}{V_m}\right)^2}.$$

1.46 Show that the coefficient of thermal expansion of a gas that obeys the equation of state:

$$V_m = \frac{RT}{P} + B(T)$$

is

$$\alpha = \frac{1}{T}\left\{\frac{RT + TB'P}{RT + BP}\right\}$$

where $B' = dB/dT$.

The coefficient of thermal expansion is defined as:

$\alpha \equiv \frac{1}{V}\left(\frac{\partial V}{\partial T}\right)_P = \frac{1}{V_m}\left(\frac{\partial V_m}{\partial T}\right)_P$. With $V_m = \frac{RT}{P} + B(T)$: $\left(\frac{\partial V_m}{\partial T}\right)_P = \frac{R}{P} + B'$.

Thus: $\alpha = \frac{\frac{R}{P} + B'}{\frac{RT}{P} + B} = \frac{1}{T}\left[\frac{RT + TB'P}{RT + BP}\right]$.

1.47 The volume of water at 500 atm (relative to its volume at STP) is:

40°C:	0.9867
60°C:	0.9967
80°C:	1.0071

(a) Estimate the coefficient of thermal expansion of water at 60°C, 500 atm.
(b) Use these data together with Table 1.9 to estimate the isothermal compressibility at 60°C.

a) The coefficient of thermal expansion is defined as:

$\alpha \equiv \frac{1}{V}\left(\frac{\partial V}{\partial T}\right)_P$. The value of the derivative may be estimated using the formula (Appendix I): $\frac{df}{dx} = \frac{f(x+h) - f(x-h)}{2h}$ thus:

$$\frac{1}{V}\left(\frac{\partial V}{\partial T}\right)_P = \left(\frac{1}{0.9967}\right)\left(\frac{1.0071 - 0.9867}{40\ K}\right) .$$

$$\alpha = 5.12 \times 10^{-4}\ K^{-1}.$$

b) The isothermal compressibility is defined as:

$\kappa_T \equiv -\frac{1}{V}\left(\frac{\partial V}{\partial P}\right)_T \cong -\frac{1}{V}\left(\frac{\Delta V}{\Delta P}\right)_T$. From Table 1.9, the specific volume of water at 60°C and 1 atm is: $V(1\ atm) = 1.0164\ cm^3/g$. The specific volume of water at 60°C and 500 atm is:

$V(500\ atm) = (0.9967)(1.0002\ cm^3/g) = 0.9969\ cm^3/g$. Thus:

$$\kappa_T = -\frac{1}{V}\left(\frac{\Delta V}{\Delta P}\right) = -\frac{(0.9969 - 1.0164)}{(0.9969)(500\ atm - 1\ atm)} .$$

$$\kappa_T(60°C,\ 500\ atm) = 3.920 \times 10^{-5}\ atm^{-1} .$$

1.48 The volume of water (relative to STP) at 40°C is 0.9924 at 1 atm and 0.9867 at 500 atm. Estimate the isothermal compressibility of water at 40°C.

$$\kappa_T \equiv -\frac{1}{V}\left(\frac{\partial V}{\partial P}\right)_T \cong -\frac{1}{V}\left(\frac{\Delta V}{\Delta P}\right)_T = -\frac{1}{V}\left(\frac{V_1 - V_2}{P_1 - P_2}\right) \quad \text{where}$$

$$\bar{V} = \frac{(V_1 + V_2)}{2} = \frac{(0.9924 + 0.9867)}{2} = 0.9896 \text{ . Thus}$$

$$\kappa_T = -\frac{1}{0.9896}\left(\frac{0.9924 - 0.9867}{1 - 500}\right) = 1.15 \times 10^{-5} \text{ atm}^{-1}.$$

1.49 A tube of CCl_4 is warmed until the liquid fills the entire volume. Calculate the pressure exerted on the walls of the tube if the temperature is raised 1°C more.

From Eq. (1.64), $\Delta P \cong \frac{\alpha}{\kappa_T}\Delta T$. Using data from Table 1.8 for CCl_4,

$$\Delta P = \frac{(1.236 \times 10^{-3} \text{ K}^{-1})}{(91.0 \times 10^{-6} \text{atm}^{-1})}(1 \text{ K}) = 13.6 \text{ atm} .$$

1.50 Prove that the coefficient of bulk expansion (α) is three times the coefficient of linear expansion:

$$k = \frac{1}{l}\left(\frac{\partial l}{\partial T}\right)_P$$

From Eq. (1.59), $\alpha = \frac{1}{V}\left(\frac{\partial V}{\partial T}\right)_P$. With $V = l^3$, $\alpha = \frac{1}{l^3}\left(\frac{\partial l^3}{\partial T}\right)_P$ or

$$\alpha = \frac{1}{l^3}\left(3l^2 \frac{\partial l}{\partial T}\right)_P = \frac{3}{l}\left(\frac{\partial l}{\partial T}\right)_P = 3 \text{ K} .$$

1.51 Estimate the molar volume of benzene at 1000 atm from data in Table 1.8.

From Eq. (1.62), $V(P) = V_0[1 - \kappa_T(P - P_0)]$. Using data from Table 1.8,

$$V_m = 89\ \text{cm}^3[1 - (63.5 \times 10^{-6}\ \text{atm}^{-1})(1000 - 1)\text{atm}] = 83\ \text{cm}^3 .$$

1.52 Use the five-point differential formula of Appendix I and the specific volumes in Table 1.9 to calculate the coefficient of thermal expansion of water at 30°C.

Using data from Table 1.9 and Eq. (AI.21c) of Appendix I,

$$\left(\frac{\partial V}{\partial T}\right)_P = \frac{[1.0017 - 8(1.0027) + 8(1.0056) - 1.0074]\text{cm}^3/\text{g}}{(12)(15\ \text{K})}$$

$$\left(\frac{\partial V}{\partial T}\right)_P = 2.9 \times 10^{-4}\ \text{cm}^3\ \text{g}^{-1}\ \text{K}^{-1} .$$

2

The First Law of Thermodynamics

2.1 For He(gas), considered as an ideal gas, calculate q, w, and ΔU if one gram is heated from 300 to 400 K (a) at constant volume, (b) at constant pressure (1 atm).

a) $\Delta U = \int_{T_1}^{T_2} C_v dT = nC_{vm}(T_2 - T_1) = 314$ J. There is no PV - work thus $w = 0$. Since $q = \Delta U - w$, $q = 314$ J.

b) For an ideal gas at constant pressure

$\Delta U = nC_{vm}(T_2 - T_1) = 314$ J. $-w = \int_{V_1}^{V_2} P_{ex} dV$ where

$P_{ex} = P = 1$ atm. Using the ideal gas law,

$$-w = P(V_2 - V_1) = nR(T_2 - T_1) = 208 \text{ J.}$$

$$q = \Delta U - w = 314 \text{ J} + 208 \text{ J} = 521 \text{ J.}$$

2.2 Calculate ΔU for heating one mole of Cl_2(gas) from 400 to 1600 K at constant volume from the data:

T/K	$C_{vm}/(J/K)$
400	26.99
600	28.29
800	28.89
1000	29.19
1200	29.42
1400	29.69
1600	29.78

At constant V, $\Delta U = \int_{T_1}^{T_2} C_{vm} dT$. From Eq. (AI.11b)

$$\int_{T_1}^{T_2} C_{vm} dT = \left[\frac{26.99}{2} + 28.29 + 28.89 + 29.19 + 29.42 + 29.69 + \frac{29.78}{2}\right](200) = 34.77 \text{ J.}$$

2.3 Calculate the heat required to raise the temperature of 50 g CO_2 from 0°C to 1000°C at constant volume using the data:

t/°C	C_{vm}/(J/K)
0	27.74
100	29.95
400	35.49
1000	42.58

At constant volume, $q = \Delta U = n\int_{T_1}^{T_2} C_{vm}dT$. Using the trapezoidal rule for each temperature interval

$$\int_0^{100} C_{vm}dT \cong \frac{1}{2}(27.74 + 29.95)(100 - 0) = 2.885 \times 10^3 \text{ J.}$$

$$\int_{100}^{400} C_{vm}dT \cong 9.816 \times 10^3 \text{ J}, \quad \int_{400}^{1000} C_{vm}dT \cong 23.42 \times 10^3 \text{ J.}$$

Then $q = \left(\frac{50 \text{ g}}{44.01 \text{ g}}\right)(2.885 \times 10^3 \text{ J} + 9.816 \times 10^3 \text{ J} + 23.42 \times 10^3 \text{ J})$

or $q = 4.104 \times 10^4$ J.

2.4 Use the van der Waals relationship:

$$\left(\frac{\partial U}{\partial V}\right)_T = \frac{a}{V_m^2}$$

to calculate ΔU for an isothermal expansion of one mole of Ar from 50 atm to 1 atm, at T = 250 K.

Since $dU = \left(\frac{\partial U}{\partial V}\right)_T dV$ at constant T,

$$\Delta U = \int_{U_1}^{U_2} dU = an^2\int_{V_1}^{V_2} \frac{1}{V^2}\, dV = an^2\left(\frac{1}{V_1} - \frac{1}{V_2}\right).$$

From the van der Waals eq., $V_m = \dfrac{RT}{P + \left(\frac{a}{V_m^2}\right)} + b$. Using the ideal gas law as a first approximation of V_m on the r.h.s., we use successive approximation to get V_{m1}(1 atm) and V_{m2}(50 atm). Thus $V_{m1} = 20.48 \text{ dm}^3$, $V_{m2} = 0.3773 \text{ dm}^3$ and $\Delta U = 355$ J.

2.5 (a) Calculate the internal pressure, $(\partial U/\partial V)_T$, for CCl_4(liquid) at 293 K, 1 atm.
(b) Repeat this calculation for NH_3(gas) at STP (use van der Waals, and V_m = 22264 cm^3).

a) The internal pressure is $\left(\frac{\partial U}{\partial V}\right)_T = T\left(\frac{\partial P}{\partial T}\right)_V - P$ or for a liquid or solid, $\left(\frac{\partial U}{\partial V}\right)_T = T\left(\frac{\alpha}{\kappa_T}\right) - P$. For CCl_4,

$$\left(\frac{\partial U}{\partial V}\right)_T = 293\ K\left(\frac{1.236 \times 10^{-3}\ K^{-1}}{91.0 \times 10^{-6}\ atm^{-1}}\right) - 1\ atm = 403\ MPa.$$

b) For a van der Waals gas, $\left(\frac{\partial U}{\partial V}\right)_T = \frac{a}{V_m^2}$. Thus for NH_3,

$$\left(\frac{\partial U}{\partial V}\right)_T = \frac{4.17\ dm^6\ atm}{(22.264\ dm^3)^2} = 8.41 \times 10^{-3}\ atm = 852\ Pa.$$

2.6 Show that the Redlich-Kwong equation gives:

$$\left(\frac{\partial U}{\partial V}\right)_T = \frac{3a}{2T^{\frac{1}{2}}V_m(V_m + b)}$$

Use the relation: $\left(\frac{\partial U}{\partial V}\right)_T = T\left(\frac{\partial P}{\partial T}\right)_V - P$. For the Redlich - Kwong equation of state: $P = \frac{RT}{V_m - b} - \frac{a}{T^{1/2}V_m(V_m + b)}$

so that $\left(\frac{\partial P}{\partial T}\right)_V = \frac{R}{V_m - b} + \frac{a}{2T^{3/2}V_m(V_m + b)}$. Thus:

$$\left(\frac{\partial U}{\partial V}\right)_T = \frac{3a}{2T^{1/2}V_m(V_m + b)}.$$

2.7 (a) Use the one-term virial equation:

$$P = \frac{RT}{V_m}\left(1 + \frac{B}{V_m}\right)$$

to derive the formula:

$$\left(\frac{\partial U}{\partial V}\right)_T = \frac{RT^2B'}{V_m^2}$$

(b) Evaluate $(\partial U/\partial V)_T$ for CO_2 at STP using the Berthelot virial coefficient; compare this to the van der Waals result [Eq. (2.15)]. (Use V_m = 22.296 dm^3 for both cases.)

a) From Eq. (2.13), $\left(\frac{\partial U}{\partial V}\right)_T = T\left(\frac{\partial P}{\partial T}\right)_V - P$. From the virial equation, $\left(\frac{\partial P}{\partial T}\right)_V = \frac{R}{V_m}\left(1 + \frac{B}{V_m}\right) + \frac{RT}{V_m}\left(\frac{B'}{V_m}\right)$, where $B' = \frac{dB}{dT}$.

Thus $\left(\frac{\partial U}{\partial V}\right)_T = \frac{RT}{V_m}\left(1 + \frac{B}{V_m}\right) + \frac{RT^2}{V_m}\left(\frac{B'}{V_m}\right) - P = \frac{RT^2B'}{V_m^2}$.

b) From Eq. (1.17), $B' = \frac{9RT_c}{128P_c}\left(\frac{12T_c^2}{T^3}\right)$. For CO_2 $B' = 0.0131$ dm^3 K^{-1}. Substituting into the above

$$\left(\frac{\partial U}{\partial V}\right)_T = \frac{(0.08206 \text{ dm}^3 \text{ atm K}^{-1})(273.15 \text{ K})^2(0.0131 \text{ dm}^3 \text{ K}^{-1})}{(22.296 \text{ dm}^3)^2}$$

$$\left(\frac{\partial U}{\partial V}\right)_T = 1631 \text{ Pa.}$$

For the van der Waals result, $\left(\frac{\partial U}{\partial V}\right)_T = \frac{a}{V_m^2}$,

$$\left(\frac{\partial U}{\partial V}\right)_T = \frac{3.59 \text{ dm}^3 \text{ atm}}{(22.296 \text{ dm}^3)^2} = 732 \text{ Pa.}$$

2.8 To 1 kg of argon (considered as an ideal gas), 2000 J of heat is added at constant $P = 1$ atm. Calculate ΔU, ΔH, ΔT, and ΔV of the gas, and the work. (Use $C_{vm} = 1.5R$, $C_{pm} = 2.5R$.)

At constant pressure,

$$\Delta T = \frac{q}{nC_{pm}} = \frac{2000 \text{ J}}{\left(\frac{10^3 \text{ g}}{39.95 \text{ g}}\right)(2.5)(8.3145 \text{ J K}^{-1})} .$$

Thus $\Delta T = 3.84$ K. Since $\Delta U = nC_{vm}\Delta T$, we have

$$\Delta U = \left(\frac{10^3 \text{ g}}{39.95 \text{ g}}\right)(1.5)(8.3145 \text{ J K}^{-1})(3.84 \text{ K}) = 1.20 \times 10^3 \text{ J}.$$

The work at constant pressure will be

$$-w = \int_{V_1}^{V_2} P_{ex}dV = P\Delta V = nR\Delta T = \left(\frac{10^3 \text{ g}}{39.95 \text{ g}}\right)(8.3143 \text{ J K}^{-1})(3.84 \text{ K})$$

or $w = -800$ J. Then $\Delta V = \frac{-w}{P} = \left(\frac{800 \text{ J}}{1\text{atm}}\right)\left(\frac{1 \text{ atm}}{101325 \text{ Pa}}\right) = 7.90 \text{ dm}^3$.

Also, $q = \Delta H = 2000$ J.

2.9 (a) Use the heat capacity from Table 2.2 to calculate ΔH when one mole of Cl_2(gas) is heated from 400 to 800 K at constant pressure.
(b) How much heat must be supplied per gram of the gas to effect this temperature change?

a) Using Eq. (2.27a), $C^{\theta}_{pm} = a + bT + \frac{c}{T^2}$ and Eq. (2.25)

$$\Delta H = n\int_{T_1}^{T_2} C_{pm}dT = n\int_{400}^{800}\left(37.08 + (0.67 \times 10^{-3})T - \frac{2.85 \times 10^{-5}}{T^2}\right)dT$$

$$\Delta H = (1)\left[37.03T + \frac{1}{2}(0.67 \times 10^{-3}T^2) + \frac{2.85 \times 10^5}{T}\right]\Bigg|_{400}^{800} = 14.6 \text{ kJ}.$$

b) heat/gram $= \frac{14600 \text{ J}}{70.90 \text{ g}} = 206$ J/g.

2.10 Calculate ΔH for heating three moles of Al(solid), at constant pressure, from 300 to 600 K. Use heat capacity from Table 2.2.

Using Eqs. (2.27a) + (2.25),

$$\Delta H = n\int_{T_1}^{T_2}\left(a + bT + \frac{c}{T^2}\right)dT = n\left[aT + \frac{bT^2}{2} - \frac{c}{T}\right] .$$

$$\Delta H = 3\left(20.67T + \frac{1}{2}(12.38 \times 10^{-3})T^2\right)\Big|_{300}^{600} = 23.6 \text{ kJ}.$$

2.11 Calculate ΔH for heating one mole of copper from 10 to 100 K at constant pressure from the specific heats below:

T/K	c_p/(J K^{-1} g^{-1})	T/K	c_p/(J K^{-1} g^{-1})
10	0.00086	60	0.137
20	0.0077	70	0.173
30	0.027	80	0.205
40	0.060	90	0.232
50	0.099	100	0.254

At constant pressure: $\Delta H = n\int_{T_1}^{T_2} C_{pm} dT$. Because C_{pm} is a function of T, we use the trapezoidal rule from Appendix AI.4:

$$\int_{x_0}^{x_n} f(x)dz = \left(\frac{f_0}{2} + f_1 + f_2 \ldots f_{n-1} + \frac{f_n}{2}\right)h$$ where h is the interval size.

Thus, with h = 10 K:

$$\int_{T_1}^{T_2} C_{pm} dT = \Delta H = \left[\frac{0.00086}{2} + 0.0077 + 0.027 + 0.060 + 0.099 + 0.137 + 0.173 + 0.205 + 0.232 + 0.254\right] \text{J K}^{-1} \text{g}^{-1} \times (63.546 \text{ g mol}^{-1})(10 \text{ K})$$

$$\Delta H = 679 \text{ J}.$$

2.12 Calculate ΔH for heating 100 g of acetone (CH_3COCH_3) from 57°C to 400°C. Use heat capacity from Table 2.3.

From Table 2.3: $C^{\theta}_{pm} = a' + b'T + c'T^2 + d'T^3 \ (J\ K^{-1})$.

For acetone: $a' = 8.468$

$b' = 269.45 \times 10^{-3}$

$c' = -143.45 \times 10^{-6}$

$d' = 29.63 \times 10^{-9}$

With $\Delta H = \int_{T_1}^{T_2} C_{pm} dT$ we may integrate directly to find:

$$\Delta H = n\left[a'T + \frac{b'T^2}{2} + \frac{c'T^3}{3} + \frac{d'T^4}{4}\right]\Bigg|_{T_1}^{T_2} .$$

Using $n = \dfrac{100\ g}{(58.08\ g\ mol^{-1})} = 1.722\ mol$, $T_1 = 330\ K$ and

$T_2 = 673\ K$: $\Delta H = 37.83\ kJ\ mol^{-1}$.

2.13 From the data table below, calculate ΔH for heating one mole of benzene (solid) from 200 K to its melting point, 278.69 K.

T/K	C_{pm}/(J/K)
200	83.7
240	104.1
260	116.1
278.69	128.7

From Eq. (2.25), $\Delta H = \int_{T_1}^{T_2} C_{pm} dT$. Using Eq. (AI.11a)

$$\int_{200}^{240} C_{pm} dT = \tfrac{1}{2}(83.7 + 104.1)(240 - 200) = 3756\ J.$$

$$\int_{240}^{260} C_{pm} dT = 2202\ J, \quad \int_{260}^{278.69} C_{pm} dT = 2288\ J.$$

Then summing the above, $\Delta H = 8.25\ kJ$.

2.14 Calculate the change in the enthalpy per mole for benzene (liquid) if the pressure is increased by 10 atm at 298 K.

From Eq. (2.24), $dH = nC_{pm}dT + nV_m(1 - \alpha T)dP$. At constant T,

$dH = nV_m(1 - \alpha T)dP$. Assuming V_m and α are constants,

$\Delta H = nV_m(1 - \alpha T)\Delta P$. Using data from Table 1.8,

$$\Delta H = (1)(89\ cm^3)(1 - [1.237 \times 10^{-3}\ K^{-1}][298\ K])(10\ atm).$$

$$\Delta H = (8.9 \times 10^{-5}\ m^3)(0.631)(10\ atm)\left(\frac{101325\ Pa}{1\ atm}\right) = 57\ J.$$

2.15 Calculate the change of the molar enthalpy of argon when it is isothermally compressed at 300 K from 1.0 to 6.0 atm, using T_c = 151 K, P_c = 48.0 atm.

From Eq. (2.29), $dH = n[B - TB']dP$, where $B' = \frac{9RT_c}{128P_c}\left(\frac{12T_c^2}{T^3}\right)$

and $B(T) = \frac{9RT_c}{128P_c}\left(1 - \frac{6T_c^2}{T^2}\right)$. For Ar, $B' = 1.84 \times 10^{-4}\ dm^3\ K^{-1}$,

$B(T) = -0.00944\ dm^3$. Thus,

$$\Delta H = n(B - TB')\Delta P = [-9.44 \times 10^{-3} - (300\ K)(1.84 \times 10^{-4})](5)\ .$$

$$\Delta H = -0.323\ dm^3\ atm = -33\ J.$$

2.16 (a) Show that the Beattie-Bridgeman second virial coefficient gives:

$$B' = \frac{A_0}{RT^2} + \frac{3c}{T^4}$$

(b) Use this result to derive:

$$\left(\frac{\partial H}{\partial P}\right)_T = B_0 - \frac{2A_0}{RT} - \frac{4c}{T^3}$$

(c) Calculate ΔH for the isothermal compression of one mole of Ar at 300 K from 1.0 to 6.0 atm.

a) From Eq. (1.16), $B(T) = B_0 - \frac{A_0}{RT} - \frac{c}{T^3}$, thus $B' = \frac{A_0}{RT^2} + \frac{3c}{T^4}$.

b) From Eq. (2.29), $dH = nC_{pm}dT + n[B - TB']dP$ or

$\left(\frac{\partial H_m}{\partial P}\right)_T = [B - TB']$. Thus,

$$\left(\frac{\partial H_m}{\partial P}\right)_T = B_0 - \frac{A_0}{RT} - \frac{c}{T^3} - T\left(\frac{A_0}{RT^2} + \frac{3c}{T^4}\right)$$

$$\left(\frac{\partial H_m}{\partial P}\right)_T = B_0 - \frac{2A_0}{RT} - \frac{4c}{T^3}.$$

c) $\Delta H = \left(B_0 - \frac{2A_0}{RT} - \frac{4c}{T^3}\right)\Delta P$. Using data from Table 1.2,

$$\Delta H = -38 \text{ J}.$$

2.17 Calculate the molar enthalpy of NH_3 relative to its enthalpy at 25.0°C, 1.00 atm, when $T = 1000$ K, $P = 100$ atm.

We break this process into two steps:

$$(T_1, P_1) \xrightarrow{1} (T_2, P_1) \xrightarrow{2} (T_2, P_2).$$

For the first step we have

$$\Delta H_{1m} = \int_{T_1}^{T_2} C_{pm}dT = \int_{298}^{1000}\left(a + bT + \frac{c}{T^2}\right)dT = \left(aT + \frac{bT^2}{2} - \frac{c}{T}\right)\Bigg|_{298}^{1000}.$$

Using data from Table 2.2, $\Delta H_{1m} = 33.5$ kJ.

In the second step we use Eq. (2.31)

$$\Delta H_{2m} = \frac{9RT_c}{128P_c}\left(1 - \frac{18T_c^2}{T^2}\right)\Delta P \ .$$

Using data from Table 1.1, with $\Delta P = 99$ atm, $\Delta H_{2m} = -412$ J. Thus

$$\Delta H = \Delta H_{1m} + \Delta H_{2m} = 33.1 \text{ kJ}.$$

2.18 (a) Calculate C_{pm} of CH_4 at 51.00°C, $P = 0$ (Table 2.2).
(b) Estimate C_{pm} of CH_4 at 51°C, 10 atm, from its critical constants, $T_c = 190.6$ K, $P_c = 45.8$ atm.

a) 51°C = 324.15 K, so that, from Table 2.2:

$$C^{\theta}_{pm} = 23.67 + (47.86 \times 10^{-3})(324.15) - \frac{1.92 \times 10^5}{(324.15)^2} \ .$$

$$C^{\theta}_{pm} = 37.35 \text{ J K}^{-1} \text{ mol}^{-1} \ .$$

b) $$C_{pm}(T, P) = C^{\theta}_{pm}(T) + \frac{81R}{32}\left(\frac{T_c}{T}\right)^3\left(\frac{P}{P_c}\right) \ .$$

For CH_4, $T_c = 190.6$ K and $P_c = 45.8$ atm, so that

$$C_{pm}(T, P) = 37.35 + \frac{81}{32}(8.3145 \text{ J K}^{-1} \text{ mol}^{-1})\left(\frac{190.6}{324.1}\right)^3\left(\frac{10}{45.8}\right) \ .$$

$$C_{pm}(51°\text{C}, 10 \text{ atm}) = 38.30 \text{ J K}^{-1} \text{ mol}^{-1} \ .$$

2.19 (a) Show that if the Beattie-Bridgeman form of the second virial coefficient is used, the dependence of C_p on pressure is:

$$\left(\frac{\partial C_{pm}}{\partial P}\right)_T = \frac{2A_0}{RT^2} + \frac{12c}{T^4}$$

(b) With constants of Table 1.2, what are the units of this equation?
(c) Calculate C_{pm} of CH_4 at 51°C, 10 atm.

a) From Eq. (2.29), $\left(\frac{\partial H}{\partial P}\right)_T = n[B - TB']$. Since

$\frac{\partial C_P}{\partial P} = \frac{\partial}{\partial P}\left(\frac{\partial H}{\partial T}\right) = \frac{\partial}{\partial T}\left(\frac{\partial H}{\partial P}\right)$, then $\frac{\partial C_P}{\partial P} = \frac{\partial}{\partial T}(n[B - TB'])$. From

Eq. (1.16), $B(T) = B_0 - \frac{A_0}{RT} - \frac{c}{T^3}$ and $B' = \frac{A_0}{RT^2} + \frac{3c}{T^4}$, so

$$\frac{\partial C_P}{\partial P} = n\frac{\partial}{\partial T}\left(B_0 - \frac{2A_0}{RT} - \frac{4c}{T^3}\right) = n\left(\frac{2A_0}{RT} + \frac{12c}{T^4}\right) .$$

b) A_0 has units of atm dm^6, B_0 has units of dm^3 mol^{-1} and c has units of K^3 dm^3 mol^{-1}. Thus $\frac{\partial C_P}{\partial P}$ [=] dm^3 K^{-1}.

c) At T = 324 K, P = 1 atm, we calculate C_P from

$C_{pm} = C^{\theta}_{pm} - TB''(P)$ where $B'' = \frac{-2A_0}{RT^3} - \frac{12c}{T^5}$ and

$C^{\theta}_{pm} = a + bT + \frac{c}{T^2}$. Using data from Tables 1.2 and 2.2,

$$C_{pm} = 38 \text{ J K}^{-1}.$$

2.20   Prove that:

$$\left(\frac{\partial C_v}{\partial V}\right)_T = T\left(\frac{\partial^2 P}{\partial T^2}\right)_V$$

Evaluate this quantity for a van der Waals gas.

C_v is $C_v = \left(\frac{\partial U}{\partial T}\right)_V$.   Since U is a state function

$$\left(\frac{\partial C_v}{\partial V}\right)_T = \frac{\partial}{\partial V}\left(\frac{\partial U}{\partial T}\right)_V = \frac{\partial}{\partial T}\left(\frac{\partial U}{\partial V}\right)_T .$$

From Eq. (2.13), $\left(\frac{\partial U}{\partial V}\right)_T = T\left(\frac{\partial P}{\partial T}\right)_V - P$.

Then $\left(\frac{\partial C_v}{\partial V}\right)_T = \frac{\partial}{\partial T}\left[T\left(\frac{\partial P}{\partial T}\right)_V - P\right] = T\left(\frac{\partial^2 P}{\partial T^2}\right)_V .$

For a van der Waals gas $P = \frac{RT}{V_m - b} - \frac{a}{V_m^2}$, thus $\left(\frac{\partial^2 P}{\partial T^2}\right)_V = 0.$

Then $\left(\frac{\partial C_v}{\partial V}\right)_T = T\left(\frac{\partial^2 P}{\partial T^2}\right)_V = 0.$

2.21   Acetylene (gas) at 15°C, 1 atm, has $C_{pm} = 41.73$ J/K. Calculate C_{vm} from its critical constants, $T_c = 309$ K, $P_c = 62$ atm (the observed value is 31.16 J/K, Table 2.1). What would C_{vm} be if this gas were ideal?

From Eq. (2.40), $C_{vm} = C_{pm} - R\left[1 + \left(\frac{B'P}{R}\right)\right]^2$, where

$\frac{B'P}{R} = \frac{27}{32}\left(\frac{T_c}{T}\right)^3\left(\frac{P}{P_c}\right)$.   For acetylene then

$$C_{vm} = 41.73\ J\ K^{-1} - 8.3145\ J\ K^{-1}\left[1 + \frac{27}{32}\left(\frac{309}{288}\right)^3\left(\frac{1}{62}\right)\right]^2$$

$$C_{vm} = 33.13\ J\ K^{-1} .$$

For an ideal gas, $C_{vm} = C_{pm} - R = 41.73 - 8.3145 = 33.42\ J\ K^{-1}.$

2.22 (a) Show that for a van der Waals gas:

$$C_{pm} - C_{vm} = \frac{R}{1 - \dfrac{2a(V_m - b)^2}{RTV_m^3}}$$

(b) Evaluate this difference for SO_2 at 15°C, 1 atm (V_m = 23.83 dm^3; compare Table 2.1).

a) From Eq. (2.36), $C_p = C_v + \left[P + \left(\frac{\partial U}{\partial V}\right)_T\right]\left(\frac{\partial V}{\partial T}\right)_P$. For a van der Waals gas, $P = \frac{RT}{V_m - b} - \frac{a}{V_m^2}$. Then

$$\left(\frac{\partial V}{\partial T}\right)_P = \frac{1}{\left(\frac{\partial T}{\partial V}\right)_P} = \left[\frac{P}{R} + \frac{a}{RV_m^2} - \frac{2a(V_m - b)}{RV_m^3}\right]^{-1}.$$

$\left(\frac{\partial U}{\partial T}\right)_V$ is given by $\left(\frac{\partial U}{\partial V}\right)_T = T\left(\frac{\partial P}{\partial T}\right)_V - P$. For a v.d.W. gas $\left(\frac{\partial U}{\partial V}\right)_T = \frac{a}{V_m^2}$. Then

$$C_{pm} - C_{vm} = \left[P + \frac{a}{V_m^2}\right]\left[\frac{1}{\frac{P}{R} + \frac{a}{RV_m^2} - \frac{2a(V_m - b)}{RV_m^3}}\right] \text{ or}$$

$$C_{pm} - C_{vm} = \frac{R}{\left\{1 - \dfrac{2a(V_m - b)^2}{RTV_m^3}\right\}}$$

b) Using data from Table 1.1, $C_{pm} - C_{vm} = 8.52 \text{ J K}^{-1}$.

2.23 Use the square-well potential constants (Table 1.7) for argon at 300 K to estimate $C_{pm} - C_{vm}$ at $P = 1$ and 10 atm [use Eq. (2.40)].

From Eq. (2.40), $C_{pm} = C_{vm} + R\left[1 + \left(\frac{B'P}{R}\right)\right]^2$. From Eq. (1.49),

$$B(T) = b_0\left[1 - (R^3 - 1)(e^{\epsilon/kT} - 1)\right] \text{ and}$$

$$B' = b_0\left[(R^3 - 1)\left(\frac{\epsilon}{kT^2}\right)e^{\epsilon/kT}\right].$$

Using data from Table 1.7 with P = 1 atm:

$$C_{pm} - C_{vm} = 82.06 \text{ cm}^3 \text{ atm K}^{-1} \times$$

$$\left[1 + 39.8 \text{ cm}^3 \frac{\left[(1.85^3 - 1)\ \frac{69.4}{300^2}\ e^{69.4/300}\right](1 \text{ atm})}{0.08206 \text{ dm}^3 \text{ atm}}\right]^2$$

$C_{pm} - C_{vm} = 1.005$ R.

For P = 10 atm, $C_{pm} - C_{vm} = 1.051$ R.

2.24 Calculate the work when an ideal gas, initially at $P = 10$ atm, $V = 2.0$ dm^3, $T = 293$ K, is expanded isothermally to $P = 1.0$ atm, if: (a) the expansion occurs vs. $P_{ex} = 1$ atm; (b) the opposing pressure is reduced in nine steps, $P_{ex} = 9, 8, 7, 6, \ldots, 2, 1$; (c) the expansion is done reversibly.

a) n and V_2 may be calculated using PV = nRT:

$$n = \frac{(10\ \text{atm})(2\ \text{dm}^3)}{(0.08206\ \text{dm}^3\ \text{atm}\ \text{K}^{-1})(293\ \text{K})} = 0.832\ \text{mol}\ ,$$

$$V_2 = \frac{(0.832)(0.08206\ \text{dm}^3\ \text{atm}\ \text{K}^{-1})(293\ \text{K})}{1\ \text{atm}} = 20\ \text{dm}^3\ .$$

The work is given by ($P_{ex} = 1$ atm)

$$-w = \int_{V_1}^{V_2} P_{ex} dV = P(V_2 - V_1)$$

$$= 1\ \text{atm}\left(\frac{101325\ \text{Pa}}{1\ \text{atm}}\right)(20 - 2\ \text{dm}^3)\left(\frac{1\ \text{m}^3}{10^3\ \text{dm}^3}\right)$$

or w = -1800 J.

b) In each step, P_{ex} = constant, so we may break the integral into steps, calculating V_2 for each integral with the ideal gas law:

$\int_{2.00}^{2.22} (9\ \text{atm})dV = 201$ J, $\int_{2.22}^{2.50} (8\ \text{atm})dV = 227$ J, and so on. Then summing the results

$$-w = 201 + 227 + 255 + 286 + 340 + 405 + 508 + 674 + 1013$$
$$= 3.9\ \text{kJ}$$

or w = -3.9 kJ.

c) For a reversible process, $-w_{max} = nRT\int_{V_1}^{V_2} \frac{dV}{V} = nRT \ln\left(\frac{V_2}{V_1}\right)$.

From part a), $V_2 = 20$ dm^3, thus

$$-w_{max} = 8.3145\ \text{J K}^{-1}(293\ \text{K})\left[\ln\left(\frac{20}{2}\right)\right](0.832) = 4670\ \text{J}$$

or w = -4670 J.

2.25 Calculate the work done by a reversible isothermal expansion of 5.00 moles of an ideal gas at 273 K from 0.025 m^3 to 0.112 m^3.

From Eq. (2.41), $-w_{max} = nRT \ln\left(\frac{V_2}{V_1}\right)$. Substituting

$$-w_{max} = (5\ \text{mol})(8.3145\ \text{J K}^{-1}\ \text{mol}^{-1})(273\ \text{K})\left[\ln\left(\frac{0.112}{0.025}\right)\right] = 17\ \text{kJ}$$

or $w_{max} = -17$ kJ.

2.26 (a) Show that the work for a reversible isothermal expansion of a van der Waals gas is:

$$-w = nRT\ \ln\left(\frac{V_2 - nb}{V_1 - nb}\right) + n^2a\left(\frac{1}{V_2} - \frac{1}{V_1}\right)$$

(b) Calculate the work of an isothermal, reversible expansion of 6.00 moles of SO_2 from 10.0 dm^3 to 150 dm^3 at 30°C using the ideal gas and van der Waals equations.

a) We have $-w = \int_{V_1}^{V_2} P_{ex}dV$. For a reversible process,

$P_{ex} = P$, and for a van der Waals gas $P = \frac{nRT}{V - nb} - \frac{an^2}{V^2}$. Then

$$-w = \int_{V_1}^{V_2}\left(\frac{nRT}{V - nb} - \frac{an^2}{V^2}\right)dV$$

$$-w = nRT\ \ln\left[\frac{(V_2 - nb)}{(V_1 - nb)}\right] + an^2\left(\frac{1}{V_2} - \frac{1}{V_1}\right).$$

b) For an ideal gas,

$$w_{max} = -nRT\ \ln\left(\frac{V_2}{V_1}\right) = (6\ \text{mol})(8.3145\ \text{J K}^{-1}\ \text{mol}^{-1})(303.15\ \text{K}) \times \ln\left(\frac{150}{10}\right).$$

$w_{max} = -41.0$ kJ.

For a van der Waals gas, SO_2, with $a = 6.71\ \text{dm}^6\ \text{atm mol}^{-2}$ and $b = 0.0564\ \text{dm}^3\ \text{mol}^{-1}$:

$$-w = (6\ \text{mol})(8.3145\ \text{J K}^{-1}\ \text{mol}^{-1})(303.15\ \text{K})\ \ln\left[\frac{150 - 6(0.0564)}{10 - 6(0.0564)}\right] +$$

$$(6.71\ \text{dm}^6\ \text{atm mol}^{-2})(6\ \text{mol})^2\left(\frac{1}{150\ \text{dm}^3} - \frac{1}{10\ \text{dm}^3}\right) \times$$

$$\left(\frac{1\ \text{J}}{9.869 \times 10^{-3}\ \text{dm}^3\ \text{atm}}\right).$$

$-w = (41{,}439.98 - 2284.49)\text{J} = 39.16$ kJ.

2.27 Show, using the Redlich-Kwong equation of state, that the work of an isothermal reversible expansion is:

$$-w = nRT \ln\left(\frac{V_2 - nb}{V_1 - nb}\right) + \frac{na}{bT^{\frac{1}{2}}} \ln\left[\frac{(V_2 + nb)V_1}{(V_1 + nb)V_2}\right]$$

For an isothermal reversible expansion: $-w = \int_{V_1}^{V_2} PdV$.

Using the Redlich - Kwong equation:

$$-w = \int_{V_1}^{V_2}\left[\frac{nRT}{(V - nb)} - \frac{an^2}{T^{1/2}V(V + nb)}\right]dV .$$

Now, $\frac{1}{V(V + nb)} = \frac{1}{nb}\left(\frac{1}{V} - \frac{1}{(V + nb)}\right)$ so that

$$-w = \int_{V_1}^{V_2}\frac{nRT}{(V - nb)} dV - \int_{V_1}^{V_2}\frac{an}{bT^{1/2}V} dV + \int_{V_1}^{V_2}\frac{an}{bT^{1/2}(V + nb)} dV .$$

Thus:

$$-w = nRT \ln(V - nb)\Big|_{V_1}^{V_2} - \frac{an}{bT^{1/2}}[\ln V - \ln(V + nb)]\Big|_{V_1}^{V_2} .$$

$$-w = nRT \ln\left(\frac{V_2 - nb}{V_1 - nb}\right) + \frac{an}{bT^{1/2}} \ln\left[\frac{(V_2 + nb)V_1}{(V_1 + nb)V_2}\right] .$$

2.28 Calculate the final temperature for an adiabatic reversible expansion from $T_1 = 600$ K, $V_m = 1.00$ dm^3 to a final $V_m = 23.0$ dm^3, if (a) the gas is argon, (b) the gas is methane. (Assume ideal gas.)

a) From Eq. (2.44), $\ln\left(\frac{T_2}{T_1}\right) = -\frac{R \ln\left(\frac{V_2}{V_1}\right)}{C_{vm}} = -\frac{8.3145}{12.55} \ln\left(\frac{23}{1}\right)$

or $T_2 = 75.2$ K.

b) We use Table 2.2 to estimate C_{pm} at 450 K, an intermediate T:

$$C^{\theta}_{pm} = a + bT + \frac{c}{T^2} = 44.26 \text{ J K}^{-1} .$$

For an ideal gas $C_{pm} - C_{vm} = R$, then

$C_{vm} = C_{pm} - R = 44.26 - 8.3145 = 35.94$ J K^{-1}. Substituting into the eq. for T_2 above, we get $T_2 = 290$ K. We now use $T = 445$ K, the mid-range T to find C_{pm}, $C_{pm} = 44.00$ J K^{-1}. This gives $C_{vm} = 35.68$ J K^{-1} and $T_2 = 289$ K.

2.29 Adiabatic temperature drops are often a convenient method for measuring heat capacities. A certain gas, when expanded adiabatically and reversibly from 380 K, 3 atm to 1 atm, had a final $T = 278$ K. Calculate its C_{pm}. (Assume ideal gas.)

From Eq. (2.45b), $\ln\left(\frac{T_2}{T_1}\right) = \frac{R}{C_{pm}} \ln\left(\frac{P_2}{P_1}\right)$. Thus

$$C_{pm} = \frac{8.3145 \text{ J K}^{-1} \ln\left(\frac{1}{3}\right)}{\ln\left(\frac{278}{380}\right)} = 29.2 \text{ J K}^{-1}.$$

2.30 A quantity of nitrogen gas at 10 atm is expanded adiabatically and reversibly to 10 times its initial volume. What is the final pressure? (Assume ideal gas.)

From Eq. (2.49), $\frac{P_2}{P_1} = \left(\frac{V_1}{V_2}\right)^{\gamma}$ where $\gamma = \frac{C_p}{C_v}$. Then

$\frac{P_2}{10 \text{ atm}} = \left(\frac{1}{10}\right)^{1.404}$, or $P = 10 \text{ atm}(0.0394) = 0.394$ atm.

2.31 An ideal gas with C_{pm} = 33.26 J/K (presumed independent of T) is expanded adiabatically from 400 K, P = 5.00 atm to P = 1.00 atm. Calculate the final temperature if (a) the expansion is reversible, (b) the expansion is vs. a constant P_{ex} = 1.00 atm, (c) the expansion is into a vacuum. [You need to derive an equation for part (b).]

a) From Eq. (2.45b), $\bar{C}_{pm} \ln\left(\frac{T_2}{T_1}\right) = R \ln\left(\frac{P_2}{P_1}\right)$.

Thus T_2 = 268 K.

b) For dq = 0, $dU = -dw = -C_V dT = -P_{ex}dV$. Integrating and using the ideal gas law for V,

$$C_V(T_2 - T_1) = -P_{ex}(V_2 - V_1) = -P_{ex}\left(\frac{nRT_1}{P_1} - \frac{nRT_2}{P_2}\right) \text{, thus}$$

$$C_{vm} = \frac{-P_{ex}R}{(T_2 - T_1)}\left(\frac{T_1}{P_1} - \frac{T_2}{P_2}\right) = C_{pm} - R = 24.95 \text{ J K}^{-1} .$$

Solving for T_2, T_2 = 320 K.

c) For an expansion into a vacuum dw = 0 and $dU = C_V dT = 0$, thus $dT = 0$ and $T_1 = T_2$ = 400 K.

2.32 (a) Show that, for an adiabatic reversible expansion of a van der Waals gas:

$$\bar{C}_{vm} \ln\left(\frac{T_2}{T_1}\right) = -R \ln\left(\frac{V_{2m} - b}{V_{1m} - b}\right)$$

(b) Compare this to the ideal gas result [Eq. (2.43)] for the compression of Ar from V_m = 20 dm^3, T = 500 K to V_m = 2.0 dm^3.

a) $dU = dw = -PdV$. With $dU = \left(\frac{\partial U}{\partial T}\right)_V dT + \left(\frac{\partial U}{\partial V}\right)_T dV$, $\left(\frac{\partial U}{\partial T}\right)_V = C_V$, and $\left(\frac{\partial U}{\partial V}\right)_T = T\left(\frac{\partial P}{\partial T}\right)_V - P$ we have:

$$C_{vm}dT + \left[T\left(\frac{\partial P}{\partial T}\right)_V - P\right]dV = -PdV \text{ which becomes:}$$

$$C_{vm}dT = -T\left(\frac{\partial P}{\partial T}\right)_V dV .$$

For a van der Waals gas, $\left(\frac{\partial P}{\partial T}\right)_V = \frac{R}{V_m - b}$ so that

$$C_{vm}dT = \frac{-RT}{V_m - b}\,dV.$$

Integrating between (T_1, V_{1m}) and (T_2, V_{2m}) gives the result:

$$\bar{C}_{vm} \ln\left(\frac{T_2}{T_1}\right) = -R \ln\left(\frac{V_{2m} - b}{V_{1m} - b}\right).$$

b) For Ar b = 0.03219 $dm^3\ mol^{-1}$, C_v = 12.59 J $K^{-1}\ mol^{-1}$.

Using the above T_2 = 108 K. From Eq. (2.43), T_2 = 109 K.

2.33 One mole of an ideal gas with C_{pm} = 30.0 J/K, C_{vm} = 20.7 J/K (both considered constant) is expanded from 400 K, 5 atm to P = 1 atm. Calculate the work if (a) the expansion is reversible and isothermal, (b) the expansion is reversible and adiabatic.

a) From Eq. (2.41), $-w_{max} = nRT \ln\left(\frac{V_2}{V_1}\right)$. Using the ideal gas law, $\frac{V_2}{V_1} = \frac{P_1}{P_2} = \frac{5}{1} = 5$. Thus

$$-w_{max} = (1)(8.3145\ J\ K^{-1})(400\ K)\ \ln(5) = 5.4\ kJ$$

or w = -5.4 kJ.

b) From Eq. (2.45b), $\bar{C}_{pm} \ln\left(\frac{T_2}{T_1}\right) = R \ln\left(\frac{P_2}{P_1}\right)$. Solving $\ln\left(\frac{T_2}{400\ K}\right) = \frac{8.3145\ J\ K^{-1}}{30.0\ J\ K^{-1}} \ln\left(\frac{1}{5}\right)$, we have T_2 = 256 K. Also $dW = nC_{vm}dT$, or $w = nC_{vm}(T_2 - T_1)$, so that

$$w = (1)(20.7\ J\ K^{-1})(256 - 400\ K) = -3.0\ kJ.$$

2.34 When air is compressed, as with a bicycle pump, the temperature rises. You can readily observe this phenomenon by feeling the coupling at the pump's air outlet. You are pumping air at 22°C, 1 atm, into a bicycle tire with 1 dm^3 volume at a pressure of 65 psig. Calculate the temperature of the air in the tire, assuming the process is adiabatic and reversible.

Converting to atm, P = 5.42 atm. From Eq. (2.45b), $\bar{C}_{pm} \ln\left(\frac{T_2}{T_1}\right) = R \ln\left(\frac{P_2}{P_1}\right)$. For $\bar{C}_{pm}$, $\bar{C}_{pm} = a + bT + \frac{c}{T^2}$.

Thus for N_2, $\bar{C}_{pm} = 29.16\ J\ K^{-1}$ and for O_2, $\bar{C}_{pm} = 29.36\ J\ K^{-1}$.

Then for air, $\bar{C}_{pm} = (0.21)(29.36) + (0.79)(29.16) = 29.20\ J\ K^{-1}$.

Thus, $\ln\left(\frac{T_2}{295\ K}\right) = \frac{8.3145\ J\ K^{-1}}{29.20\ J\ K^{-1}} \ln\left(\frac{5.42}{1}\right)$ or $T_2 = 477\ K = 204°C$.

2.35 Five moles of an ideal gas ($C_{pm} = 22\ J\ K^{-1}$) initially at 300 K, 1 atm, are compressed reversibly to 10 atm. The gas and its container are in thermal contact with a water bath, and the total heat capacity (gas, container, bath) is 9000 J K^{-1}. Calculate the final temperature if the whole system is adiabatic.

From Eq. (2.45b), $\bar{C}_p \ln\left(\frac{T_2}{T_1}\right) = nR \ln\left(\frac{P_2}{P_1}\right)$. We use the total heat capacity of the system for $\bar{C}_p$. Then

$$\ln\left(\frac{T_2}{300\ K}\right) = (5\ mol)\frac{8.3145\ J\ K^{-1}\ mol^{-1}}{9000\ J\ K^{-1}} \ln\left(\frac{10}{1}\right)$$

or $T_2 = 303\ K$.

2.36 Use the van der Waals relation:

$$\left(\frac{\partial U}{\partial V}\right)_T = \frac{a}{V_m^2}$$

to calculate the temperature change in a Joule expansion ($P_{ex} = 0$, adiabatic) if one mole of CO_2 is expanded from 5 dm^3 to 25 dm^3. (Use $C_{vm} = 28.1$ J/K.)

From Eq. (2.51), $\left(\frac{\partial T}{\partial V}\right)_U = -\frac{1}{C_v}\left(\frac{\partial U}{\partial V}\right)_T$. Using the v.d.W. relation,

$\left(\frac{\partial T}{\partial V}\right)_U = -\frac{1}{nC_{vm}}\frac{a}{V_m^2} = -\frac{1}{nC_{vm}}\frac{an^2}{V^2}$ or $dT = -\frac{an^2}{nC_{vm}V^2}dV$. Integration

gives $(T_2 - T_1) = \frac{an}{C_{vm}}\left(\frac{1}{V_2} - \frac{1}{V_1}\right)$. For CO_2

$$\Delta T = \frac{(1\ mol)(3.59\ dm^6\ atm\ mol^{-2})}{28.1\ J\ K^{-1}\ mol^{-1}}\left(\frac{1}{25\ dm^3} - \frac{1}{5\ dm^3}\right) = -2\ K\ .$$

2.37 Estimate the low-pressure Joule-Thomson coefficient of CO_2 at 400 K from its critical constants. Use this value to estimate the temperature drop if CO_2 at 400 K, 50 atm, is expanded to 1 atm.

From Eq. (2.56), $\mu C_{pm}^{\theta} = TB' - B$. Using Eq. (1.17)

$B(T) = \frac{9RT_c}{128P_c}\left(1 - \frac{6T_c^2}{T^2}\right)$ and $B' = \frac{9RT_c}{128P_c}\left(\frac{12T_c^2}{T^3}\right)$. Then

$$\mu = \frac{1}{C_{pm}^{\theta}}\left(\frac{81RT_c^3}{64P_cT^2} - \frac{9RT_c}{128P_c}\right).$$

Substituting in data for CO_2,

$$\mu = \frac{1}{42.36\ J\ K^{-1}}\left(\frac{81(0.08206\ dm^3\ atm\ K^{-1})(304.2\ K)^3}{64(73\ atm)(400\ K)^2} - \right.$$

$$\left.\frac{9(0.08206\ dm^3\ atm\ K^{-1})(304.2\ K)}{128(73\ atm)}\right).$$

$\mu = 0.54\ K\ atm^{-1}$.

Since $\mu \cong \frac{\Delta T}{\Delta P}$, then $\Delta T \sim \Delta P\mu = (-49\ atm)(0.54\ K\ atm^{-1}) = -26\ K.$

2.38 Since the Joule-Thomson coefficient is a function of both T and P, calculation of ΔT for a given ΔP could be complicated. Show that if C_p can be considered constant (independent of P and T), the final temperature of a Joule-Thomson expansion is:

$$T_2 = T_1 - \int_0^P \mu(T_1, P)\,dP$$

We have $dH = \left(\frac{\partial H}{\partial P}\right)_T dP + \left(\frac{\partial H}{\partial T}\right)_P dT$. Consider the process to be done in two steps: 1) pressure change at constant T, 2) temperature change at constant P. Since the process is isenthalpic, dH = 0. Thus $0 = \left(\frac{\partial H}{\partial P}\right)_T dP + \left(\frac{\partial H}{\partial T}\right)_P dT$ or $0 = -\mu C_p dP + C_p dT$. Since μ corresponds to step 1, $\int_P^0 \mu(T_1, P) C_p dP = \int_{T_1}^{T_2} C_p dT = C_p(T_2 - T_1)$. Assuming C_p is independent of P and T, $T_2 - T_1 = -\int_0^P \mu(T_1, P)dP$.

2.39 Use the results of Problem 2.38 to calculate the temperature change when CO_2 at 350 K, 100 atm, undergoes a Joule-Thomson expansion to 1 atm, given (for CO_2, 350 K) $\mu = 0.8187 - (3.276 \times 10^{-3})P - (5.66 \times 10^{-6})P^2$ (units: K/atm).

From problem 2.38, $\Delta T = -\int_0^P \mu(T_1, P)dP$. Substituting

$$\Delta T = -\int_{1\ \text{atm}}^{100\ \text{atm}} (0.8187 - (3.276 \times 10^{-3})P - (5.66 \times 10^{-6})P^2)dP$$

$\Delta T = -63$ K.

2.40 (a) Show that the van der Waals second virial coefficient, $B = b - a/RT$, gives:

$$\mu C_{pm} = \left(\frac{2a}{RT} - b\right)$$

(b) Use this result to calculate μ of N_2 at 0°C and 100°C (compare Table 2.4).
(c) Use this result to calculate the inversion temperature of nitrogen (compare Table 2.5).

a) $\mu C^{\ominus}_{pm} = TB' - B$ with $B = b - \frac{a}{RT}$, $B' = \frac{dB}{dT} = \frac{a}{RT^2}$. Thus

$$\mu C^{\ominus}_{pm} = T\left(\frac{a}{RT^2}\right) - \left(b - \frac{a}{RT}\right) \text{ and } \mu C^{\ominus}_{pm} = \frac{2a}{RT} - b .$$

b) For N_2, $a = 1.39\ dm^6\ atm\ mol^{-2}$ and $b = 0.0391\ dm^3\ mol^{-1}$.

At 0°C,

$$C^{\ominus}_{pm} = 28.58 + (3.77 \times 10^{-3})(273.15) - \frac{(0.50 \times 10^5)}{(273.15)^2} .$$

$$C^{\ominus}_{pm}(0°C) = 28.94\ J\ K^{-1}\ mol^{-1}.$$

Thus

$$\mu = \left(\frac{1}{28.94\ J\ K^{-1}\ mol^{-1}}\right)\left(\frac{1\ J}{9.869 \times 10^{-3}\ dm^3\ atm}\right)$$

$$\times \left[\frac{2(1.39\ dm^6\ atm\ mol^{-2})}{(0.08206\ dm^3\ atm\ mol^{-1}\ K^{-1})(273.15\ K)} - 0.0391\ dm^3\ mol^{-1}\right]$$

$\mu(0°C) = 0.297\ K\ atm^{-1}$, $\mu(0°C, expt) = 0.2655\ K\ atm^{-1}$.

At 100°C, $C^{\ominus}_{pm}(100°C) = 29.63\ J\ K^{-1}\ mol^{-1}$ so that

$\mu(100°C) = 0.177\ K\ atm^{-1}$. Experimentally,

$\mu(100°C, expt) = 0.1291\ K\ atm^{-1}$.

c) The Joule - Thomson inversion temperature T_i occurs when $\mu = 0$, so that $T_i = \frac{2a}{Rb} = 866\ K$. From Table 2.5, the inversion temperature of N_2 is 621 K.

2.41 The gas $CHCl_2F$ (Genetron-21) is used as a refrigerant, solvent, and propellant. The following data apply:

$$M = 102.93 \text{ g}, \qquad T_c = 451.7 \text{ K}, \qquad P_c = 51 \text{ atm}$$

$$B(331 \text{ K}) = -528 \text{ cm}^3/\text{mol}, \qquad B(339 \text{ K}) = -446 \text{ cm}^3/\text{mol},$$

$$B(366 \text{ K}) = -403 \text{ cm}^3/\text{mol}$$

(a) Use the $B(T)$ data to calculate B' and μC_p at 339 K. When calculating the derivative, use the three-point formula of Appendix I with $1/T$ as the independent variable.
(b) Calculate the same quantities using the Berthelot virial coefficient.

a) The three-point formula is: $\dfrac{df}{dx} = \dfrac{f(x + h) - f(x - h)}{2h}$.

Here we have f = B, $(x + h) = \dfrac{1}{331 \text{ K}} = 3.021 \times 10^{-3} \text{ K}^{-1}$,

$(x - h) = \dfrac{1}{366 \text{ K}} = 2.732 \times 10^{-3} \text{ K}^{-1}$, so that

$h = 1.446 \times 10^{-4} \text{ K}^{-1}$ and

$$\frac{dB}{d\left(\frac{1}{T}\right)} = \frac{-528 \text{ cm}^3 + 403 \text{ cm}^3}{2(1.446 \times 10^{-4} \text{ K}^{-1})} = -4.323 \times 10^5 \text{ cm}^3 \text{ K} .$$

Also:

$$\frac{dB}{dT} = -\frac{1}{T^2}\left(\frac{dB}{d\left(\frac{1}{T}\right)}\right) = \frac{(4.323 \times 10^5 \text{ cm}^3 \text{ K})}{(399 \text{ K})^2} = 3.762 \text{ cm}^3 \text{ K}^{-1} .$$

With $\mu C^{\ominus}_{pm} = TB' - B$,

$$\mu C^{\ominus}_{pm} = (339 \text{ K})(3.762 \text{ cm}^3 \text{ K}^{-1}) + 446 \text{ cm}^3 = 1721 \text{ cm}^3 = 1.72 \text{ dm}^3 .$$

b) For $CHCl_2F$,

$$B' = \frac{27RT_c^3}{32P_cT^3} = \frac{27(0.08206 \text{ dm}^3 \text{ atm K}^{-1}\text{mol}^{-1})(451.7 \text{ K})^3}{32(51 \text{ atm})(339 \text{ K})^3} \quad \text{or}$$

$$B' = 3.21 \text{ cm}^3 \text{ K}^{-1} \text{ mol}^{-1}.$$

Then $\mu C^{\ominus}_{pm} = (339 \text{ K})(3.21 \text{ cm}^3 \text{ K}^{-1}) + 446 \text{ cm}^3 = 1.53 \text{ dm}^3$.

2.42 Calculate the Joule-Thomson coefficient of ethylene (C_2H_4) at 15°C from its square-well potential constants (Table 1.7). (Use the heat capacity of Table 2.1.)

From Eq. (1.49), $B(T) = b_0\left[1 - (R^3 - 1)\left(e^{\epsilon/kT} - 1\right)\right]$ thus

$$B' = b_0\left(\frac{\epsilon}{kT^2}\right) e^{\epsilon/kT} \ (R^3 - 1) .$$

For C_2H_4, $B(T) = -152.2 \text{ cm}^3$ and $B' = 0.9938 \text{ cm}^3 \text{ K}^{-1}$. From Eq. (2.56), $\mu = \frac{1}{C^{\ominus}_{pm}} [TB' - B]$. From Table 2.1,

$C^{\ominus}_{pm} = 42.17 \text{ J K}^{-1}$. Thus $\mu = 1.05 \text{ K atm}^{-1}$.

2.43 (a) Show that, in terms of the Beattie-Bridgeman constants:

$$\mu C_{pm} = -B_0 + \frac{2A_0}{RT} + \frac{4c}{T^3}$$

(b) Calculate μ for N_2 at 0°C. Use $C_{pm} = 29.10$ J/K.
(c) Calculate the inversion temperature of N_2 using this formula.

a) From Eq. (1.16), $B(T) = B_0 - \frac{A_0}{RT} - \frac{c}{T^3}$ and $B' = \frac{A_0}{RT^2} + \frac{3c}{T^4}$.

From Eq. (2.56), $\mu C^{\ominus}_{pm} = TB' - B$ thus $\mu C^{\ominus}_{pm} = \frac{2A_0}{RT} + \frac{4c}{T^3} - B_0$.

b) For N_2 at 0°C,

$$\mu = \frac{101.33 \text{ J atm}^{-1} \text{ dm}^{-3}}{29.10 \text{ J K}^{-1}}\left(\frac{2(1.3445 \text{ atm dm}^6)}{(0.08206 \text{ dm}^3 \text{ atm K}^{-1})(273 \text{ K})} + \frac{4(4.20 \times 10^4 \text{ dm}^3 \text{ K})}{(273 \text{ K})^3} - 0.05046 \text{ dm}^3\right)$$

$\mu = 0.271 \text{ K atm}^{-1}$.

c) Since C_{pm} is a positive constant, T_i occurs when

$B_0 - \frac{2A_0}{RT_i} - \frac{4c}{T_i^{\,3}} = 0$. Use Newton's method (Appendix I) to find the root: $T_i = 657$ K.

2.44 (a) Show that for a van der Waals gas:

$$U_m(T, V) - U_m^{\ominus}(T) = \frac{a}{V_m}$$

(b) Calculate this quantity for O_2 when $V_m = 5\ \text{dm}^3$.
(c) Derive the equivalent expression for the enthalpy.

a) $$U_m(T, V) = U_m^{\theta}(T) - \int_{\infty}^{V_m}\left[P - T\left(\frac{\partial P}{\partial T}\right)_V\right]dV_m .$$

For a van der Waals gas: $\left(\frac{\partial P}{\partial T}\right)_V = \frac{R}{V_m - b}$. Thus:

$$U_m(T, V) = U_m^{\theta}(T) - \int_{\infty}^{V_m}\left[\frac{RT}{V_m - b} - \frac{a}{V_m^2} - \frac{RT}{V_m - b}\right]dV_m$$

$$= U_m^{\theta}(T) + \int_{\infty}^{V_m}\frac{a}{V_m^2}\,dV_m$$

$$U_m(T, V) = U_m^{\theta}(T) - \frac{a}{V_m}$$

b) For O_2, $a = 1.36\ \text{dm}^6\ \text{atm}$, so that

$$U_m(T, 5\ \text{dm}^3) - U_m^{\theta}(T) = -\left(\frac{1.36\ \text{dm}^6\ \text{atm}}{5\ \text{dm}^3}\right)\left(\frac{1\ \text{J}}{9.869 \times 10^{-3}\ \text{dm}^3}\right) .$$

$$U_m(T, 5\ \text{dm}^3) - U_m^{\theta}(T) = -27.56\ \text{J}.$$

c) $H = U + PV$, so that $H_m - H_m^{\theta} = U_m - U_m^{\theta} + PV_m - PV_m^{\theta}$.

With $PV_m = \frac{V_m RT}{V_m - b} - \frac{a}{V_m}$ and $PV^{\theta}{}_m = RT$, we have:

$$H_m - H_m^{\theta} = \frac{V_m RT}{V_m - b} - \frac{2a}{V_m} - RT = \frac{bRT}{V_m - b} - \frac{2a}{V_m} .$$

2.45 Show that for a Redlich-Kwong gas:

$$U_m(T,V) = U^{\ominus}(T) - \frac{3a}{2bT^{\frac{1}{2}}}\ln\left(\frac{V_m + b}{V_m}\right)$$

$U_m(T, V) = U_m^{\theta}(T) - \int_{\infty}^{V_m}\left[P - T\left(\frac{\partial P}{\partial T}\right)_V\right]dV_m$. The Redlich - Kwong equation of state gives:

$$\left(\frac{\partial P}{\partial T}\right)_V = \frac{R}{V_m - b} + \frac{a}{2T^{3/2}V_m(V_m + b)} .$$

Thus:

$$U_m(T, V) = U_m^{\theta}(T) - \int_{\infty}^{V_m}\left[\frac{RT}{V_m - b} - \frac{a}{T^{1/2}V_m(V_m + b)} - \frac{RT}{V_m - b} - \frac{a}{2T^{1/2}V_m(V_m + b)}\right] dV_m$$

$$= U_m^{\theta}(T) - \int_{\infty}^{V_m}\frac{3a}{2T^{1/2}V_m(V_m + b)} dV_m .$$

With $\frac{1}{V_m(V_m + b)} = \frac{1}{bV_m} - \frac{1}{b(V_m + b)}$ we have:

$$U_m(T, V) = U_m^{\theta}(T) + \int_{\infty}^{V_m} \frac{3a}{2T^{1/2}}\left[\frac{1}{bV_m} - \frac{1}{b(V_m + b)}\right]dV_m .$$

$$U_m(T, V) = U_m^{\theta}(T) + \frac{3a}{2bT^{1/2}}\left[\ln V_m - \ln(V_m + b)\right]_{\infty}^{V_m} .$$

$$U_m(T, V) = U_m^{\theta}(T) - \frac{3a}{2bT^{1/2}} \ln\left(\frac{V_m + b}{V_m}\right) .$$

3

The Second Law of Thermodynamics

3.1 The vapor pressure of water (steam pressure) is 1 atm at 100°C, but 15.3 atm (210 psig) at 200°C. Compare the work obtainable by a steam engine from fuel providing 10^6 J of heat at these temperatures. Assume a condensing temperature of 27°C.

a) From Eq. (3.2), $-w = \left(\frac{T_2 - T_1}{T_2}\right)q_2$. For $T_2 = 373$ K,

$T_1 = 300$ K, $w = -1.96 \times 10^5$ J.

b) For $T_2 = 473$ K, $T_1 = 300$ K, $w = -3.66 \times 10^5$ J.

3.2 Calculate the efficiency of an engine operating at 1 atm pressure (*i.e.*, at the normal boiling point) if the working substance is (a) H_2O, (b) Hg, (c) Na. In parts (a) and (b), assume a condenser temperature of 30°C; use 100°C for (c). (Why wouldn't you use 30°C for Na?)

a) From Eq. (3.2), $e = \frac{T_2 - T_1}{T_2}$. For H_2O, $T_2 = 373$ K,

$$e = \frac{373 - 303}{373} = 0.188 = 19\% \ .$$

b) For Hg, $T_2 = 630$ K, $e = \frac{630 - 303}{630} = 0.519 = 52\%$.

c) For Na, $T_2 = 1156$ K, $e = \frac{1156 - 303}{1156} = 0.677 = 68\%$.

3.3 Assume a house loses (or gains) heat at a rate of 500 J s^{-1} for each degree Celsius temperature difference. If the outside temperature is 30°C, calculate the power required for an air conditioner to keep the house at (a) 25°C, (b) 20°C. The actual power would be several times this, but the ratios are reasonable.

From Eq. (3.4), $w = \left(\frac{T_2 - T_1}{T_1}\right) q_1$. Since power $= \frac{\text{work}}{\text{time}}$,

$P = \left(\frac{T_2 - T_1}{T_1}\right)\frac{q_1}{t} = \frac{\Delta T}{T_1}\left(\frac{q_1}{t}\right)$. Using $\frac{q_1}{t} = 500\ \text{J sec}^{-1}\ \text{K}^{-1}(\Delta T)$,

$$P = \frac{\Delta T(500\ \text{J sec}^{-1}\ \text{K}^{-1})}{T_1}\ \Delta T\ .$$

a) For $T_2 = 303$ K, $T_1 = 298$ K,

$$P = \frac{(5\ \text{K})^2(500\ \text{J sec}^{-1}\ \text{K}^{-1})}{298\ \text{K}} = 42\ \text{W}.$$

b) For $T_2 = 303$ K, $T_1 = 293$ K,

$$P = \frac{(10\ \text{K})^2(500\ \text{J sec}^{-1}\text{K}^{-1})}{293\ \text{K}} = 171\ \text{W}.$$

3.4 (a) The rate of heat loss from a warm body is proportional to the temperature gradient. Show that the power required for a heat pump is proportional to the *square* of the temperature difference; that is, it takes four times as much power to keep a house at 20°C when the outside is 0°C than when the outside is 10°C. (b) Calculate the power needed for an "ideal" heat pump to heat a house with 1000 m^2 of wall area if the inside temperature is 20°C and the outside is 10° or 0°C. Assume that the walls are 10 cm thick and have a thermal conductivity of 0.05 J K^{-1} m^{-1} s^{-1}. The actual power required would be much larger.

a) Since $w = \frac{\Delta T}{T_1} q_1$, $P = \frac{w}{t} = \frac{\Delta T}{T_1}\left(\frac{q_1}{t}\right)$. Since $\frac{q}{t} \cong \frac{dq}{dt} = c\Delta T$,

$P = \frac{(\Delta T)^2 c}{T_1}$ where c is a constant.

b) $\frac{dq}{dt} = \frac{(\text{area of walls})(\text{thermal conductivity})\Delta T}{(\text{wall thickness})}$. Thus

$$P = \frac{(10\ \text{K})^2(1000\ \text{m}^2)(0.05\ \text{J K}^{-1}\ \text{m}^{-1}\ \text{sec}^{-1})}{293\ \text{K}(0.1\ \text{m})} = 171\ \text{W}.$$

For $\Delta T = 20$ K,

$$P = \frac{(20\ \text{K})^2(1000\ \text{m}^2)(0.05\ \text{J K}^{-1}\ \text{m}^{-1}\ \text{sec}^{-1})}{293\ \text{K}(0.1\ \text{m})} = 683\ \text{W}.$$

3.5 Draw a diagram of a Carnot cycle on a *T* vs. *S* plot. What is the significance of the area inside a Carnot-cycle *PV* plot (Figure 3.2) and the plot (*TS*) you have just made?

For step 1 of the Carnot cycle, $q_2 = RT_2 \ln\left(\frac{V_2}{V_1}\right)$, thus $\Delta S_1 = \frac{q_2}{T_2} = R \ln\left(\frac{V_2}{V_1}\right)$. For step 2, w = ΔU, thus dq = 0 and $\Delta S_2 = 0$. For step 3, $\Delta S_3 = R \ln\left(\frac{V_4}{V_3}\right) = \frac{q_1}{T_1}$ and for step 4, $\Delta S_4 = 0$. In a P - V plot, the area enclosed represents the work done. For the ΔS vs. T plot, the area represents the net heat since $dq = TdS$.

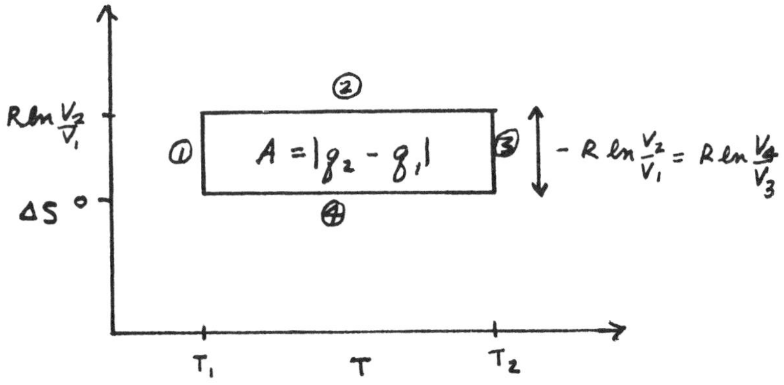

3.6 Calculate the entropy change when 1 kg of water is heated at constant pressure from 10°C to 60°C.

From Eq. (3.11a), $\Delta S = n\int_{T_1}^{T_2} \frac{C_{pm}}{T}\, dT = nC_{pm} \ln\left(\frac{T_2}{T_1}\right)$. For 1 kg of liquid water, $n = \frac{10^3 \text{ g}}{18.015 \text{ g mol}^{-1}} = 55.51$ moles. From Table 2.2, $C_{pm} = 75.48 \text{ J K}^{-1} \text{ mol}^{-1}$. Thus

$$\Delta S = 55.51 \text{ mol}(75.48 \text{ J K}^{-1} \text{ mol}^{-1}) \ln \frac{333 \text{ K}}{283 \text{ K}} = 682 \text{ J K}^{-1}.$$

3.7 Calculate the entropy change when one mole of CO_2(gas) is heated at constant pressure from 300 to 1000 K. Use the heat capacity of Table 2.2.

From Eq. (3.11a), $\Delta S = n\int_{T_1}^{T_2} \frac{C_{pm}}{T}\, dT$. From Table 2.2,

$C_{pm} = a + bT + \frac{c}{T^2}$. Thus

$$\Delta S = n\int_{T_1}^{T_2} \frac{\left(a + bT + \frac{c}{T^2}\right)}{T}\, dT$$

$$= n\left[a \ln\left(\frac{T_2}{T_1}\right) + b(T_2 - T_1) - \frac{c}{2}\left(\frac{1}{T_2^2} - \frac{1}{T_1^2}\right)\right] .$$

Substituting values for CO

$$\Delta S = (1)\left[44.23 \text{ J K}^{-1} \ln\left(\frac{1000}{300}\right) + 8.79 \times 10^{-3} \text{ J K}^{-2}(700 \text{ K})\right.$$

$$\left. + \frac{8.62 \times 10^5 \text{ J K}}{2}\left(\frac{1}{(1000 \text{ K})^2} - \frac{1}{(300 \text{ K})^2}\right)\right] .$$

$$\Delta S = 55.05 \text{ J K}^{-1} .$$

3.8 Use the heat capacity of Table 2.3 to calculate the change in entropy when 1 gram of sulfur dioxide is heated from 300 K to 1200 K (at constant pressure).

At constant pressure, $\Delta S = n\int_{T_1}^{T_2} \frac{C_{pm}}{T}\, dT$. From Table 2.3 for sulfur dioxide:

$$C^{\theta}_{pm} = a' + b'T + c'T^2 + d'T^3 \quad \left(\frac{J}{K}\right)$$

with $a' = 25.72$

$b' = 57.923 \times 10^{-3}$

$c' = -38.09 \times 10^{-6}$

$d' = 8.606 \times 10^{-9}$

Integrating, we find:

$$\Delta S = n\left(a' \ln T + b'T + \frac{c'T^2}{2} + \frac{d'T^3}{3}\right)\Bigg|_{300\ K}^{1200\ K} .$$

With $n = \left(\frac{1\ g}{64.06\ g\ mol^{-1}}\right) = 1.561 \times 10^{-2}$ mol we find:

$$\Delta S = 1.561 \times 10^{-2}(35.66 + 52.13 - 25.71 + 4.88) J\ K^{-1}$$

$$\Delta S = 1.045\ J\ K^{-1} .$$

3.9 Use the heat capacities for copper given below to calculate ΔH and ΔS when 1 kg of copper is heated from 25 K to 200 K at constant P.

T/K	C_{pm}/(J/K)
25	1.00
50	6.28
100	16.15
150	20.54
200	22.68

$\Delta H = \int_{T_1}^{T_2} C_{pm} dT \cong \bar{C}_{pm} \Delta T$. If we break the temperature range into small intervals, $\Delta H = \sum_i \bar{C}_{pmi} \Delta T_i$ and similarly $\Delta S = \sum_i \bar{C}_{pmi} \ln\left(\frac{T_{2i}}{T_{1i}}\right)$. From the given data

$\bar{C}_{pm}$ (J K^{-1})	ΔT (K)	$\ln \frac{T_2}{T_1}$
3.64	25	0.6931
11.22	50	0.6931
18.35	50	0.4055
21.61	50	0.2877

$\Delta H = (3.64)(25) + (11.22)(50) + (18.35)(50) + (21.61)(50)$

$\Delta H = 2650 \text{ J mol}^{-1}$.

For 1 kg of Cu, $n = \dfrac{10^3}{63.456 \text{ g mol}^{-1}} = 15.76$ mol. Then $\Delta H = 41.7$ kJ. For ΔS ,

$\Delta S = (3.64)(0.6931) + (11.22)(0.6931) + (18.35)(0.4055) + (21.61)(0.2877)$

or $\Delta S = 23.96 \text{ J K}^{-1} \text{ mol}^{-1}$. For 15.76 moles, $\Delta S = 377 \text{ J K}^{-1}$.

3.10 (a) A mole of an ideal gas is heated at constant pressure from 310 to 420 K. Assume C_{pm} = 30 J/K and calculate q, w, ΔU, ΔH, and ΔS for this process. (b) Do the same for a process of heating (310 to 420 K) at constant volume.

a) $\Delta H = nC_{pm}\Delta T = (1)(30\ \text{J K}^{-1})(420 - 310\ \text{K}) = 3.3\ \text{kJ}$. Also,

$\Delta U = nC_{vm}\Delta T$, where for an ideal gas $C_{pm} - R = C_{vm}$.

$$\Delta U = (1)(30\ \text{J K}^{-1} - 8.314\ \text{J K}^{-1})(420 - 310\ \text{K}) = 2.4\ \text{kJ}.$$

$$\Delta S = nC_{pm} \ln \frac{T_2}{T_1} = (1)(30\ \text{J K}^{-1}) \ln \frac{420}{310} = 9.1\ \text{J K}^{-1} .$$

Assuming only PV work and $P_{ex} = P$,

$$-w = \int P dV = \int \frac{nRT}{V}\, dV = \int_{T_1}^{T_2} nR\, dT = nR(T_2 - T_1) .$$

$$w = -(1)(8.3143\ \text{J K}^{-1})(420 - 310\ \text{K}) = -0.9\ \text{kJ}.$$

$$q = \Delta U - w = 3.3\ \text{kJ}.$$

b) As before $\Delta H = 3.3$ kJ, $\Delta U = 2.4$ kJ. $\Delta S = nC_{vm} \ln \frac{T_2}{T_1}$ or $\Delta S = 6.59\ \text{J K}^{-1}$. $w = 0$ and $q = \Delta U = 2.4$ kJ.

3.11 One kg of iron (specific heat $c_p = 0.47\ \text{J K}^{-1}\ \text{g}^{-1}$) at 100°C is placed in 1 kg of water ($c_p = 4.19\ \text{J K}^{-1}\ \text{g}^{-1}$) at 0°C. Calculate the final temperature and the entropy change.

$$\Delta S = \Delta S_{Fe} + \Delta S_{H_2O} = m_{Fe} \int_{373\ \text{K}}^{T_f} \frac{C_p(Fe)}{T}\, dT + m_{H_2O} \int_{273\ \text{K}}^{T_F} \frac{C_p(H_2O)}{T}\, dT .$$

T_F may be found by a heat balance:

$$m_{Fe}C_p(Fe)(373 - T_F) = m_{H_2O}C_p(H_2O)(T_F - 273) .$$

$$(1000\ \text{g})(0.47\ \text{J K}^{-1}\ \text{g}^{-1})(373 - T_F) = (1000\ \text{g}) \times$$

$$(4.19\ \text{J K}^{-1}\ \text{g}^{-1})(T_F - 273)$$

Solving for T_F, we find $T_F = 283\ K = 10^\circ C$. Assuming that C_p is constant, integration gives

$$\Delta S = (1000\ g)\left[(0.47\ J\ K^{-1}\ g^{-1})\ \ln\left(\frac{283}{373}\right)\right.$$

$$\left. + \left(4.19\ J\ K^{-1}\ g^{-1}\right)\ \ln\left(\frac{283}{273}\right)\right].$$

$$\Delta S = 20.95\ J\ K^{-1}.$$

3.12 Calculate the entropy change when one mole of an ideal gas is compressed isothermally from 1 atm to 2.5 atm.

From Eq. (3.14b),

$$\Delta S = -nR\ \ln\frac{P_2}{P_1} = -1(8.3145\ J\ K^{-1})\ \ln(2.5) = -7.62\ J\ K^{-1}.$$

3.13 Calculate the entropy of mixing for 1 kg of air (O_2, 21%; N_2, 79% mole).

From Eq. (3.15), $\Delta_{mix}S = -R(n_A \ln X_A + n_B \ln X_B)$ where $X_{O_2} = 0.21$ and $X_{N_2} = 0.79$. Air has a molecular weight $\overline{M}_{air} = 28.85$ g, thus $n_{O_2} = \left(\frac{1000\ g}{28.85\ g}\right)(0.21) = 7.28$ mol and $n_{N_2} = 27.38$ mol.

$$\Delta_{mix}S = -8.3145\ J\ K^{-1}(7.28\ \ln(0.21) + 27.38\ \ln(0.79)).$$

$$\Delta_{mix}S = 148\ J\ K^{-1}.$$

3.14 Chlorine has two isotopes, mass 35 (75.53%) and mass 37 (24.47%). Calculate the contribution to the molar entropy of Cl_2 from the mixing of the various isotopic species.

For Cl_2 we have three possible combinations of isotopes:
$^{35}Cl - ^{35}Cl$, $^{37}Cl - ^{35}Cl$ ($^{35}Cl - ^{37}Cl$), and $^{37}Cl - ^{37}Cl$.

The mole fraction of each of these is:

35 - 35	(0.7553)(0.7553)	= 0.5705	$= X_1$
35 - 37	2(0.7553)(0.2447)	= 0.3696	$= X_2$
37 - 37	(0.2447)(0.2447)	= 0.0599	$= X_3$
		1.0000	

From Eq. (3.15), $\Delta_{mix}S = -R(n_1 \ln X_1 + n_2 \ln X_2 + n_3 \ln X_3)$

For 1 mole of Cl_2,

$$\Delta_{mix}S = -(8.3145 \text{ J K}^{-1}) \times$$

$$(0.5705 \ln(0.5705) + 0.3696 \ln(0.3696) + 0.0599 \ln(0.0599))$$

$$\Delta_{mix}S = 7.12 \text{ J K}^{-1} \text{ mol}^{-1} .$$

3.15 An ideal monatomic gas expands adiabatically from 800 K, 8 atm, to 1 atm final pressure. Calculate ΔS, ΔU, and q for the process if it is (a) reversible, (b) irreversible, doing 3000 J of work, (c) irreversible against zero pressure.

a) We find the final temperature from Eq. (2.45b),

$C_{pm}\ln\left(\frac{T_2}{T_1}\right) = R\ \ln\left(\frac{P_2}{P_1}\right)$. For an ideal monatomic gas,

$C_{pm} = \frac{5}{2}R$, thus $T_2 = 348$ K.

$\Delta U = nC_{vm}\Delta T = \frac{3}{2}nR\Delta T = \frac{3}{2}(8.3145\ \text{J K}^{-1})(348\ \text{K} - 800\ \text{K}) = -5640$ J.

Since $dq_{rev} = 0$, $dS = 0$ and $\Delta S = 0$.

b) Since $q = 0$, $\Delta U = q + w = w = -3000\ \text{J} = nC_{vm}\Delta T$.

The final T is then found to be

$$T_2 = \frac{-3000\ \text{J}}{\frac{3}{2}(8.3145\ \text{J K}^{-1})} + 800\ \text{K} = 559\ \text{K} .$$

Since $dH = TdS + VdP$, $dS = \frac{dH}{T} - \frac{VdP}{T} = \frac{dH}{dT}\frac{dT}{T} - \frac{nRdP}{P}$.

Integrating, $\Delta S = C_p\ \ln\frac{T_2}{T_1} - nR\ \ln\frac{P_2}{P_1}$ where $C_p = \frac{5}{2}$ R .

Then $\Delta S = 9.84\ \text{J K}^{-1}\ \text{mol}^{-1}$.

c) $w = 0$. Since $q = 0$, $\Delta U = q + w = 0$. Since $\Delta U = C_v\Delta T$,

$T_1 = T_2 = 800$ K . $\Delta S = -nR\ \ln\frac{P_2}{P_1} = 17.29\ \text{J K}^{-1}\ \text{mol}^{-1}$.

3.16 One mole of an ideal monatomic gas initially at STP is put through each of the reversible steps below, in each case starting at STP. Calculate w, q, ΔU, ΔH, and ΔS for each case.
(a) Cooling at constant volume to −100°C.
(b) Isothermal compression to 100 atm.
(c) Constant pressure heating to 100°C.
(d) Adiabatic expansion to 0.1 atm.

a) $w = 0$, so that

$$\Delta U = q = C_v \Delta T = \frac{3}{2}(8.3145 \text{ J K}^{-1})(173 - 273 \text{ K}) = -1.25 \text{ kJ}.$$

$$\Delta H = C_p \Delta T = \frac{5}{2}(8.3145 \text{ J K}^{-1})(173 - 273 \text{ K}) = -2.08 \text{ kJ}.$$

From Eq. (3.13),

$$\Delta S = C_v \ln \frac{T_2}{T_1} = \frac{3}{2}(8.3145 \text{ J K}^{-1}) \ln \frac{173}{273} = -5.69 \text{ J K}^{-1} .$$

b) From Eq. (2.41),

$$-w_{max} = nRT \ln\left(\frac{V_2}{V_1}\right) = nRT \ln\left(\frac{P_1}{P_2}\right) = -10.45 \text{ kJ}$$

or $w = 10.45$ kJ. Since the process is isothermal $\Delta U = C_v \Delta T = 0$.

$$q = \Delta U - w = -w = -10.45 \text{ kJ}. \quad \Delta H = C_p \Delta T = 0 .$$

$$\Delta S = -RT \ln\left(\frac{P_2}{P_1}\right) = -38.3 \text{ J K}^{-1} .$$

c) For a constant pressure reversible process

$$-w = \int P dV = \int_{T_1}^{T_2} nRdT = nR(T_2 - T_1) = 831 \text{ J or } w = -0.83 \text{ kJ}.$$

$$\Delta H = q = C_p \Delta T = \frac{5}{2}(8.3145 \text{ J K}^{-1})(373 - 273 \text{ K}) = 2.08 \text{ kJ}.$$

$$\Delta U = q + w = 2080 \text{ J} - 831 \text{ J} = 1.25 \text{ kJ}.$$

$$\Delta S = C_p \ln\left(\frac{T_2}{T_1}\right) = 6.5 \text{ J K}^{-1} .$$

d) $q = 0$. From Eq. (2.45b), the final temperature is

$$C_p \ln\left(\frac{T_2}{T_1}\right) = R \ln\left(\frac{P_2}{P_1}\right) , \quad T_2 = 109 \text{ K} . \quad \text{Then } \Delta U = C_v \Delta T = -2.05 \text{ kJ}$$

and $w = -2.05$ kJ. $\Delta H = C_p\Delta T = \frac{5}{2} R\Delta T = -3.41$ kJ and

$$\Delta S = \frac{q_{rev}}{T} = 0 .$$

3.17 One mole of an ideal monatomic gas, initially at 300 K, 1 atm, is compressed and heated to 400 K, 2 atm. Calculate ΔU, ΔH and ΔS for this change.

Step A: Heat from 300 K to 400 K at constant p = 1 atm. For an ideal gas: $\Delta U_A = n\int_{300}^{400} C_{vm}dT$. With n = 1 and $C_{vm} = \frac{3}{2}$ R:

$$\Delta U_A = \tfrac{3}{2}(8.3145\ \text{J K}^{-1})(100\ \text{K}) = 1247\ \text{J} .$$

Also: $\Delta H_A = n\int_{300}^{400} C_{pm}dT$. With n = 1 and $C_{pm} = \frac{5}{2}$ R:

$$\Delta H_A = 2079\ \text{J} .$$

Finally: $\Delta S_A = n\int_{300}^{400} \frac{C_{pm}}{T}\, dT$.

$$\Delta S_A = \tfrac{5}{2}(8.3145\ \text{J K}^{-1})\ \ln\left(\frac{400}{300}\right) = 5.980\ \text{J K}^{-1} .$$

Step B: Compress from 1 to 2 atm at constant T = 400 K. For an ideal gas, ΔU and ΔH are functions of temperature only, so that

$$\Delta U_B = \Delta H_B = 0 .$$

$$\Delta S_B = \int_{V_1}^{V_2} nR\, \frac{dV}{V} = -nR\ \ln\left(\frac{P_2}{P_1}\right) .$$

$$\Delta S_B = -(8.3145\ \text{J K}^{-1})\ \ln(2) = -5.763\ \text{J K}^{-1} .$$

Thus:

$$\Delta U = \Delta U_A + \Delta U_B = 1247\ \text{J}$$

$$\Delta H = \Delta H_A + \Delta H_B = 2079\ \text{J}$$

$$\Delta S = \Delta S_A + \Delta S_B = 0.217\ \text{J K}^{-1} .$$

3.18 Tin melts at 231.9°C with a heat of fusion of 7070 J mol^{-1}. The heat capacities are C_{pm}(solid) = 28.1 J K^{-1}, C_{pm}(liq) = 30.2 J K^{-1}.
(a) Calculate ΔS of fusion at 231.9°C.
(b) Calculate ΔS when tin, supercooled 55°C below the normal mp, is frozen.
(c) Calculate ΔS(surroundings) and ΔS(isolated) for (b).

a) $\Delta_f S = \frac{\Delta_f H}{T} = \frac{7070\ J}{505.1\ K} = 14.0\ J\ K^{-1}$.

b) For heating to the melting point,

$$\Delta S_1 = C_p \ln\left(\frac{T_2}{T_1}\right) = (30.2\ J\ K^{-1})\ \ln\left(\frac{505.1}{450.1}\right) = 3.49\ J\ K^{-1}\ .$$

For freezing at the melting point,

$$\Delta S_2 = -14.0\ J\ K^{-1}\ .$$

For cooling the solid,

$$\Delta S_3 = (28.1\ J\ K^{-1})\ln\left(\frac{450.1}{505.1}\right) = -3.24\ J\ K^{-1}\ .$$

$$\Delta S = \Delta S_1 + \Delta S_2 + \Delta S_3 = -13.7\ J\ K^{-1}\ .$$

c) $\Delta H_{sys} = (30.2\ J\ K^{-1})(55\ K) - 7070\ J - (28.1\ J\ K^{-1})(55K)$.

$$\Delta H_{sys} = -6954.5\ J = -\Delta H_{surr}\ .$$

$$\Delta S_{surr} = \frac{\Delta H_{surr}}{T} = \frac{6954.5\ J}{450.1\ K} = 15.4\ J\ K^{-1}\ .$$

$$\Delta S_{isol} = \Delta S_{surr} + \Delta S_{sys} = 15.4\ J\ K^{-1} - 13.7\ J\ K^{-1} = 1.7\ J\ K^{-1}\ .$$

3.19 (a) Show that the entropy change of a van der Waals gas for an isothermal change $V_1 \rightarrow V_2$ is:

$$\Delta S = nR \ln\left(\frac{V_2 - nb}{V_1 - nb}\right)$$

(b) Calculate ΔS for expanding one mole of NH_3 from 2 dm^3 to 20 dm^3 at 25°C. Compare this to the ideal gas result.

a) From Eq. (3.7), $dU = TdS - PdV$ or $dS = \frac{dU}{T} + \frac{PdV}{T}$. Also

$dU = \left(\frac{\partial U}{\partial T}\right)_V dT + \left(\frac{\partial U}{\partial V}\right)_T dV$. Since $dT = 0$ and from Eq. (2.15),

$dU = \frac{an^2}{V^2}\, dV$, then $dS = \left(\frac{an^2}{V^2} + P\right)\frac{dV}{T}$.

Using $P = \frac{nRT}{V - nb} - \frac{an^2}{V^2}$, $dS = \left(\frac{nRT}{V - nb}\right)\frac{dV}{T} = \left(\frac{nR}{V - nb}\right)dV$.

Integrating, $\Delta S = \int_{V_1}^{V_2}\left(\frac{nR}{V - nb}\right)dV = nR \ln\left(\frac{V_2 - nb}{V_1 - nb}\right)$.

b) For NH_3,

$$\Delta S = (1)(8.3143 \text{ J K}^{-1}) \ln\left(\frac{20 - 1(0.0371)}{2 - 1(0.0371)}\right) = 19.28 \text{ J K}^{-1}.$$

For an ideal gas, $\Delta S = (1)(8.3145 \text{ J K}^{-1}) \ln\left(\frac{20}{2}\right) = 19.14 \text{ J K}^{-1}$.

3.20 (a) Show that the entropy change of a gas, isothermally expanded from V_1 to V_2 is, according to the Redlich-Kwong equation of state:

$$\Delta S = nR \ln\left[\frac{(V_2 - nb)}{(V_1 - nb)}\right] + \frac{na}{2bT^{3/2}} \ln\left[\frac{V_2(V_1 + nb)}{V_1(V_2 + nb)}\right]$$

(b) Using the Redlich-Kwong equation, calculate ΔS for expanding one mole of NH_3 from 2 dm^3 to 20 dm^3 at 25°C. Compare this to the ideal gas result.

$\left(\frac{\partial S}{\partial V}\right)_T = \left(\frac{\partial P}{\partial T}\right)_V$. For an isothermal expansion:

$$\Delta S = \int_{V_1}^{V_2}\left(\frac{\partial S}{\partial V}\right)_T dV = \int_{V_1}^{V_2}\left(\frac{\partial P}{\partial T}\right)_V dV .$$

For a Redlich - Kwong gas: $P = \frac{nRT}{V - nb} - \frac{an^2}{T^{1/2}V(V + nb)}$.

Thus: $\left(\frac{\partial P}{\partial T}\right)_V = \frac{nR}{V - nb} - \frac{an^2}{2T^{3/2}V(V + nb)}$.

$$\Delta S = \int_{V_1}^{V_2}\left[\frac{nR}{V - nb} - \frac{an^2}{2T^{3/2}V(V + nb)}\right]dV .$$

With $\frac{1}{V(V + nb)} = \frac{1}{nb}\left(\frac{1}{V} - \frac{1}{V + nb}\right)$ we may integrate to find:

$$\Delta S = \left[nR \ln(V - nb) + \frac{an}{2bT^{3/2}} \ln\left(\frac{V}{V + nb}\right)\right]_{V_1}^{V_2} .$$

Finally:

$$\Delta S = nR \ln\left(\frac{V_2 - nb}{V_1 - nb}\right) + \frac{an}{2bT^{3/2}} \ln\left(\frac{V_2(V_1 + nb)}{V_1(V_2 + nb)}\right) .$$

3.21 Calculate ΔA and ΔG for the isothermal compression of one mole of an ideal gas from 1 atm to 2.5 atm at 27°C.

From Eq. (3.21), $dA = -SdT - PdV$. Since $dT = 0$, $dA = -PdV$.

For an ideal gas, $dA = \frac{-nRT}{V} dV$ or integrating,

$$\Delta A = -nRT \ln \frac{V_2}{V_1} = nRT \ln \frac{P_2}{P_1}$$

$$\Delta A = (1)(8.3145\ J\ K^{-1})(300\ K) \ln\left(\frac{2.5}{1}\right) = 2286\ J .$$

From Eq. (3.22), $dG = -SdT + VdP$ or $dG = VdP = \frac{nRTdP}{P}$ at constant T. Integrating,

$$\Delta G = nRT \ln \frac{P_2}{P_1} = (1)(8.3145 \text{ J K}^{-1})(300 \text{ K}) \ln\left(\frac{2.5}{1}\right)$$

$$\Delta G = 2286 \text{ J} = \Delta A .$$

3.22 Calculate ΔA and ΔG for compressing one mole of NH_3 from 1 atm to 2.5 atm at 27°C using the van der Waals equation. The volume changes from 24.497 dm^3 to 9.718 dm^3.

At constant T, $dA = -PdV$. For a van der Waals gas,

$P = \frac{nRT}{V - nb} - \frac{an^2}{V^2}$. Then $dA = \left(\frac{nRT}{V - nb} - \frac{an^2}{V^2}\right)dV$ or

$$\Delta A = nRT \ln\left(\frac{V_2 - nb}{V_1 - nb}\right) + an^2\left(\frac{1}{V_2} - \frac{1}{V_1}\right) .$$

Using $b = 0.0371 \text{ dm}^3 \text{ mol}^{-1}$, $a = 4.17 \text{ dm}^6 \text{ atm mol}^{-2}$,

$\Delta A = 2286$ J .

For an isothermal process, $dG = VdP$. Using $VdP = d(PV) - PdV$ and $dA = -PdV$, $dG = d(PV) + dA$ or $\Delta G = P_2V_2 - P_1V_1 + \Delta A$. Then

$\Delta G = 2265$ J .

3.23 A useful objective is to write thermodynamic variables (H, U, S, and so on) in terms of measurable parameters. We have seen (Ch. 2) that the Joule-Thomson coefficient is measurable. Derive the following equation from the basic equations and definitions:

$$dH = C_p dT - \mu C_p dP$$

$dH = \left(\frac{\partial H}{\partial T}\right)_P dT + \left(\frac{\partial H}{\partial P}\right)_T dP$. Since $C_p = \left(\frac{\partial H}{\partial T}\right)_P$ and from the cyclic rule, $\left(\frac{\partial H}{\partial P}\right)_T = -\left(\frac{\partial T}{\partial P}\right)_H \left(\frac{\partial H}{\partial T}\right)_P$, $dH = C_p dT - \left(\frac{\partial T}{\partial P}\right)_H C_p dP$.

Recognizing $\mu = \left(\frac{\partial T}{\partial P}\right)_H$, $dH = C_p dT - \mu C_p dP$.

3.24 Derive the equation:

$$\frac{\kappa_T}{\kappa_S} = \frac{C_p}{C_v}$$

from the basic equations (Table 3.1) and definitions.

From the definition of the heat capacities:

$C_P = \left(\frac{\partial H}{\partial T}\right)_P = T\left(\frac{\partial S}{\partial T}\right)_P$ and $C_V = \left(\frac{\partial U}{\partial T}\right)_V = T\left(\frac{\partial S}{\partial T}\right)_V$. Thus

$\frac{C_P}{C_V} = \frac{\left(\frac{\partial S}{\partial T}\right)_P}{\left(\frac{\partial S}{\partial T}\right)_V}$. We now use the cyclic rule to obtain

$\left(\frac{\partial S}{\partial T}\right)_P = \frac{-1}{\left(\frac{\partial T}{\partial P}\right)_S\left(\frac{\partial P}{\partial S}\right)_T}$ and $\left(\frac{\partial S}{\partial T}\right)_V = \frac{-1}{\left(\frac{\partial T}{\partial V}\right)_S\left(\frac{\partial V}{\partial S}\right)_T}$. Then

$\frac{C_P}{C_V} = \frac{\left(\frac{\partial T}{\partial V}\right)_S\left(\frac{\partial V}{\partial S}\right)_T}{\left(\frac{\partial T}{\partial P}\right)_S\left(\frac{\partial P}{\partial S}\right)_T} = \frac{\left(\frac{\partial V}{\partial P}\right)_T}{\left(\frac{\partial V}{\partial P}\right)_S}$. Since $\kappa_T \equiv -\frac{1}{V}\left(\frac{\partial V}{\partial P}\right)_T$ and

$\kappa_S \equiv -\frac{1}{V}\left(\frac{\partial V}{\partial P}\right)_S$ then $\frac{C_P}{C_V} = \frac{\kappa_T}{\kappa_S}$.

3.25 Some properties of liquids are relatively easy to measure—for example, C_p, α, and κ_S (from the velocity of sound). Other properties are more difficult to measure because liquids are not very compressible—for example, C_v and κ_T.

(a) Derive the equation:

$$\kappa_T = \kappa_S + \frac{TV\alpha^2}{C_p}$$

(b) Calculate κ_S, κ_T, γ, and C_{vm} for benzene at 25°C from these data: $C_{pm} = 134$ J K^{-1}, $V_m = 89.8$ cm^3, $M = 78.11$ g/mole, $c = 1295$ m s^{-1}, $\alpha = 1.24 \times 10^{-3}$ K^{-1}.

a) From Eq. (AII.11), $\left(\frac{\partial V}{\partial P}\right)_T = \left(\frac{\partial V}{\partial P}\right)_S + \left(\frac{\partial V}{\partial S}\right)_P\left(\frac{\partial S}{\partial P}\right)_T$.

$\left(\frac{\partial V}{\partial S}\right)_P = \left(\frac{\partial V}{\partial T}\right)_P\left(\frac{\partial T}{\partial S}\right)_P = \frac{TV\alpha}{C_P}$. Using Maxwell's relation,

$\frac{1}{V}\left(\frac{\partial V}{\partial P}\right)_T = \frac{1}{V}\left(\frac{\partial V}{\partial P}\right)_S - \frac{TV^2\alpha^2}{C_P}\left(\frac{1}{V}\right)$ or $\kappa_T = \kappa_S + \frac{TV\alpha^2}{C_P}$.

b) $\kappa_T - \kappa_S = \dfrac{T\alpha^2 V}{C_p}$

$$= \dfrac{(298 \text{ K})(1.24 \times 10^{-3} \text{ K}^{-1})^2(89.8 \text{ cm}^3)}{134 \text{ J K}^{-1}} \left(\dfrac{1 \text{ J}}{9.869 \text{ cm}^3 \text{ atm}} \right)$$

$$= 3.11 \times 10^{-5} \text{ atm}^{-1} \ .$$

Since $\kappa_S = \dfrac{1}{C^2 \rho}$ where $\rho = \dfrac{M}{V_m} = 8.70 \times 10^5 \text{ g m}^{-3}$, then

$\kappa_S = 6.85 \times 10^{-13} \text{ g}^{-1} \text{ sec}^2 \text{ m} = 6.94 \times 10^{-5} \text{ atm}$. κ_T is then

$$\kappa_T = \kappa_S + 3.11 \times 10^{-5} \text{ atm}^{-1} = 1.01 \times 10^{-4} \text{ atm}^{-1} \ .$$

Using the eq. derived in problem 3.24,

$$C_v = \dfrac{C_p \kappa_S}{\kappa_T} = \dfrac{(134 \text{ J K}^{-1})(6.945 \times 10^{-5} \text{ atm}^{-1})}{(1.01 \times 10^{-4} \text{ atm}^{-1})} = 92.1 \text{ J K}^{-1} \ .$$

From Eq. (3.33), $\gamma = \dfrac{C_p}{C_v} = 1.45$.

3.26 Derive the equation:

$$\left(\dfrac{\partial H}{\partial T} \right)_V = C_v + \dfrac{V\alpha}{\kappa_T}$$

From Table 3.1, $H = U + PV$. Then $\dfrac{dH}{dT} = \dfrac{dU}{dT} + \dfrac{d(PV)}{dT}$ and

$\left(\dfrac{\partial H}{\partial T} \right)_V = \left(\dfrac{\partial U}{\partial T} \right)_V + V\left(\dfrac{\partial P}{\partial T} \right)_V$. Since $C_v = \left(\dfrac{\partial U}{\partial T} \right)_V$ and from the

cyclic rule $\left(\dfrac{\partial P}{\partial T} \right)_V = \dfrac{-1}{\left(\dfrac{\partial T}{\partial V} \right)_P \left(\dfrac{\partial V}{\partial P} \right)_T} = - \dfrac{\left(\dfrac{\partial V}{\partial T} \right)_P}{\left(\dfrac{\partial V}{\partial P} \right)_T}$, then

$\left(\dfrac{\partial H}{\partial T} \right)_V = C_v - V \dfrac{\left(\dfrac{\partial V}{\partial T} \right)_P}{\left(\dfrac{\partial V}{\partial P} \right)_T}$. Using $\alpha = \dfrac{1}{V}\left(\dfrac{\partial V}{\partial T} \right)_P$ and $\kappa_T = -\dfrac{1}{V}\left(\dfrac{\partial V}{\partial P} \right)_T$

we have $\left(\dfrac{\partial H}{\partial T} \right)_V = C_v + \dfrac{V\alpha}{\kappa_T}$.

3.27 Show that the temperature change on adiabatic compression is:

$$\left(\frac{\partial T}{\partial P}\right)_S = \frac{\alpha V_m T}{C_{pm}}$$

Calculate the temperature change when 10 atm pressure is applied adiabatically to benzene at 25°C. Assume incompressibility.

From Table 3.1, $dS = \frac{C_P}{T}\,dT - \left(\frac{\partial V}{\partial T}\right)_P dP$. With $dS = 0$,

$$\left(\frac{\partial T}{\partial P}\right)_S = \left(\frac{\partial V}{\partial T}\right)_P \frac{T}{C_P} \text{ . Using } \alpha = \frac{1}{V}\left(\frac{\partial V}{\partial T}\right)_P, \left(\frac{\partial T}{\partial P}\right)_S = \frac{V\alpha T}{C_P} = \frac{V_m \alpha T}{C_{pm}} \text{ .}$$

Using data from Tables 1.8 and 3.3,

$$\left(\frac{\partial T}{\partial P}\right)_S = \frac{(89 \times 10^{-6}\ m^3)(1.237 \times 10^{-3}\ K^{-1})(298\ K)}{136\ J\ K^{-1}}$$

$$\left(\frac{\partial T}{\partial P}\right)_S = 2.41 \times 10^{-7}\ m^3\ K\ J^{-1} \text{ .}$$

Assuming $\left(\frac{\partial T}{\partial P}\right)_S \cong \frac{\Delta T}{\Delta P}$, $\Delta T = \Delta P(2.41 \times 10^{-7}\ m^3\ K\ J^{-1})$ or

$$\Delta T = 10\ atm\left(\frac{2.41 \times 10^{-7}\ m^3\ K}{J}\right)\left(\frac{1\ J}{9.869\ cm^3\ atm}\right) \times \left(\frac{10^6\ cm^3}{1\ m^3}\right) = 0.24\ K \text{ .}$$

3.28 Aluminum ($V_m = 10\ cm^3$, $C_{pm} = 25.4\ J\ K^{-1}$, $\alpha = 2.6 \times 10^{-5}\ K^{-1}$) initially at 25°C, is struck by a force of 10 tons (U.S.) on one square inch. Calculate the maximum temperature rise (use the equation derived in the previous problem).

From problem 3.27, $\frac{\Delta T}{\Delta P} \cong \left(\frac{\partial T}{\partial P}\right)_S = \frac{\alpha V_m T}{C_{pm}}$. Since

10 tons/in = 1.38×10^8 Pa,

$$\Delta T = \frac{(1.38 \times 10^8\ Pa)(2.6 \times 10^{-5}\ K^{-1})(298.15\ K)}{25.4\ J\ K^{-1}\left(\frac{100\ cm}{m}\right)^3} = 0.42\ K \text{ .}$$

3.29 Calculate the standard entropy of H_2 (gas) at 500 K from the value at 25°C given in Table 3.2.

The standard entropy at 500 K is: $$S^\ominus = S^\ominus(298\text{ K}) + \int_{298}^{500} \frac{C_p^\ominus \, dT}{T} .$$

From Table 2.2:

$$C_p^\ominus = \left[27.28 + (3.26 \times 10^{-3})T + \frac{(0.50 \times 10^5)}{T^2}\right] \text{J K}^{-1}\text{ mol}^{-1} .$$

Performing the integration gives:

$$\int_{298}^{500} \frac{C_p^\ominus \, dT}{T} = 14.96 \text{ J K}^{-1}\text{ mol}^{-1} .$$

From Table 3.2, $S^\ominus(298\text{ K}) = 130.684\text{ J K}^{-1}\text{ mol}^{-1}$ so that

$$S^\ominus(500\text{ K}) = 145.64\text{ J K}^{-1}\text{ mol}^{-1} .$$

3.30 Use the data below to calculate the standard entropy of ammonia at 298.15 K (units: cal or cal/K, all for one mole).

T	C_{pm}	T	C_{pm}	T	C_{pm}
15	0.175	80	4.954	150	9.272
20	0.368	90	5.612	160	9.846
30	1.033	100	6.246	170	10.42
40	1.841	110	6.877	180	11.03
50	2.663	120	7.497	190	11.71
60	3.474	130	8.120	195.42	11.98
70	4.232	140	8.699		

Melts 195.42, $\Delta_f H$ = 1351.6, C_{pm}(liq.) = 17.89 (ave.), boils 239.74, $\Delta_v H$ = 5581.

T	C_{pm} (gas)
239.74	8.36
298.15	8.49

From Eq. (3.36), $S(T) = S_0 + \int_0^T \frac{C_p}{T}\, dT$. For the solid NH_3 we break the integral above into intervals according to the given temperatures. For each interval we find an average C_p and integrate:

$$\Delta S_{\substack{\text{interval}\\ T_1 \to T_2}} = \overline{C}_p \ln \frac{T_2}{T_1} \ . \quad \text{Summing} \ , \ \Delta S_{15 \to 195.42\ K} = 10.2 \text{ cal K}^{-1} \ .$$

For the phase change,

$$\Delta S = \frac{\Delta_f H}{T_f} = \frac{1351.6 \text{ cal}}{195.42 \text{ K}} = 6.9 \text{ cal K}^{-1} \ .$$

For heating the liquid to 239.74 K, we have

$$\Delta S = (17.89 \text{ cal K}^{-1}) \ln \frac{239.74}{195.42} = 3.66 \text{ cal K}^{-1} \ .$$

For the liquid to gas change,

$$\Delta S = \frac{5581 \text{ cal}}{239.74 \text{ K}} = 23.28 \text{ cal K}^{-1} \ .$$

For heating the gas to 298.15 K,

$$\Delta S = (8.43 \text{ cal K}^{-1}) \ln \frac{298.15}{239.74} = 1.8 \text{ cal K}^{-1} \ .$$

Then $\quad \Delta S = 10.2 + 6.9 + 3.7 + 23.3 + 1.8 = 45.9 \text{ cal K}^{-1}$

$$\Delta S = 192.2 \text{ J K}^{-1} \ .$$

To get $S_m^\ominus$ we add in the correction for nonideality

$$S_m^\ominus = S_m(P = 1 \text{ atm}) + \frac{27R}{32}\left(\frac{T_c}{T}\right)^3\left(\frac{P^\ominus}{P_c}\right)$$

$$S_m^\ominus = 192.2 \text{ J K}^{-1} + 0.2 \text{ J K}^{-1} = 192.4 \text{ J K}^{-1} .$$

3.31 The refrigerant gas, $CHCl_2F$, has a virial coefficient $B = -354 \text{ cm}^3$ and $B' = 1.66 \text{ cm}^3 \text{ K}^{-1}$ at 394 K. Calculate ΔS for isothermal compression of this gas at 394 K from 1 atm to 2.5 atm.

From Eq. (3.39), $S_m(P_2) - S_m(P_1) = -R \ln\left(\frac{P_2}{P_1}\right) - B'(P_2 - P_1)$ or

$$\Delta S = -(8.3143 \text{ J K}^{-1}) \ln(2.5) - (1.66 \text{ cm}^3 \text{ K}^{-1})(2.5 - 1)\text{atm}$$

$$\Delta S = -7.87 \text{ J K}^{-1} .$$

3.32 Calculate the entropy of NH_3 (gas) at 25°C, 10 atm pressure, assuming (a) ideal gas, (b) the Berthelot virial coefficient.

a) For an ideal gas: $S_m(P_2) = S_m(P_1) - R \ln\left(\frac{P_2}{P_1}\right)$.

From Table 3.2, $S_m^\theta(298 \text{ K}, 1 \text{ atm}) = 192.45 \text{ J K}^{-1} \text{ mol}^{-1}$ so that

$$S_m^\theta(298 \text{ K}, 10 \text{ atm}) = [192.45 - (8.3143) \ln(10)] \text{J K}^{-1} \text{ mol}^{-1}$$

$$S_m^\theta(298 \text{ K}, 10 \text{ atm}) = 173.31 \text{ J K}^{-1} \text{ mol}^{-1} .$$

b) $S_m(T, P) = S_m^\theta(T) - R \ln\left(\frac{P}{P^\theta}\right) - B'P$. For ammonia gas:

$$B'(T) = \frac{27R}{32}\left(\frac{T_c}{T}\right)^3\left(\frac{1}{P_c}\right)$$

$$= \frac{27(8.3145 \text{ J K}^{-1} \text{ mol}^{-1})}{32}\left(\frac{405.5}{298}\right)^3\left(\frac{1}{111.5 \text{ atm}}\right)$$

$$= 0.1585 \text{ J K}^{-1} \text{ atm}^{-1} \text{ mol}^{-1} .$$

Thus:

$$S_m(298 \text{ K}, 10 \text{ atm}) = 173.31 \text{ J K}^{-1} \text{ mol}^{-1} - 1.585 \text{ J K}^{-1}\text{mol}^{-1}$$

$$S_m(298 \text{ K}, 10 \text{ atm}) = 171.72 \text{ J K}^{-1} \text{ mol}^{-1} .$$

3.33 Calculate the entropy of benzene (liq.) under 1000 atm pressure at 25°C.

For condensed phases $\left(\frac{\partial S}{\partial P}\right)_T = -V\alpha$ or at constant T: $\Delta S = -V\alpha\Delta P$,

$S_m(1000 \text{ atm}) = S_m^\theta(1 \text{ atm}) - V\alpha\Delta P$. Using data from Tables 1.8 and 3.2,

$$S_m = 173\ \mathrm{J\ K^{-1}\ mol^{-1}} - (89\ \mathrm{cm^3})(1.237 \times 10^{-3}\ \mathrm{K^{-1}})(999\ \mathrm{atm}) \times \left(\frac{1\ \mathrm{J}}{9.869\ \mathrm{atm\ cm^3}}\right)$$

$$S_m = 162\ \mathrm{J\ K^{-1}}\ .$$

3.34 Propane (gas) has a standard entropy at 25°C of 270 J K^{-1}.
(a) Calculate ΔS° when propane at 25°C is burned to form products at 25°C:

$$C_3H_8 + 5\,O_2 = 3\,CO_2 + 4\,H_2O\ \text{(liq.)}$$

(b) When burned, a mole of propane provides 2.108×10^6 J of heat (that is, the ΔH° for the above reaction is -2.108×10^6 J). Calculate the maximum work available if this heat is used in an engine operating between 300 and 450 K.
(c) A fuel cell is a device that produces an electrical current from a reaction. Calculate the maximum electrical work available if propane is reacted in fuel cell.

a) $\Delta_r S^{\ominus} = S^{\ominus}(\text{products}) - S^{\ominus}(\text{reactants})$. Using Table 3.2

$$\Delta_r S^{\ominus} = 3(213.72\ \mathrm{J\ K^{-1}}) + 4(70.00\ \mathrm{J\ K^{-1}}) - 270\ \mathrm{J\ K^{-1}} - 5(205.06\ \mathrm{J\ K^{-1}})$$

$$\Delta_r S^{\ominus} = -374\ \mathrm{J\ K^{-1}}\ .$$

b) From Eq. (3.3),

$$w = \frac{T_2 - T_1}{T_2}(-q_2) = \frac{450\ \mathrm{K} - 300\ \mathrm{K}}{450\ \mathrm{K}}(2.108 \times 10^6\ \mathrm{J}) = 7.03 \times 10^5\ \mathrm{J}.$$

c) The maximum electrical work is $-\Delta G$. $\Delta G = \Delta H - T\Delta S$ or

$$\Delta G = -2.108 \times 10^6\ \mathrm{J} - (298\ \mathrm{K})(-374\ \mathrm{J\ K^{-1}}) = -1.997 \times 10^6\ \mathrm{J} = -w$$

$$w = 2.0 \times 10^6\ \mathrm{J}\ .$$

3.35 (a) The statistical theory of rubber (refs. 3 and 5) gives the following formula for the stress (σ) of a rubber as a function of the length:

$$\sigma = \frac{\rho RT}{zM}\left(\frac{l}{l_0} - \frac{l_0^2}{l^2}\right)$$

where ρ = density, M = molecular weight of the monomer unit, and z = number of monomer units between cross-links. Show that the work per unit volume for stretching the rubber from l_0 ($\varepsilon = 0$) to l (ε) is:

$$\frac{w}{V} = \int_0^\varepsilon \sigma\, d\varepsilon = \frac{\rho RT}{zM}\frac{\varepsilon^2(\varepsilon + 3)}{2(\varepsilon + 1)}$$

(b) Calculate the work for stretching a 10 cm × (0.05 cm²) rubber band to 50 cm. Assume the rubber is isoprene, that it is an ideal rubber, 1.25% cross-linking, and 25°C.

a) From Eq. (3.44), $w = \int f\, dl$. From Eq. (3.47), $\sigma = \frac{f}{A_0}$,

thus $w = \int \sigma A_0\, dl$. Then $\frac{w}{V} = \int_{l_0}^{l} \frac{\sigma A_0 dl}{l_0 A_0} = \int_{l_0}^{l} \frac{\sigma}{l_0}\, dl$.

From Eq. (3.48), $\epsilon = \frac{l - l_0}{l_0}$, then $\frac{d\epsilon}{dl} = \frac{1}{l_0}$ and $dl = l_0 d\epsilon$.

Then $\frac{w}{V} = \int_0^\epsilon \sigma\, d\epsilon$. Also

$$\sigma = \frac{\rho RT}{zM}\left(\frac{l}{l_0} - \frac{l_0^2}{l^2}\right) = \frac{\rho RT}{zM}\left(1 + \epsilon - \frac{1}{(1 + \epsilon)^2}\right).$$

$$\frac{w}{V} = \int_0^\epsilon \frac{\rho RT}{zM}\left(1 + \epsilon - \frac{1}{(1 + \epsilon)^2}\right)d\epsilon = \frac{\rho RT}{zM}\left[\epsilon \Big|_0^\epsilon + \frac{1}{2}\epsilon^2 \Big|_0^\epsilon + \frac{1}{1 + \epsilon}\Big|_0^\epsilon\right]$$

$$\frac{w}{V} = \frac{\rho RT}{zM}\left[\frac{\epsilon^2(\epsilon + 3)}{2(1 + \epsilon)}\right].$$

b) $\epsilon = 4$. For isoprene M = 0.068 kg. V = 0.5 x 10^{-6} m³ and ρ = 970 kg m^{-3} (Table 3.4). If the % crosslinking is 1.25, then 1.25 in 100 units are cross-linked. The number of monomer units in 100 units is then $\frac{100}{1.25}$ = 80 = z. Then

$$\frac{w}{V} = \frac{(970 \text{ kg m}^{-3})(8.3145 \text{ J K}^{-1})(298 \text{ K})}{80(0.068 \text{ kg})}\left[\frac{16(7)}{2(5)}\right] = 4.948 \times 10^6 \text{ J}$$

and w = 2.47 J.

3.36 Calculate the specific heat at constant volume of natural rubber from its specific heat at constant pressure.

From Eq. (2.39), $C_v = C_p - \frac{TV\alpha^2}{K_T}$.

$V = \frac{M}{\rho} = \frac{68 \text{ g}}{0.970 \text{ g cm}^{-3}} = 7.01 \times 10^{-5} \text{ m}^3$. Thus for 1 mole,

$$C_v = 1.828 \text{ J K}^{-1} \text{ g}^{-1}(68 \text{ g}) - \frac{(298 \text{ K})(7.01 \times 10^{-5} \text{ m}^3)(6.6 \times 10^{-4} \text{ K}^{-1})^2}{5.14 \times 10^{-10} \text{ Pa}^{-1}} .$$

$C_v = 106.6 \text{ J K}^{-1}$ or $C_v = 1.568 \text{ J K}^{-1} \text{ g}^{-1}$.

3.37 (a) Use the statistical formula for σ (Problem 3.35) to show that the initial modulus of the rubber (also called Young's modulus, the initial slope of the stress-strain curve) is:

$$\left(\frac{d\sigma}{d\varepsilon}\right)_{l_0} = \frac{3\rho RT}{zM}$$

(b) Calculate the percent cross-linking of chloroprene from the initial modulus listed in Table 3.4. (Note that Table 3.4 lists a "typical" value, and this obviously could vary.)

a) From the chain rule, $\frac{d\sigma}{d\epsilon} = \frac{d\sigma}{dl} \cdot \frac{dl}{d\epsilon}$. Then

$$\frac{d\sigma}{d\epsilon} = \frac{\rho RT}{zM}\left(\frac{l^3 + 2l_0^{\,3}}{l_0 l^3}\right)(l_0) = \frac{\rho RT}{zM}\left(\frac{l^3 + 2l_0^{\,3}}{l^3}\right) .$$

At $l = l_0$, $\left(\frac{d\sigma}{d\epsilon}\right)_{l_0} = \frac{\rho RT}{zM}\left(\frac{l_0^{\,3} + 2l_0^{\,3}}{l_0^{\,3}}\right) = \frac{3\rho RT}{zM}$

b) Using data from Table 3.4, $z = \frac{3\rho RT}{M\left(\frac{d\sigma}{d\epsilon}\right)_{l_0}}$

$$z = \frac{3(1.320 \text{ g cm}^{-3})(298 \text{ K})(0.08206 \text{ dm}^3 \text{ atm K}^{-1})\left(\frac{10^3 \text{ cm}^3}{1 \text{ dm}^3}\right)}{86 \text{ g}(1.6 \times 10^6 \text{ Pa})\left(\frac{1 \text{ atm}}{101325 \text{ Pa}}\right)} = 71.3 .$$

The % crosslinking is $\frac{1}{z}(100) = \frac{100}{71.3} = 1.40\%$.

3.38 Calculate ΔT when a 10 cm $\times$ (2 mm $\times$ 3 mm) rubber band is adiabatically stretched to 20 cm. Assume that the rubber is SBR and use Hooke's law with $\sigma/Pa = 3 \times 10^6 \varepsilon$.

From problem 3.35, $\frac{w}{V} = \int_0^\epsilon \sigma \, d\epsilon$. With $\sigma = (3 \times 10^6 \epsilon) \, Pa^{-1}$,

$$\frac{w}{V} = 3 \times 10^6 \left(\frac{1}{2} \epsilon^2 \right)\Big|_0^\epsilon = 1.5 \times 10^6 \epsilon^2 .$$

$$V = 10 \ cm \left(\frac{1 \ m}{10^2 \ cm} \right)(6 \ mm^2)\left(\frac{1 m^2}{10^6 \ mm^2} \right) = 6 \times 10^{-7} \ m^3 .$$

$\epsilon = \frac{20 - 10}{10} = 1$. Then $w = (6 \times 10^{-7})(1.5 \times 10^6)(1) = 0.90 \ J$.

Since $dq = 0$, $dU = dw$ and $C_v dT = dw$. Then $\Delta T = \frac{w}{C_v} \cong \frac{w}{C_p}$.

The weight of the band is

$$\rho V = 9.8 \times 10^5 \ g \ m^{-3}(6 \times 10^{-7} \ m^3) = 0.588 \ g .$$

Then $\Delta T = \dfrac{0.90 \ J}{(1.828 \ J \ K^{-1} \ g^{-1})(0.588 \ g)} = 0.84 \ K$.

3.39 In our discussion of the effect of heat on the length of a rubber band under tension, we neglected the effect of thermal expansion. Assume the coefficient of linear expansion is one-third the volume coefficient (α) and calculate this effect for a 15-cm band and $\Delta T = 100°C$.

The coefficient of linear expansion is $\frac{1}{3}\alpha = \frac{1}{l}\left(\frac{\partial l}{\partial T} \right)_P$ by

analogy to the coefficient of thermal expansion. Then

$\Delta l \cong \frac{1}{3}\alpha l \Delta T$. Using a typical α value from Table 3.4,

$$\Delta l = \frac{1}{3}(6.6 \times 10^{-4} \ K^{-1})(15 \ cm)(100 \ K) = 0.3 \ cm .$$

3.40 The stress (σ) on vulcanized natural rubber was measured at constant elongation as a function of temperature; the result was linear with (370% stretching) $\sigma/\text{Pa} = 1.47 \times 10^6 + 1.09 \times 10^4\, t$ (t in °C). Calculate $(\partial U/\partial l)_T$ (per unit volume) for this rubber at 0°C. (Assume A_0 is independent of T.)

From Eq. (3.54), $\left(\frac{\partial U}{\partial l}\right)_T = f - T\left(\frac{\partial f}{\partial T}\right)_l$ where $f = A_0\sigma$.

Then $\left(\frac{\partial f}{\partial T}\right)_l = A_0\left(\frac{\partial \sigma}{\partial T}\right)_l + \left(\frac{\partial A_0}{\partial T}\right)_l \sigma$. Assuming $\left(\frac{\partial A_0}{\partial T}\right)_l = 0$,

$\frac{1}{A_0}\left(\frac{\partial U}{\partial l}\right)_T = \sigma - T\left(\frac{\partial \sigma}{\partial T}\right)_l$. From the given equation,

$\left(\frac{\partial \sigma}{\partial T}\right)_l = 1.09 \times 10^4 \text{ Pa K}^{-1}$. Then

$$\frac{1}{A_0}\left(\frac{\partial U}{\partial l}\right)_T = 1.47 \times 10^6 \text{ Pa} + (1.09 \times 10^4 \text{ Pa K}^{-1})(273 \text{ K}) - (1.09 \times 10^4 \text{ Pa K}^{-1})(273 \text{ K}) .$$

$$\frac{1}{A_0}\left(\frac{\partial U}{\partial l}\right)_T = 1.47 \times 10^6 \text{ Pa} = 1.47 \times 10^6 \text{ J m}^{-3} .$$

3.41 Prove:

$$\left(\frac{\partial S}{\partial T}\right)_l = \frac{C_l}{T}$$

where C_l is the heat capacity at constant length.

$dU = TdS + fdl = \left(\frac{\partial U}{\partial T}\right)_l dT + \left(\frac{\partial U}{\partial l}\right)_T dl$. Using $\left(\frac{\partial U}{\partial T}\right)_l = C_l$ and letting $dl = 0$, $TdS = C_l dT$ or $\left(\frac{\partial S}{\partial T}\right)_l = \frac{C_l}{T}$.

3.42 Prove that C_l, the specific heat at constant length, is equal to C_v for an ideal rubber.

$dU = \left(\frac{\partial U}{\partial l}\right)_T dl + \left(\frac{\partial U}{\partial T}\right)_l dl$. For an ideal rubber $\left(\frac{\partial U}{\partial l}\right)_T = 0$,

then $dU = \left(\frac{\partial U}{\partial T}\right)_l dT = C_l dT$. Also $dU = \left(\frac{\partial U}{\partial V}\right)_T dV + \left(\frac{\partial U}{\partial T}\right)_V dT$.

Since by the chain rule $\left(\frac{\partial U}{\partial V}\right)_T = \left(\frac{\partial U}{\partial l}\right)_T \left(\frac{\partial l}{\partial V}\right)_T$ and for an ideal

rubber $\left(\frac{\partial U}{\partial l}\right)_T = 0$, $\left(\frac{\partial U}{\partial V}\right)_T = 0$. Thus

$$dU = \left(\frac{\partial U}{\partial T}\right)_V dT = C_v dT \text{ and } C_l dT = C_v dT \text{ or } C_l = C_v .$$

3.43 (a) Assuming bond lengths (C=C) 1.07×10^{-8} cm and (C—C) 1.09×10^{-8} cm and a C=C—C bond angle of 120°, calculate the length of an isoprene monomer unit. (*Ans:* 3.25×10^{-8} cm.)
(b) In Chapter 9 it is shown that a random walk of N steps of length L will have an rms length of $\sqrt{N}\,L$. Assuming a random walk, calculate the mean length of an 80-unit isoprene chain. Assume the "links" are rigid units with the length calculated in (a).
(c) Assume the isoprene links to be arranged in a three-dimensional cube, estimate the density of rubber from the answer in (b).

a) Using the given bond lengths and angles, x is given by

$$x = (1.09 \times 10^{-8}\text{ cm})\sin[120° - 90°] = 5.45 \times 10^{-9}\text{ cm}$$

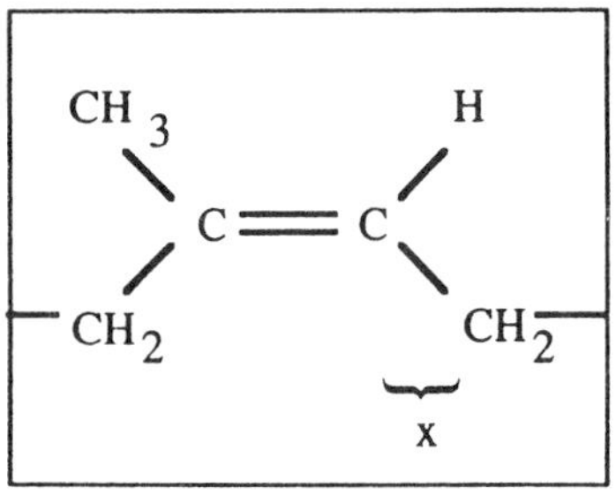

The length of the unit is then

$$l = 1.07 \times 10^{-8}\text{ cm} + 2(5.45 \times 10^{-9}\text{ cm}) + 1.09 \times 10^{-8}\text{ cm}$$

$$l = 3.25 \times 10^{-8}\text{ cm} .$$

b) The mean length is $\bar{l} = \sqrt{80}\,(3.25 \times 10^{-8}\text{ cm}) = 2.91 \times 10^{-7}\text{ cm}$.

c) The volume of the cell is

$$V = (2.91 \times 10^{-7}\text{ cm})^3 = 2.46 \times 10^{-20}\text{ cm}^3 .$$

The weight of the cell is $\frac{1}{4}$(wgt 12 chains) = wgt 3 chains since each of the 12 sides are shared by 4 cubes. The weight of 3 chains is

$$W = 3(80\text{ units})\left(\frac{68\text{ g mol}^{-1}\text{ unit}}{6.022 \times 10^{23}\text{ mol}^{-1}}\right) = 2.71 \times 10^{-20}\text{ g} .$$

Thus $\rho = \frac{W}{V} = \frac{2.71 \times 10^{-20}\text{ g}}{2.46 \times 10^{-20}\text{ cm}^3} = 1.10\text{ g cm}^{-3}$.

3.44 So, there you are—in the middle of the desert with a warm can of soda and a powerful rubber band. You stretch the rubber band and let it equilibrate in the air, then release it adiabatically around the can. How much will the temperature drop, and how many times must you do this to make the soda drinkable? Use V_0(rubber) = 10^{-5} m^3, C_p(rubber) = 20 J K^{-1}, C_p(can) = 2000 J K^{-1}. Assume Hooke's law with $\sigma/\text{Pa} = 2 \times 10^6\ \varepsilon$ and $\varepsilon = 8$ for the stretch (you have powerful arms as well).

$$\frac{w}{V} = \int_0^{\epsilon} \sigma\, d\epsilon\ ,\quad w = \tfrac{1}{2}(2 \times 10^{-6})\epsilon^2 V_0 = \tfrac{1}{2}(2 \times 10^{-6})(8)^2(10^{-5}) = 640\text{ J} .$$

For an adiabatic expansion, $-w = C_V \Delta T$. Assuming $C_V = C_p$, for the rubber band, $\Delta T_b = \frac{-640\text{ J}}{20\text{ J K}^{-1}} = -32\text{ K}$. The temperature change of the can per rubber band pull is then

$-(32\text{ K})(20\text{ J K}^{-1}) = \Delta T(2000\text{ J K}^{-1})$, or $\Delta T_c = -0.32$ K. 100°F is 40°C, which we assume to be the starting temperature of the can. To cool it to 5°C (drinkable) would require $\frac{35}{0.32} = 109$ flips.

4

Equilibrium in Pure Substances

4.1 Calculate the activity of water (V_m = 18 cm^3/mol) at 100 atm and 25°C.

Assuming water to behave as an incompressible liquid:

$$a = \exp\left[\frac{V_m(P - P^\theta)}{RT}\right] .$$

At 25°C and 100 atm:

$$a = \exp\left[\frac{(18\ \text{cm}^3\ \text{mol}^{-1})(100\ \text{atm} - 1\ \text{atm})}{(82.057\ \text{cm}^3\ \text{atm mol}^{-1}\ \text{K}^{-1})(298.15\ \text{K})}\right] = 1.076 .$$

4.2 Show that the change of the Helmholtz free energy with temperature is given by:

$$\left(\frac{\partial(A/T)}{\partial(1/T)}\right)_V = U$$

A = U - TS so that $\frac{A}{T} = \frac{U}{T} - S$ and

$$\left[\frac{\partial\left(\frac{A}{T}\right)}{\partial\left(\frac{1}{T}\right)}\right]_V = U + \frac{1}{T}\left[\frac{\partial U}{\partial\left(\frac{1}{T}\right)}\right]_V - \left[\frac{\partial S}{\partial\left(\frac{1}{T}\right)}\right]_V .$$

Because $d\left(\frac{1}{T}\right) = -\frac{1}{T^2}\,dT$, we have:

$$\left[\frac{\partial\left(\frac{A}{T}\right)}{\partial\left(\frac{1}{T}\right)}\right]_V = U - T\left(\frac{\partial U}{\partial T}\right)_V + T^2\left(\frac{\partial S}{\partial T}\right)_V .$$

But dU = TdS - PdV so that $\left(\frac{\partial U}{\partial T}\right)_V = T\left(\frac{\partial S}{\partial T}\right)_V$.

Thus: $$\left[\frac{\partial\left(\frac{A}{T}\right)}{\partial\left(\frac{1}{T}\right)}\right]_V = U .$$

4.3 From data given in an example in Section 3.3, the ΔG of the process:

$$\text{water}(-10°\text{C}) \longrightarrow \text{ice}(-10°\text{C})$$

can be calculated as:

$$\Delta G = \Delta H - T\Delta S = -5610 - 263.15(-20.5) = -215 \text{ J/mole}$$

At $-10°$C, ice has a vapor pressure of 1.950 torr, while super-cooled water has a vapor pressure of 2.149 torr. Use these data to calculate ΔG for freezing water at $-10°$C.

From Eq. (4.20b), $\Delta_{vap}G^{\theta} = -RT \ln\left(\frac{p^0}{p^{\theta}}\right)$. For sublimation

$\Delta_{sub}G^{\theta} = -RT \ln\left(\frac{p^0}{p^{\theta}}\right)$. Since $\Delta_{vap}G^{\theta} = G^{\theta}_{vap} - G^{\theta}_{liq}$ and

$\Delta_{sub}G^{\theta} = G^{\theta}_{vap} - G^{\theta}_{solid}$, then

$\Delta_{fus}G^{\theta} = G^{\theta}_{liq} - G^{\theta}_{solid} = \Delta_{sub}G^{\theta} - \Delta_{vap}G^{\theta}$ and

$$\Delta_{fus}G^{\theta} = RT \ln\left(\frac{p^0(\text{liq})}{p^0(\text{solid})}\right) = (8.3143 \text{ J K}^{-1})(263.15 \text{ K}) \ln\left(\frac{2.149}{1.950}\right)$$

$\Delta_{fus}G^{\theta} = 213 \text{ J mol}^{-1}$.

Then $\Delta G^{\theta}(\text{water} \rightarrow \text{ice}) = -\Delta_{fus}G^{\theta} = -213$ J .

4.4 Use data in Table 4.2 to estimate the vapor pressure of CCl_2F_2 at 200 K.

For constant Δ_vH^{θ}, we use Eq. (4.23)

$$P_2^0 = P_1^0 \exp\left[\frac{-\Delta_vH^{\theta}}{R}\left(\frac{1}{T_2} - \frac{1}{T_1}\right)\right]$$

$$P_2^0 = (760 \text{ torr})\exp\left[\frac{-19970 \text{ J}}{8.3143 \text{ J K}^{-1}}\left(\frac{1}{200 \text{ K}} - \frac{1}{243.4 \text{ K}}\right)\right]$$

$P_2^0 = 89.4$ torr .

4.5 Methyl mercaptan (CH_3SH) has vapor pressures $P° = 100$ torr at $-34.8°C$, $P° = 400$ torr at $-7.9°C$.
(a) Calculate the enthalpy of vaporization.
(b) Estimate the normal boiling point.

a) From Eq. (4.23),

$$\Delta_v H = -R\left(\frac{1}{T_2} - \frac{1}{T_1}\right)^{-1} \ln\left(\frac{P_2^0}{P_1^0}\right)$$

$$\Delta_v H = -(8.3143 \text{ J K}^{-1})\left(\frac{1}{265.3 \text{ K}} - \frac{1}{238.4 \text{ K}}\right)^{-1} \ln\left(\frac{400}{100}\right) = 27.10 \text{ kJ} .$$

b) $$T_b = \left\{\frac{1}{T_1} - \frac{R}{\Delta_v H} \ln\left(\frac{760 \text{ torr}}{P_1^0}\right)\right\}^{-1}$$

$$T_b = \left\{\frac{1}{265.3} - \frac{8.3143 \text{ J K}^{-1}}{27.10 \text{ kJ}} \ln\left(\frac{760}{400}\right)\right\}^{-1}$$

$$T_b = 279.92 \text{ K} = 6.77°C .$$

4.6 The vapor pressure of water is 149.38 torr at 60°C and 233.7 torr at 70°C. Calculate the enthalpy of vaporization.

From Eq. (4.23),

$$\Delta_v H = -R\left(\frac{1}{T_2} - \frac{1}{T_1}\right)^{-1} \ln\left(\frac{P_2^0}{P_1^0}\right)$$

$$\Delta_v H = -(8.3145 \text{ J K}^{-1})\left(\frac{1}{343.15 \text{ K}} - \frac{1}{333.15 \text{ K}}\right)^{-1} \ln\left(\frac{233.7}{149.38}\right)$$

$$\Delta_v H = 42.54 \text{ kJ} .$$

4.7 At the top of Mount Everest, the atmospheric pressure is about 1/3 atm. Calculate the boiling point of water at the top of that mountain.

Assuming $\Delta_v H$ is a constant, the integrated form of the Clausius - Clapeyron equation may be written as:

$$T_2 = \left[\frac{1}{T_1} - \frac{R}{\Delta_v H^\theta}\left(\ln \frac{P_2^0}{P_1^0}\right)\right]^{-1} .$$

With $T_1 = 100°C = 373.15$ K, $\Delta_v H^\theta = 44.8$ kJ mol^{-1} and $\frac{P_2^0}{P_1^0} = \frac{1}{3}$,

we find $T_2 = 346.77$ K $= 73.6°C$.

4.8 Use the vapor pressures of ClF_3 given below to calculate the enthalpy of vaporization. Use a graphical method or linear regression.

t/°C	$P°$/torr	t/°C	$P°$/torr
−46.97	29.06	−33.14	74.31
−41.51	42.81	−30.75	86.43
−35.59	63.59	−27.17	107.66

From Eq. (4.21a), $\frac{d(\ln P^0)}{d\left(\frac{1}{T}\right)} = -\frac{\Delta_v H^\theta}{R}$. If $\Delta_v H^\theta$ is a constant,

a plot of $\ln P^0$ vs. $\frac{1}{T}$ should be a line with slope $= -\frac{\Delta_v H^\theta}{R}$.

Linear regression gives $-\frac{\Delta_v H^\theta}{R} = -3.682 \times 10^3$ K , thus

$\Delta_v H^\theta = 30.61$ kJ with $\sigma(\Delta_v H^\theta) = 0.11$ kJ and $r = 0.99998$.

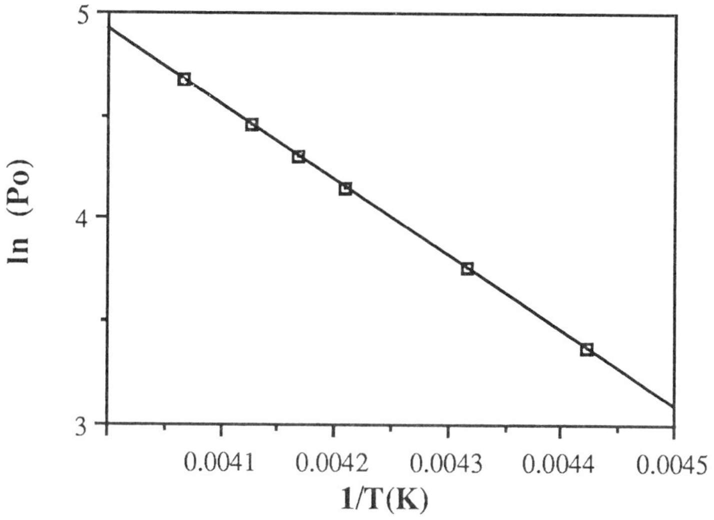

4.9 Use the vapor-pressure data below to calculate the enthalpy of vaporization of 1-butene.

T/K	$P°$/atm
273.15	1.268
277.60	1.490
283.15	1.810

As in problem 4.8, a plot of ln P^0 vs. $\frac{1}{T}$ has slope $= -\frac{\Delta_v H^\theta}{R}$.

From linear regression $-\frac{\Delta_v H^\theta}{R} = -2.760 \times 10^3$ K , $\Delta_v H^\theta = 22.9$ kJ

with $\sigma(\Delta_v H^\theta) = 0.06$ kJ and $r = -1.0000$.

4.10 Vapor pressures of Cl_2 are given below. Make a graph of ln P vs. $1/T$ and determine the enthalpy of vaporization by either a graphical or a least-squares method.

T/K	$P°$/atm	T/K	$P°$/atm
227.6	0.585	283.15	4.934
238.7	0.982	294.3	6.807
249.8	1.566	305.4	9.173
260.9	2.388	316.5	12.105
272.0	3.483	327.6	15.676

From Eq. (4.21a), $\frac{d(\ln P^0)}{d\left(\frac{1}{T}\right)} = -\frac{\Delta_v H^\theta}{R}$. A plot of ln P^0 vs. $\frac{1}{T}$

is shown below. We find $-\frac{\Delta_v H^\theta}{R} = -(2.44 \pm 0.08) \times 10^3$ K so that

$\Delta_v H^\theta = 20.29$ kJ with $\sigma(\Delta_v H^\theta) = 0.07$ kJ and $r = -0.99995$.

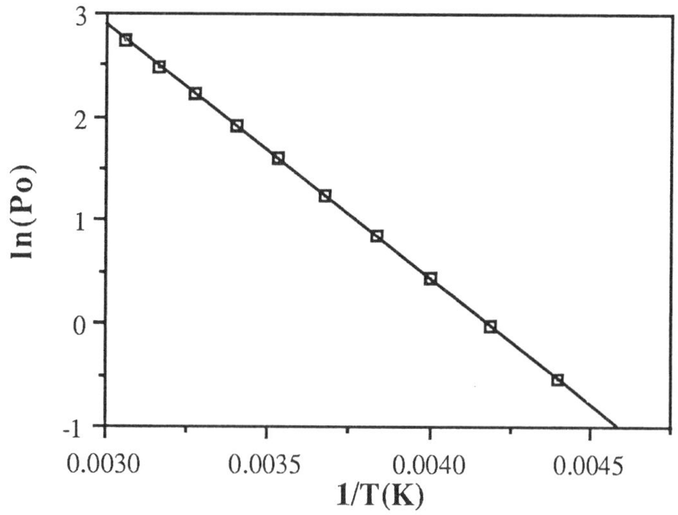

4.11 Use the vapor pressures of ice given below to calculate the enthalpy of sublimation at −30°C.

t/°C	$P°$/torr
−28	0.351
−30	0.2859
−32	0.2318

As in the previous three problems, a linear regression of

$\ln P^0$ vs. $\frac{1}{T}$ gives $-\frac{\Delta_v H^\theta}{R} = -6.100 \times 10^3 \pm 40.2$ K so that

$\Delta_v H^\theta = 50.72$ kJ with $\sigma(\Delta_v H^\theta) = 0.33$ kJ , $r = -0.99998$.

4.12 The vapor pressure of carbonyl sulfide (OCS) is given by the following empirical formula (for 162–224 K):

$$\log_{10}(P°/\text{torr}) = \frac{-1318.260}{T} + 10.15309 - (1.4778 \times 10^{-2})T + (1.8838 \times 10^{-5})T^2$$

(a) Determine the vapor pressure and heat of vaporization of this substance at 200 K.
(b) Calculate the temperature for which $P° = 50$ torr.

a) Plug in T = 200 K to find $\log_{10}(P^0/\text{torr}) = 1.3597$ or

$P^0 = 22.89$ torr. From the given equation, we get

$$\left(\frac{d \log_{10} P^0}{dT}\right) = \left(\frac{1318.26}{T^2} - 1.4778 \times 10^{-2} + 2(1.8838 \times 10^{-5})T\right)$$

or at T = 200 K, $\left(\frac{d \log_{10} P^0}{dT}\right) = 0.0257\ K^{-1}$. Since

$$\Delta_v H^{\theta} = 2.303RT^2\left(\frac{d \log_{10} P^0}{dT}\right), \quad \Delta_v H^{\theta} = 19.68 \text{ kJ}.$$

b) Use the Newton - Raphson iteration Eq. (AI.9) with

$$T_{n+1} = T_n - \frac{f(T_n)}{f'(T_n)} \quad \text{where}$$

$$f(T_n) = \log_{10}\left(\frac{P^0}{\text{torr}}\right) + \frac{1318.26}{T} - 10.15309 + (1.4778 \times 10^{-2})T$$

$$- (1.8838 \times 10^{-5})T^2$$

and $f'(T_n) = -\frac{1318.26}{T^2} + (1.4778 \times 10^{-2}) - 2(1.8838 \times 10^{-5})T$.

With $P^0 = 50$ torr, $T^{(1)} = 200$ K, then $T^{(2)} = 213.2$ K,

$T^{(3)} = 214.2$ K and $T^{(4)} = 214.2$ K .

4.13 Liquid nitrogen, normal boiling point 77.33 K, is a convenient cryoscopic bath for use in the laboratory. If a lower temperature is required, it can be obtained by reducing the pressure over the boiling nitrogen. Use data from Table 4.2 to estimate the temperature of boiling N_2 when P = 100 torr.

From Eq. (4.23),

$$T_2 = \left\{\frac{1}{T_1} - \frac{R}{\Delta_v H^{\ominus}} \ln\left(\frac{P_2^0}{P_1^0}\right)\right\}^{-1}$$

$$T_2 = \left\{\frac{1}{77.33\ \mathrm{K}} - \frac{8.3143\ \mathrm{J\ K^{-1}}}{5.577 \times 10^3\ \mathrm{J}} \ln\left(\frac{100}{760}\right)\right\}^{-1} = 62.68\ \mathrm{K}\ .$$

4.14 The heat of vaporization of N_2 has been given as (units: J K^{-1} mol^{-1}):

$$\Delta_v H = 8070 - 32.07T$$

(a) Derive a formula for the vapor pressure of liquid nitrogen as a function of T; the normal bp is 77.33 K.
(b) Calculate the boiling temperature for P = 100 torr; contrast your answer to that from the previous problem, which was calculated by a less accurate method.

a) From Eq. (4.21b), $\dfrac{d \ln P^0}{dT} = \dfrac{\Delta_v H^{\ominus}}{RT^2}$ or

$d \ln P^0 = \left(\dfrac{8070}{RT^2} - \dfrac{32.07}{RT}\right)dT$. Integrating

$$\ln P^0 = \int_{77.33}^{T}\left(\frac{8070}{RT^2} - \frac{32.07}{RT}\right)dT$$

$$\ln P^0 = 970.65\left(\frac{1}{77.33} - \frac{1}{T}\right) - 3.857 \ln\left(\frac{T}{77.33}\right)$$

where T is in K and P^0 in atm. Rewriting,

$\ln(P^0/\mathrm{torr}) = 35.956 - \dfrac{970.65}{T} - 3.857 \ln T$, where T is in K.

b) $T = 970.65(35.956 - \ln(P^0/\mathrm{torr}) - 3.857 \ln T)^{-1}$. With $T^{(1)} = 77.33$ and P^0 = 100 torr, $T^{(2)} = 66.57$, $T^{(3)} = 64.03$, $T^{(4)} = 63.41$, $T^{(5)} = 63.25$ and $T^{(6)} = 63.21$ K.

4.15 The following data apply to $CHClF_2$ (Freon-22) at 300 K. $\Delta H_v = 15.65$ kJ/mol, $P° =$ 10.86 atm, C_{pm}(liq) = 121.2 J/K, C_{pm}(vap) = 55.0 J/K.
(a) Derive the following formula for the heat of vaporization:

$$\Delta_v H = R(4270 - 7.96T)$$

(State any assumptions explicitly.)
(b) Use this result to derive the formula for the vapor pressure:

$$\ln (P°/\text{atm}) = 62.02 - 7.96 \ln T - \frac{4270}{T}$$

(c) Estimate the normal boiling temperature of this gas using the results of part (b).

a) The heat capacity is $C_p \equiv \left(\frac{\partial H}{\partial T}\right)_P$. Thus $C_{pm}(\text{liq}) = \left(\frac{\partial H_{liq}}{\partial T}\right)_P$

and $C_{pm}(\text{vap}) = \left(\frac{\partial H_v}{\partial T}\right)_P$ so that $C_{pm}(\text{vap}) - C_{pm}(\text{liq}) = \left(\frac{\partial H_v}{\partial T}\right)_P$.

Assuming constant C_{pm},

$$\Delta_v H \Big|_{\Delta_v H^0}^{\Delta_v H} = T\left(C_{pm}(\text{vap}) - C_{pm}(\text{liq})\right) \Big|_{T^0}^{T}$$

$$\Delta_v H \Big|_{\Delta_v H^0}^{\Delta_v H} = 66.2(300 - T)\text{J K}^{-1} + 15.65 \times 10^3 \text{ J} = R(4271 - 7.96T).$$

b) Using the Clausius - Clapeyron eq.,

$d(\ln P^0) = \left(\frac{4271}{T^2} - \frac{7.96}{T}\right)dT$. Integrating from $P^0 = 10.86$ atm

at T = 300 K to P^0 at T gives $\ln P^0 = 62.02 - 7.96(\ln T) - \frac{4271}{T}$.

c) Using the Newton - Raphson iteration [Eq. (AI.9)],

$$T^{(1)} = 300 \text{ K}, \ldots, T^{(6)} = 226.53 \text{ K}.$$

4.16 The heat of vaporization of Zn (nbp 907°C) is given by (units: J):

$$\Delta_v H = 1.286 \times 10^5 - 8.87T - 2.41 \times 10^{-3} T^2$$

Zinc (gas) is monatomic with $C_{pm} = 2.5R$. Use these data to calculate the heat capacity of Zn (liq) at the normal bp.

$C_{pm}(\text{vap}) - C_{pm}(\text{liq}) = \left(\frac{\partial \Delta_v H}{\partial T}\right)_P$. Assuming C_{pm} is constant w.r.t. T and with $\Delta_v H = 1.286 \times 10^5 - 8.87T - 2.41 \times 10^{-3}T^2$,

$$C_{pm}(\text{liq}) = C_{pm}(\text{vap}) + 8.87 + 4.82 \times 10^{-3}T$$

$$C_{pm}(\text{liq}) = 2.5R + 8.87 + 4.82 \times 10^{-3}(1180.15\ \text{K}) = 35.3\ \text{J K}^{-1} .$$

4.17 Ammonia (NH_3) at 0°C has a vapor pressure of 4.2380 atm and a specific volume of 1.5660 cm^3/g. Calculate the vapor pressure of ammonia at this temperature under an excess pressure of 100 atm.

From Eq. (4.24), $P = P^0 \exp\left(\frac{V_m P_x}{RT}\right)$. Since

$$V_m = (1.566\ \text{cm}^3\ \text{g}^{-1})(17.03\ \text{g})\left(\frac{1\ \text{dm}^3}{1000\text{cm}^3}\right) = 2.667 \times 10^{-2}\ \text{dm}^3 ,$$

$$P = (4.2380\ \text{atm})\exp\left(\frac{(2.667 \times 10^{-2}\ \text{dm}^3)(100\ \text{atm})}{(0.08206\ \text{dm}^3\ \text{atm K}^{-1})(273.15\ \text{K})}\right)$$

$$P = 4.7735\ \text{atm} .$$

4.18 The normal vapor pressure of thallium at 1200 K is 8.26 torr; its density at that temperature is approximately 10.4 g/cm^3. Calculate its vapor pressure under 1000 atm of an inert gas.

From Eq. (4.24), $P = P^0 \exp\left(\frac{V_m P_x}{RT}\right)$. Since

$V_m = \frac{M}{\rho} = \frac{204.37\ \text{g}}{1.04 \times 10^4\ \text{g dm}^{-3}} = 1.965 \times 10^{-2}\ \text{dm}^3$, then

$$P = (8.26\ \text{torr}) \exp\left(\frac{(1.965 \times 10^{-2}\ \text{dm}^3)(1000\ \text{atm})}{(0.08206\ \text{dm}^3\ \text{atm K}^{-1})(1200\ \text{K})}\right)$$

$$P = 10.08\ \text{torr} .$$

4.19 Use data in Table 4.3 to calculate the surface free energy, surface energy, and surface entropy of ethanol at 20°C.

From Table 4.3, $A_s = \gamma = 22.8 \times 10^{-3}$ J m^{-2}. From Eq. (4.31), $U_s = \gamma - T\left(\frac{\partial \gamma}{\partial T}\right)_V$. Using the 3-point differential method of Eq. (AI.19b) and Table 4.3,

$$\left(\frac{\partial \gamma}{\partial T}\right)_V \cong \left(\frac{21.9 - 23.6}{20 \text{ K}}\right) \times 10^{-3} \text{ J m}^{-2} = -8.50 \times 10^{-5} \text{ J K}^{-1} \text{ m}^{-2}.$$

Thus $U_s = 22.8 \times 10^{-3} - (293.15 \text{ K})(-8.50 \times 10^{-5} \text{ J K}^{-1} \text{ m}^{-2})$

or $U_s = 4.77 \times 10^{-2}$ J m^{-2}. From Eq. (4.30), $S_s = -\left(\frac{\partial \gamma}{\partial T}\right)_{V,\,A}$

or $S_s = 8.50 \times 10^{-5}$ J m^{-2} K^{-1}.

4.20 Use data in Table 4.3 to calculate the surface energy and entropy of water at 60°C. (Use the 5-point differentiation method of Appendix I.)

From Eq. (AI.21c) in the appendix,

$$\left(\frac{\partial \gamma}{\partial T}\right)_V = \frac{[f_0 - 8f_1 + 8f_3 - f_4]}{12h}$$

$$= \frac{[72.75 - 8(69.60) + 8(62.6) - 58.8] \times 10^{-3}}{12(20)}$$

$$\left(\frac{\partial \gamma}{\partial T}\right)_V = -1.75 \times 10^{-4} \text{ J K}^{-1} \text{ m}^{-2}$$

or $S_s = 1.75 \times 10^{-4}$ J K^{-1} m^{-2}. Then

$$U_s = \gamma - T\left(\frac{\partial \gamma}{\partial T}\right)_V = 66.2 \times 10^{-3} \text{ J m}^{-2} -$$

$$(333.15 \text{ K})(-1.75 \times 10^{-4} \text{ J K}^{-1} \text{ m}^{-2})$$

$$U_s = 0.125 \text{ J m}^{-2}.$$

4.21 Calculate the surface area if 5 grams of water (25°C) is dispersed into droplets with a radius of 20 nm. Calculate the work required to create this dispersion.

From Eq. (4.25), $dw = \gamma\, d\mathcal{A}$. Assuming γ is a constant, $w = \gamma\mathcal{A}$.

The surface area of a single droplet is $\mathcal{A}_0 = 4\pi r^2$ and the number of droplets is $N = \dfrac{5\ g}{\left(\frac{4}{3}\pi r^3 \rho\right)} = \dfrac{\text{total wt}}{\text{wt per droplet}}$.

Then $\mathcal{A} = N\mathcal{A}_0 = \dfrac{3(5\ g)}{\rho r} = \dfrac{3(5\ g)}{(0.997\ g\ cm^{-3})(20 \times 10^{-7}\ cm)} = 752\ m^2$

and $w = (72.0 \times 10^{-3}\ J\ m^{-2})\mathcal{A} = 54\ J$.

4.22 (a) From the data below calculate the surface energy of acetone at 20°C:

T/°C	γ/(dynes cm^{-1})
0°	26.2
20°	23.7
40°	21.2

(b) Calculate the added energy when 1 cm^3 of acetone is dispersed as droplets of 1 micron (10^{-6} m) radius.

a) From Eq. (4.31), $U_s = \gamma - T\left(\frac{\partial \gamma}{\partial T}\right)_V$. Using Eq. (AI.19b) to calculate the derivative at 20°C,

$$\left(\frac{\partial \gamma}{\partial T}\right)_V = \left(\frac{21.2 - 26.2}{40}\right) = -0.125\ \frac{\text{dynes}}{\text{cm K}} = -1.25 \times 10^{-4}\ J\ K^{-1}\ m^{-2} .$$

Then $U_s = 23.7 \times 10^{-3}\ J\ m^{-2} - (293.15\ K)(-1.25 \times 10^{-4}\ J\ K^{-1}\ m^{-2})$

or $U_s = 6.03 \times 10^{-2}\ J\ m^{-2}$.

b) The energy of dispersion is $\Delta U \cong U_s\Delta\mathcal{A} = U_s\mathcal{A}$. The total droplet area is

$$\mathcal{A} = N\mathcal{A}_0 = \left(\frac{V}{\frac{4}{3}\pi r^3}\right)(4\pi r^2) = \frac{3V}{r} = \frac{3(1\ cm)^3}{10^{-4}\ cm} = 3 \times 10^4\ cm^2 = 3\ m^2 .$$

Thus $\Delta U = 0.18\ J$.

4.23 Methanol has vapor pressure of 1.000 atm at 64.7°C; the density of the liquid is 0.7510 g/cm^3. Calculate the vapor pressure of methanol if it is dispersed as 200-nm radius droplets at this temperature.

From Eq. (4.36), $P = P^0 \exp\left(\frac{2\gamma M}{\rho r R T}\right)$ or

$P = (760 \text{ torr}) \times$

$$\exp\left(\frac{2(20.2 \times 10^{-3} \text{ J m}^{-2})(3.2042 \times 10^{-2} \text{ kg})}{(751 \text{ kg m}^{-3})(200 \times 10^{-9} \text{ m})(8.3143 \text{ J K}^{-1})(337.85 \text{ K})}\right) .$$

$P = 762$ torr .

4.24 The normal melting point of lead is 327.3°C, where its densities are ρ(liq) = 10.51 g/cm^3, ρ(solid) = 11.23 g/cm^3. Calculate its melting point at a pressure of 1000 atm. (ΔH_f = 5.10 kJ/mol. Note that you must assume no phase change for the solid when the pressure is applied.)

From Eq. (4.39), $T_f = T_f^{\theta} \exp\left\{ [V_m(\text{liq}) - V_m(\text{solid})]\frac{(P - P^{\theta})}{\Delta_f H} \right\}$.

Since $V_m(\text{liq}) = \frac{M_{Pb}}{\rho(\text{liq})} = \frac{207.2 \text{ g}}{10.51 \text{ g cm}^{-3}} = 1.97 \times 10^{-5} \text{ m}^3$ and

$V_m(\text{solid}) = \frac{M_{Pb}}{\rho(\text{solid})} = \frac{207.2 \text{ g}}{11.23 \text{ g cm}^{-3}} = 1.85 \times 10^{-5} \text{ m}^3$, then

$T_f = (600.45 \text{ K}) \times$

$$\exp\left\{ (1.97 \times 10^{-5} - 1.85 \times 10^{-5})\text{m}^3 \frac{(10^3 - 1)101325 \text{ Pa}}{5.10 \times 10^3 \text{ J}} \right\}$$

$T_f = 614.9 \text{ K} = 341.8^{\circ}\text{C}$.

4.25 Calculate the enthalpy change for heating 1 g of ice at −200°C to steam at 300°C. Use the heat capacities of Figure 2.3.

The enthalpy change is

$$\Delta H = \int_{-200^\circ C}^{0^\circ C} C_{pm}(\text{ice})dT + \Delta_f H + \int_{0^\circ C}^{100^\circ C} C_{pm}(\text{liq})dT + \Delta_v H + \int_{100^\circ C}^{300^\circ C} C_{pm}(\text{steam})dT \ .$$

From Table 4.2, $\Delta_f H = 6.01 \times 10^3$ J, $\Delta_v H = 40.66 \times 10^3$ J .

From Figure 2.3, we may calculate the integrals as the area under the C_p vs. T curve. Thus

$$\int_{-200^\circ C}^{0^\circ C} C_{pm}(\text{ice})dT = (285 \text{ J g}^{-1})(18.02 \text{ g}) = 5134.3 \text{ J mol}^{-1}$$

$$\int_{0^\circ C}^{100^\circ C} C_{pm}(\text{liq})dT = 7546.1 \text{ J mol}^{-1}$$

$$\int_{100^\circ C}^{300^\circ C} C_{pm}(\text{steam})dT = 7208.0 \text{ J mol}^{-1} \ .$$

Summing gives $\Delta H = 66.56 \text{ kJ mol}^{-1} = 3.7 \text{ kJ g}^{-1}$.

4.26 Carbon dioxide at its triple point (T = 216.5 K, P = 5.11 atm) has molar volumes 29.1 cm^3 (solid), 37.4 cm^3 (liquid). Estimate the melting point of CO_2 at 100 atm. (Use ΔH_f = 7950 J/mol.)

From Eq. (4.39), $T_f = T_f^\theta \exp\left\{ [V_m(\text{liq}) - V_m(\text{solid})]\frac{(P - P^\theta)}{\Delta_f H} \right\}$

T_f = (216.5 K) x

$$\exp\left\{[37.4 - 29.1] \times 10^{-6} \text{ m}^3 \frac{(100 - 5.11)101325 \text{ Pa}}{7950 \text{ J}}\right\}$$

T_f = 218.7 K .

4.27 The standard free energy per mole of diamond is greater than that of graphite by 2.90 kJ at 25°C. (How this could be determined will be discussed in Chapter 6.) The density of graphite is 2.260 g/cm^3 and that of diamond 3.513 g/cm^3. Estimate the pressure required to convert graphite to diamond at 25°C.

For diamond and graphite at equilibrium, $\mu_d = \mu_g$ so that

$$\mu_g^\theta + V_{mg}(P - P^\theta) = \mu_d^\theta + V_{md}(P - P^\theta) \text{ and}$$

$$\mu_g^\theta - \mu_d^\theta = (V_{md} - V_{mg})(P - P^\theta) \text{ or } P = P^\theta + \frac{(\mu_g^\theta - \mu_d^\theta)}{(V_{md} - V_{mg})} .$$

Since

$$V_{md} = \left[(3.513 \text{ g cm}^{-3})(100 \text{ cm m}^{-1})\left(\frac{1}{12.011 \text{ g}}\right)\right]^{-1} = 3.419 \times 10^{-6} \text{ m}^3$$

and $V_{mg} = 5.315 \times 10^{-6} \text{ m}^3$, then

$$P = 101325 \text{ Pa} + \frac{-2.87 \times 10^3 \text{ J}}{(3.419 - 5.315) \times 10^{-6} \text{ m}^3} = 1.51 \times 10^9 \text{ Pa}$$

$$P = 1.5 \times 10^4 \text{ atm} .$$

4.28 Use the fact that enthalpy is a state variable to derive a relationship among the enthalpies for vaporization, sublimation, and fusion.

When solid, liquid and vapor phases coexist in equilibrium,

$\Delta_{fus}H = H_m(\text{liq}) - H_m(\text{solid})$, $\Delta_{vap}H = H_m(\text{vap}) - H_m(\text{liq})$,

$\Delta_{sub}H = H_m(\text{vap}) - H_m(\text{solid})$ so that $\Delta_{sub}H = \Delta_{fus}H + \Delta_{vap}H$.

4.29 The heat of sublimation of metals is usually determined indirectly because the vapor pressures are so low. The vapor pressure of liquid Cd is:

$$\ln (P°/\text{torr}) = 28.292 - \frac{1.340 \times 10^4}{T} - 1.2572 \ln T$$

The heat of fusion at the triple point (593 K) is 6138 J/mol. Calculate the heats of vaporization and sublimation at 594 K.

From the Clausius - Clapeyron equation, $\Delta_v H^\theta = RT^2 \frac{d(\ln P^0)}{dT}$.

From the problem statement, $\frac{d(\ln P^0)}{dT} = \frac{1.340 \times 10^4}{T^2} - \frac{1.2572}{T}$.

With T = 594 K, $\frac{d(\ln P^0)}{dT} = 0.0359\ K^{-1}$, thus $\Delta H_v^\theta = 105.3$ kJ .

From problem 4.28, $\Delta_s H = \Delta_v H + \Delta_f H$ so that with $\Delta_f H = 6.14$ kJ,

$\Delta_s H = 111.4$ kJ .

4.30 The vapor pressure of ice is 1.950 torr at −10°C and 4.579 torr at 0°C. The vapor pressure of water is 9.209 torr at 10°C, 4.579 torr at 0°C. Calculate the enthalpies of vaporization, sublimation, and fusion for water at 0°C.

From Eq. (4.23),

$$\Delta_{sub}H^\theta = -R\left[\frac{1}{T_2} - \frac{1}{T_1}\right]^{-1} \ln\left(\frac{P_2{}^0}{P_1{}^0}\right)$$

$$\Delta_{sub}H^\theta = -(8.3145\ \text{J K}^{-1})\left[\frac{1}{273.15\ \text{K}} - \frac{1}{263.15\ \text{K}}\right]^{-1} \ln\left(\frac{4.579}{1.950}\right)$$

$\Delta_{sub}H^\theta = 51.01$ kJ .

For $\Delta_{vap}H^\theta$ we also use Eq. (4.23),

$$\Delta_{vap}H^\theta = -(8.3145\ \text{J K}^{-1})\left[\frac{1}{273.15\ \text{K}} - \frac{1}{283.15\ \text{K}}\right]^{-1} \ln\left(\frac{4.579}{9.209}\right)$$

$\Delta_{vap}H^\theta = 44.93$ kJ .

From problem 4.28, $\Delta_{fus}H = \Delta_{sub}H - \Delta_{vap}H$ so that

$\Delta_{fus}H = 6.08$ kJ .

4.31 The *Handbook of Chemistry and Physics* (CRC Publishing Co.) gives the following empirical formulas for NO: sublimation pressure:

$$\ln (P°/\text{torr}) = 23.136 - \frac{1975}{T}$$

and vapor pressure:

$$\ln (P°/\text{torr}) = 19.434 - \frac{1568}{T}$$

Calculate (a) ΔH(vap), (b) ΔH(sub), (c) ΔH(fus), and (d) the temperature at the triple point for this substance.

a) From Eq. (4.21b), $\Delta_{vap}H^{\theta} \cong RT^2 \frac{d(\ln P^0)}{dT}$, with $\frac{d(\ln P^0)}{dT} = \frac{1568}{T^2}$, we have $\Delta_{vap}H^{\theta} = 1568\ R = 13.04$ kJ .

b) For sublimation $\frac{d(\ln P^0)}{dT} = \frac{1975}{T^2}$, using Eq. (4.21b) we find $\Delta_{sub}H^{\theta} = 1975\ R = 16.42$ kJ .

c) From problem 4.27, $\Delta_{fus}H = \Delta_{sub}H - \Delta_{vap}H$ so that $\Delta_{fus}H = 3.38$ kJ .

d) At the triple point, the sublimation and vapor pressures are equal, so that

$23.136 - \frac{1975}{T} = 19.434 - \frac{1568}{T}$ and thus $T = 109.9$ K .

4.32 Use the data in Figure 4.2 to determine the heats of vaporization and sublimation of carbon dioxide. From these values, calculate the heat of fusion.

From Eq. (4.21a), $\Delta_v H^\theta = -R \dfrac{d(\ln P^0)}{d\left(\frac{1}{T}\right)}$. From Figure 4.2, for liquid CO_2, $\dfrac{d(\ln P^0)}{d\left(\frac{1}{T}\right)} = -2 \times 10^3\ K^{-1}$. For solid CO_2, $\dfrac{d(\ln P^0)}{d\left(\frac{1}{T}\right)} = -3.2 \times 10^3\ K^{-1}$, so that $\Delta_{vap} H^\theta = 16.6$ kJ and $\Delta_{sub} H^\theta = 26.6$ kJ . From problem 4.27, $\Delta_{fus} H = \Delta_{sub} H - \Delta_{vap} H$, so that $\Delta_{fus} H = 10.0$ kJ .

4.33 The Clapyron equation:

$$\frac{dP}{dT} = \frac{\Delta H}{T\Delta V}$$

was derived in the text by using the continuity of the chemical potential at the phase transition point. It does not apply to a second-order transition, since, for such a case, $\Delta H = 0$ and $\Delta V = 0$. For a second-order transition, use the continuity of the entropy to derive the analogous equation:

$$\frac{dP}{dT} = \frac{\Delta C_p}{TV\Delta\alpha}$$

where α is the coefficient of thermal expansion.

$dS = \left(\frac{\partial S}{\partial T}\right)_P dT + \left(\frac{\partial S}{\partial P}\right)_T dP$. Since $dH = TdS + VdP$, $T\left(\frac{\partial S}{\partial T}\right)_P = \left(\frac{\partial H}{\partial T}\right)_P = C_p$ and $\left(\frac{\partial S}{\partial T}\right)_P = \frac{C_p}{T}$. Also $\left(\frac{\partial S}{\partial P}\right)_T = -\left(\frac{\partial V}{\partial T}\right)_P = -\alpha V$ so that $dS = \frac{C_p}{T} dT - \alpha V dP$. For phases 1 and 2, $dS_1 = dS_2$, $V_1 = V_2$, so that $\frac{C_{p1}}{T} dT - \alpha_1 V dP = \frac{C_{p2}}{T} - \alpha_2 V dP$. With $\Delta C_p = C_{p2} - C_{p1}$ and $\Delta\alpha = \alpha_2 - \alpha_1$, $\Delta\alpha V dP = \frac{\Delta C_p}{T} dT$ and $\frac{dP}{dT} = \frac{\Delta C_p}{TV\Delta\alpha}$.

4.34 Use the continuity of V at a second-order phase transition to derive the Ehrenfest equation:

$$\frac{dP}{dT} = \frac{\Delta\alpha}{\Delta\kappa_T}$$

(See the discussion in the previous problem.)

$dV = \left(\frac{\partial V}{\partial T}\right)_P dT + \left(\frac{\partial V}{\partial P}\right)_T dP$. From Table 3.1, $\left(\frac{\partial V}{\partial T}\right)_P = \alpha V$ and $\left(\frac{\partial V}{\partial P}\right)_T = -\kappa_T V$ so that $dV = \alpha V dT - \kappa_T V dP$. Since V is continuous, then for phases 1 and 2,

$\alpha_1 dT - \kappa_{T_1} dP = \alpha_2 dT - \kappa_{T_2} dP$. With $\Delta\alpha = \alpha_2 - \alpha_1$ and $\Delta\kappa_T = \kappa_{T_2} - \kappa_{T_1}$, $\Delta\kappa_T dP = \Delta\alpha dT$ or $\frac{dP}{dT} = \frac{\Delta\alpha}{\Delta\kappa_T}$.

4.35 The differences between the free energies at the minima of Figure 4.15, is just:

$$\Delta_v G = G(\text{vapor}) - G(\text{liquid})$$

Calculate this quantity from the graph at 82 K and 102 K. Then use these quantities to estimate the entropy and enthalpy of vaporization (using Eqs. (4.7) and (4.18)). Compare these results to the experimental values of Table 4.1.

$$\Delta_v G = G(\text{vapor}) - G(\text{liquid}) .$$

For CH_4 at 82 K, $\Delta_v G = -6.4 - (-12) = 5.6\ \text{dm}^3\ \text{atm mol}^{-1}$. At 102 K, $\Delta_v G = -9.8 - (-4.0) = -5.8\ \text{dm}^3\ \text{atm mol}^{-1}$. With

$S = -\left(\frac{\partial G}{\partial T}\right)_{P,\,n}$ we may approximate:

$$\Delta_v S \sim -\left(\frac{\Delta G}{\Delta T}\right)_{P,\,n} = -\left(\frac{-11.4}{20}\right)\text{dm}^3\ \text{atm mol}^{-1}\ \text{K}^{-1}$$

$$\Delta_v S \sim 57.8\ \text{J K}^{-1}\ \text{mol}^{-1} \quad (73.3\ \text{Table 4.2}) .$$

Also, $\left[\frac{\partial\left(\frac{G}{T}\right)}{\partial T}\right]_P = -\frac{H}{T^2}$ so that

$$\Delta H_v \sim -T^2\left(\frac{\Delta\left(\frac{\Delta_v G}{T}\right)}{\Delta T}\right) = (92\ \text{K})^2\left[\frac{\left(\frac{-5.8}{102\ \text{K}}\right) - \left(\frac{5.6}{82\ \text{K}}\right)}{20\ \text{K}}\right]\ \text{dm}^3\ \text{atm mol}^{-1}$$

$$\Delta H_v \sim 52.96\ \text{dm}^3\ \text{atm mol}^{-1} = 5.4\ \text{kJ mol}^{-1}\quad (8.18\quad \text{Table 4.2})\ .$$

4.36 Derive equations for $U(V)$, $S(V)$ and $G(V)$, equivalent to Eqs. (4.42) through (4.44), for a gas obeying the Redlich-Kwong equation of state.

$dU = \left[T\left(\frac{\partial P}{\partial T}\right)_V - P\right]dV_m$. For a Redlich - Kwong gas:

$P = \frac{RT}{V_m - b} - \frac{a}{T^{1/2}V_m(V_m + b)}$ so that

$\left(\frac{\partial P}{\partial T}\right)_{V_m} = \frac{R}{V_m - b} + \frac{a}{2T^{3/2}V_m(V_m + b)}$ and

$dU = \left(\frac{3a}{2T^{1/2}V_m(V_m + b)}\right)dV_m$. Integrating, we find:

$U(T, V_m) = u(T) + \frac{3a}{2T^{1/2}b}\ln\left(\frac{V_m}{V_m + b}\right)$ where $u(T)$ is a constant of integration. $dS = \left(\frac{\partial P}{\partial T}\right)_V dV_m$. Substituting and integrating we find:

$$S(T, V_m) = s(T) + R\ln(V_m - b) + \frac{a}{2bT^{3/2}}\ln\left(\frac{V_m}{V_m + b}\right)\ .$$

$$G = U - TS + PV$$

$$G(T, V_m) = g(T) + \frac{a}{T^{1/2}b}\ln\left(\frac{V_m}{V_m + b}\right) - RT\ln(V_m - b) + PV_m\ .$$

5
Statistical Thermodynamics

5.1 Calculate the probability of having 1, 4, 5, or 6 heads when throwing a coin 12 times.

$W(p, q) = \left(\frac{1}{2}\right)^N \frac{N!}{p!\ q!}$ where $W(p, q)$ is the probability of having p heads and q tails in $N = p + q$ throws. Thus:

$$W(1, 11) = \left(\frac{1}{2}\right)^{12} \frac{12!}{1!\ 11!} = 0.0029 = 0.29\ \%\ .$$

Similarly,

$$W(4, 8) = \left(\frac{1}{2}\right)^{12} \frac{12!}{4!\ 8!} = 0.1208 = 12.08\ \%\ .$$

$$W(5, 7) = \left(\frac{1}{2}\right)^{12} \frac{12!}{5!\ 7!} = 19.34\ \% \text{ and } W(6,6) = 22.56\ \%\ .$$

5.2 Consider two connected 1 dm^3 containers, each containing an ideal gas at 1 torr (25°C). If N is the average number of particles in each container but the number fluctuated so that the containers had $N + \sqrt{N}$ and $N - \sqrt{N}$ particles respectively, what would be the pressure difference between the two parts of the container?

According to the ideal gas law, $P = \frac{nRT}{V}$. If we define $N = nL$, then: $P_1 = \left[\frac{N}{L} + \frac{\sqrt{N}}{L}\right]\frac{RT}{V}$ and $P_2 = \left[\frac{N}{L} - \frac{\sqrt{N}}{L}\right]\frac{RT}{V}$. Thus:

$\Delta P = P_1 - P_2 = \frac{2\sqrt{N}RT}{LV}$. Now, $N = \frac{LPV}{RT}$ so that

$$\Delta P = 2\left(\frac{PRT}{LV}\right)^{1/2}$$

$$= 2\left[\frac{\left(\frac{1}{760}\text{ atm}\right)(0.08206\text{ dm}^3\text{ atm mol}^{-1}\text{ K}^{-1})(298.15\text{ K})}{(6.022 \times 10^{23}\text{ mol}^{-1})(1\text{ dm}^3)}\right]^{1/2}$$

$$\Delta P = 4.6 \times 10^{-13}\text{ atm} = 3.51 \times 10^{-10}\text{ torr.}$$

5.3 Suppose you had a bag containing a large number of balls, 40% red and 60% green. Calculate the probability that you would draw 0, 4, or 8 red balls in 10 trials.

The probability is given by Eq. (5.9). For 0 red balls:

$$W(10,\ 0) = (0.4)^0(0.6)^{10}\ \frac{10!}{0!\ 10!} = 0.0060 = 0.6\ \%\ .$$

For 4 red balls:

$$W(10,\ 4) = (0.4)^4(0.6)^6\ \frac{10!}{4!\ 6!} = 0.2508 = 25.08\ \%\ .$$

For 8 red balls:

$$W(10,\ 8) = (0.4)^8(0.6)^2\ \frac{10!}{8!\ 2!} = 0.1060 = 1.06\ \%\ .$$

5.4 Chlorine is a mixture of isotopes, approximately 75% mass 35 and 25% mass 37. Calculate the fraction of diatomic species—35-35, 35-37 or 37-37—in chlorine gas. Calculate the entropy of mixing for these species in one mole of Cl_2 gas.

The entropy of mixing is: $\Delta_{mix}S = -R \sum_i n_i \ln X_i$. The fractions of diatomic species are:

$$W(35 - 35) = (0.75)^2 = 0.5625 .$$

$$W(35 - 37) = 2(0.75)(0.25) = 0.375 .$$

$$W(37 - 37) = 0.0625 .$$

These probabilities will represent both mole fractions and number of moles for one mole of Cl_2, so that:

$$\Delta_{mix}S = -(8.3143 \text{ J K}^{-1} \text{ mol}^{-1})\Big[0.5625 \text{ mol}(\ln 0.5625)$$

$$+ 0.375 \text{ mol}(\ln 0.375) + 0.0625 \text{ mol}(\ln 0.0625)\Big]$$

$$\Delta_{mix}S = 7.19 \text{ J K}^{-1} .$$

5.5 Natural hydrogen contains approximately 0.015% heavy hydrogen (deuterium, mass 2), but deuterium-enriched samples are readily available. Suppose you had a sample of methane whose hydrogen was 80% deuterium. List all possible species and calculate their probability. Calculate the entropy of mixing for these species.

Possible species and their probabilities are:

CD_4	$X(D_4) = (0.80)^4 = 0.4096$
CHD_3	$X(D_3) = 4(0.80)^3(0.20) = 0.4096$
CH_2D_2	$X(D_2) = 6(0.80)^2(0.20)^2 = 0.1536$
CH_3D_1	$X(D_1) = 4(0.80)(0.20)^3 = 0.0256$
CH_4	$X(D_0) = (0.20)^4 = 0.0016$

The molar entropy of mixing is:

$$\Delta_{mix}S_m = -R \sum_i X_i \ln X_i = 9.338 \text{ J K}^{-1} \text{ mol}^{-1} .$$

5.6 Compute the number of distinct permutations of the letters in the words LEAK, LEEK, MISSISSIPPI. Confirm your calculation for the first two by writing out all the possibilities.

For LEAK, the number of permutations is $4 \times 3 \times 2 \times 1 = 4! = 24$.

The possible combinations are:

LEAK	ELKA	ALEK	KLEA
LEKA	ELAK	ALKE	KLAE
LAKE	EKLA	AKEL	KEAL
LAEK	EKAL	AKLE	KELA
LKEA	EALK	AELK	KALE
LKAE	EAKL	AEKL	KAEL

For LEEK, the number of permutations is $\frac{4!}{2!} = \frac{24}{2} = 12$.

These are:

LEEK	EKLE	ELKE	KLEE
LEKE	EKEL	EELK	KELE
LKEE	ELEK	EEKL	KEEL

For MISSISSIPPI, the number of distinct permutations is

$$\frac{11!}{4!\ 4!\ 2!} = 34{,}650 \ .$$

5.7 In a SCRABBLE™ set there are (of 98 tiles), 2 P, 2 C, 2 H, 12 E, 2 M.
(a) If you drew 5 tiles at random, what is the chance that they would spell (in order) PCHEM?
(b) Is ORGANIC more probable? (8 O, 6 R, 3 G, 9 A, 6 N, 9 I, 2 C.)
(c) What is the probability of drawing the letters P, C, H, E, M in any sequence?

a) The probability of drawing the letters P-C-H-E-M is given by the product of drawing each letter from the number of tiles left. Thus

$$p = \left(\frac{2}{98}\right)\left(\frac{2}{97}\right)\left(\frac{2}{96}\right)\left(\frac{12}{95}\right)\left(\frac{2}{94}\right) = 2.36 \times 10^{-8} .$$

b) For ORGANIC,

$$p = \left(\frac{8}{98}\right)\left(\frac{6}{97}\right)\left(\frac{3}{96}\right)\left(\frac{9}{95}\right)\left(\frac{6}{94}\right)\left(\frac{9}{93}\right)\left(\frac{2}{92}\right) = 2.01 \times 10^{-9} .$$

Thus it is less probable.

c) There are 5! sequences of the 5 letters that would give us PCHEM. Then

$$p = 5!(2.36 \times 10^{-8}) = 2.83 \times 10^{-6} .$$

5.8 A flexible polymer chain can be modeled as a set of rigid links (length λ). It can be shown that for N links, the number of configurations is:

$$W = AL^2 \exp\left(-\frac{L^2}{N\lambda^2}\right)$$

where L is the end-to-end distance and A is a constant:
(a) Prove that S is a maximum when $L = \sqrt{N}\,\lambda$.
(b) Calculate ΔS for stretching the chain by 10%. Assume $N = 100$ and a mole of chains.

a) From Eq. (5.1), $S = k \ln W$. Then $S = k \ln\left[AL^2 e^{-L^2/N\lambda^2}\right]$

or $S = k\left[\ln (AL^2) - \frac{L^2}{N\lambda^2}\right]$. S will be a maximum when $\left(\frac{\partial S}{\partial L}\right) = 0$.

$\left(\frac{\partial S}{\partial L}\right) = \left[\frac{1}{AL^2}(2AL) - \frac{2L}{N\lambda^2}\right] = 0$ gives $L = \sqrt{N}\lambda$.

b) The change in entropy is given by

$$\Delta S = S(L_1 = 1.1\ L_0) - S(L_0) = k\left[\ln \frac{(1.1\ L_0)^2}{L_0^2} - \frac{(1.1\ L_0)^2 + L_0^2}{N\lambda^2}\right]$$

$$\Delta S = k\left[\ln(1.1)^2 - \frac{0.21\ L_0^2}{N\lambda^2}\right].$$

For $N = 100$, $L_0 = 10\lambda$, $\Delta S = k(-0.0194)$. For one mole,

$$\Delta S = R(-0.0194) = -0.161\ \text{J/K}.$$

5.9 Comparison of statistical and third-law entropies of CH_3D reveals a discrepancy of 11.6 J K^{-1} mol^{-1}. Explain. What would you anticipate the discrepancy in S to be for CH_2D_2?

For CH_3D, we would expect 4 orientations at 0 K. Then

$S = Lk \ln 4 = 11.53$ J K^{-1} mol^{-1}. For CH_2D_2 the number

of possible orientations is $W = \frac{4!}{2!\ 2!} = 6$, thus

$$S = R \ln 6 = 14.90\ \text{J K}^{-1}\ \text{mol}^{-1}.$$

5.10 A system containing 38 particles has three equally spaced energy levels available. Two population distributions are A: (18, 12, 8), B: (17, 14, 7). Show that both distributions have the same energy. Is either of these a Boltzmann distribution? Calculate *W* for each. Which is more probable? If the energy-level spacing ($\Delta\varepsilon$) is 10^{-22} J, what is *T*?

We label the 3 energy levels $\epsilon_1 = c$, $\epsilon_2 = 2c$, $\epsilon_3 = 3c$. Then

$$E_A = 18c + 12(2c) + 8(3c) = 66c$$

$$E_B = 17c + 14(2c) + 7(3c) = 66c .$$

From Eq. (5.27), $\frac{n_i}{n_j} = e^{-\beta(\epsilon_i - \epsilon_j)}$, thus

$\frac{n_1}{n_2} = \frac{n_2}{n_3} = \left(\frac{n_1}{n_3}\right)^{1/2} = e^{\beta c}$ for a Boltzmann distribution with evenly spaced levels. Distribution A is Boltzmann, B is not. W may be calculated as follows:

$$W_A = \frac{38!}{18!\ 12!\ 8!} = 4.230 \times 10^{15}$$

$$W_B = \frac{38!}{17!\ 14!\ 7!} = 3.349 \times 10^{15} .$$

A is more probable. For distribution A,

$\frac{n_1}{n_2} = \frac{18}{12} = \exp(10^{-22}\ \mathrm{J}/kT)$ or T = 18 K .

5.11 A molecule has three equally spaced energy levels. At equilibrium the number of molecules (out of 5550) in each level is 5000, 500, 50. Confirm that this is a Boltzmann distribution. Use Stirling's approximation to calculate ln W for this distribution and for the distribution (5001, 498, 51) (with the same total energy) to show that the Boltzmann distribution is the more probable.

We denote the 3 energy levels $\epsilon_1 = c$, $\epsilon_2 = 2c$, $\epsilon_3 = 3c$. For a Boltzmann distribution with evenly spaced levels,

$\frac{n_1}{n_2} = \frac{n_2}{n_3} = \sqrt{\frac{n_1}{n_3}}$ which is easily confirmed for the given distribution. $W = \frac{5550!}{5000!\ 500!\ 50!}$ and

$\ln W = \ln 5550! - \ln 5000! - \ln 50!$. Using Stirling's approximation, $\ln W = 1960.75$. For the other distribution

$$\ln W = \ln\left[\frac{5550!}{5001!\ 498!\ 51!}\right] = 1960.74 \ .$$

5.12 What is the probability that two blocks of a material (with $C_p = 10\ \mathrm{J\ K^{-1}}$ for each) in thermal contact will differ in temperature by 0.003 K at 300 K (when they have reached equilibrium)?

$$\Delta S = C_p \ln\left(\frac{T_f}{T_i}\right) = C_p\left[\ln\left(1+\frac{\partial T}{T}\right) + \ln\left(1 - \frac{\partial T}{T}\right)\right]$$

$$\Delta S = C_p \ln\left[1 - \left(\frac{\partial T}{T}\right)^2\right] \ .$$

If x << 1, then $\ln(1 - \epsilon) \sim -\epsilon$ so that, with $\epsilon = \left(\frac{\partial T}{t}\right)^2$:

$\Delta S \sim -C_p\left(\frac{\partial T}{T}\right)^2$. $\left(\frac{\partial T}{T}\right) = \left(\frac{0.0015}{300}\right)$ and $C_p = 10\ \mathrm{J\ K^{-1}}$, so that:

$\Delta S \sim -2.5 \times 10^{-1}\ \mathrm{J\ K^{-1}}$ and $P = e^{\Delta S/k} = \exp(-1.8 \times 10^{13})$.

5.13 The probability of a fluctuation, as given by Eq. 5.7, is very small for macroscopic amounts of material. However, over small regions of space containing a small number of molecules, such fluctuations can be quite probable. In fact, fluctuations in the density of air in the upper atmosphere, in regions with size on the order of the wavelength of light, are responsible for the light scattering that gives the sky its blue color. Consider two cubic volumes with volume V, each containing N molecules. A fluctuation of density can be created by increasing one volume by δV and decreasing the other volume by a similar amount. Show that, if $\delta V/V \ll 1$, the entropy change for this process will be:

$$\Delta S/k = -N(\delta V/V)^2$$

Blue light has a wavelength of 400 nm. Assuming a cube of this size, calculate the probability that the density will fluctuate by 1%, assuming $P = 0.01$ atm, $T = 300$ K. Repeat the calculation for red light, wavelength 750 nm. Explain how this relates to the color of the sky.

$\Delta S = Nk\Sigma \ln\left[\frac{V(\text{final})}{V(\text{initial})}\right]$. For the fluctuation:

$\Delta S = Nk\left[\ln\left(\frac{V + \partial V}{V}\right) + \ln\left(\frac{V - \partial V}{V}\right)\right]$. Let $\frac{\partial V}{V} = \epsilon$, so that

$\ln(1 + \epsilon) = \epsilon - \frac{\epsilon^2}{2} \ldots$ and $\ln(1 - \epsilon) = -\epsilon - \frac{\epsilon^2}{2} \ldots$

Hence, $\frac{\Delta S}{k} \cong -N\epsilon^2 = -N\left(\frac{\partial V}{V}\right)^2$. $V = 6.4 \times 10^{-20}$ m^3 ,

$N = \frac{PLV}{RT} = 1.57 \times 10^4$ and with $\frac{\partial V}{V} = 0.01$, $\frac{\Delta S}{k} = -1.57$. Thus

$p = \exp\left(\frac{\Delta S}{k}\right) = 0.208$. Repeating the calculation with

$V = (750 \text{ nm})^3$, $p = 3.20 \times 10^{-5}$. The sky is blue because blue light is scattered more than red.

5.14 A population of 1,000,000 particles has two energy states available to it with $\Delta\varepsilon = 4.14 \times 10^{-21}$ J.
(a) Calculate the populations of the levels for T = 10 K, 300 K, 3000 K.
(b) What will be the populations as $T \rightarrow \infty$?

a) Defining $\epsilon_1 = 0$, $\epsilon_2 = 4.14 \times 10^{-21}$ J , the population of each level is $n_i = \dfrac{Ne^{-\beta\epsilon_i}}{\sum_j e^{-\beta\epsilon_j}}$. For T = 10 K,

$$\beta = \frac{1}{kT} = \frac{1}{(10\ \text{K})(1.381 \times 10^{-23}\ \text{J K}^{-1})} = 7.25 \times 10^{21}\ \text{J}^{-1} .$$

Then

$$n_1 = \frac{(1 \times 10^6)}{1 + \exp[-(7.25 \times 10^{21})(4.14 \times 10^{-21})]} = 1 \times 10^6 .$$

$$n_2 = \frac{(1 \times 10^6)\ \exp[-(7.25 \times 10^{21})(4.14 \times 10^{-21})]}{1 + \exp[-(7.25 \times 10^{21})(4.14 \times 10^{-21})]} = 9.22 \times 10^{-8} .$$

For T = 300 K, $\beta = 2.42 \times 10^{20}\ \text{J}^{-1}$. This gives $n_1 = 7.31 \times 10^5$ and $n_2 = 2.69 \times 10^5$.

For T = 3000 K, $\beta = 2.42 \times 10^{19}\ \text{J}^{-1}$, $n_1 = 5.25 \times 10^5$ and $n_2 = 4.74 \times 10^5$.

b) As $T \rightarrow \infty$, then $\beta \rightarrow 0$ and $e^{-\beta\epsilon_i} \rightarrow 1$. Thus

$$n_1 = \frac{(1 \times 10^6)}{1 + 1} = 5 \times 10^5 \quad \text{and} \quad n_2 = \frac{(1 \times 10^6)}{1 + 1} = 5 \times 10^5 .$$

5.15 A system has two energy levels with $\varepsilon/k = 100$ K; the levels are not degenerate— that is, $g = 1$ for both. Calculate the fractional population of these levels at $T = 10$, 100, 1000 K. What would be the populations as T approached infinity?

The ratio $\frac{n_1}{n_2}$ is given by Boltzmann's law: $\frac{n_1}{n_2} = \exp[-\beta(\epsilon_1 - \epsilon_2)]$.

With $n_1 + n_2 = N$, we may calculate the fractional populations :

$$X_1 = \frac{n_1}{N} = \frac{\frac{n_1}{n_2}}{\frac{n_1}{n_2} + 1} = \frac{\exp[-\beta(\epsilon_1 - \epsilon_2)]}{1 + \exp[-\beta(\epsilon_1 - \epsilon_2)]}$$

$$X_2 = \frac{n_2}{N} = 1 - X_1 .$$

With $\beta = \frac{1}{kT}$ and $\frac{(\epsilon_1 - \epsilon_2)}{k} = 100$ K :

$$X_1(10\text{ K}) = \frac{\exp(-10)}{1 + \exp(-10)} = 4.54 \times 10^{-5}$$

$$X_2(10\text{ K}) = 0.99995 .$$

Similarly:

$$X_1(100\text{ K}) = 0.269, \quad X_2(100\text{ K}) = 0.731 .$$

$$X_1(1000\text{ K}) = 0.475 , \quad X_2(1000\text{ K}) = 0.525 .$$

As $T \to \infty$, $X_1 \to 0.5$ and $X_2 \to 0.5$.

5.16 For the system described in the previous problem, calculate the average energy $T = 10$, 20, 100, 110, 1000 and 1010 K. What is happening to the heat capacity? Why?

The average energy of the system will be $\langle\epsilon\rangle = \sum_i X_i\epsilon_i$, where X_i is the fractional population of the ith state, as calculated in the previous problem. We let $\frac{\epsilon_1}{k} = 100$ K and $\frac{\epsilon_2}{k} = 0$ K , so that:

$$\left\langle\frac{\epsilon}{k}\right\rangle = (100)(4.54 \times 10^{-5}) = 0.00454\text{ K} \quad \text{at } 10\text{ K} .$$

Similarly:

$$\left\langle\frac{\epsilon}{k}\right\rangle = 0.669 \text{ K at } 20 \text{ K}$$
$$\left\langle\frac{\epsilon}{k}\right\rangle = 26.9 \text{ K at } 100 \text{ K}$$
$$\left\langle\frac{\epsilon}{k}\right\rangle = 28.7 \text{ K at } 110 \text{ K}$$
$$\left\langle\frac{\epsilon}{k}\right\rangle = 47.50 \text{ K at } 1000 \text{ K}$$
$$\left\langle\frac{\epsilon}{k}\right\rangle = 47.53 \text{ K at } 1010 \text{ K}$$

The heat capacity is $C \equiv \frac{\partial\langle\epsilon\rangle}{\partial T} \sim \frac{\Delta\langle\epsilon\rangle}{\Delta T}$. Using the data above with the mean temperatures we find:

$$\frac{C}{k}\ (15 \text{ K}) = 0.07$$
$$\frac{C}{k}\ (105 \text{ K}) = 0.18$$
$$\frac{C}{k}\ (1005 \text{ K}) = 0.03$$

We observe that the heat capacity exhibits a maximum.

5.17 In spectroscopy, it is relatively common to observe situations in which a higher-energy state has a larger population than a lower-energy state. Such population "inversions" are important in the operation of lasers. Assuming Boltzmann's equation for state populations applied, what would you have to say about the temperature of such a system? Is it legitimate to apply this equation in such a situation—for example, could such an inversion occur at thermal equilibrium?

A population inversion would be represented by a negative temperature. Since Boltzmann's equation strictly applies to thermal equilibrium, it is not valid--but scientists often refer to negative temperatures in such cases.

5.18 Prove that:

$$C_v = Nk\beta^2 \frac{\partial^2 \ln z}{\partial \beta^2}$$

With $E = U - U_0$, $C_V = \left(\frac{\partial U}{\partial T}\right)_V = \left(\frac{\partial (E + U_0)}{\partial T}\right)_V = \left(\frac{\partial E}{\partial T}\right)_V$. Since

$E = NkT^2\left(\frac{\partial \ln z}{\partial T}\right)_V$, then

$$\left(\frac{\partial E}{\partial T}\right)_V = 2NkT\left(\frac{\partial \ln z}{\partial T}\right)_V + NkT^2\left(\frac{\partial^2 \ln z}{\partial T^2}\right)_V .$$

If $\beta = \frac{1}{kT}$, $T = \frac{1}{k\beta}$ and $\frac{\partial}{\partial T} = \frac{\partial \beta}{\partial T}\frac{\partial}{\partial \beta} = \frac{-1}{kT^2}\left(\frac{\partial}{\partial \beta}\right) = -k\beta^2\frac{\partial}{\partial \beta}$ and

$\frac{\partial^2}{\partial T^2} = k^2\beta^4\left(\frac{\partial^2}{\partial \beta^2}\right) + 2k^2\beta^3\left(\frac{\partial}{\partial \beta}\right)$. Thus

$\left(\frac{\partial E}{\partial T}\right)_V = -2Nk\beta\left(\frac{\partial \ln z}{\partial \beta}\right)_V + Nk\beta^2\left(\frac{\partial^2 \ln z}{\partial \beta^2}\right)_V + 2Nk\beta\left(\frac{\partial \ln z}{\partial \beta}\right)_V$ or

$$C_V = Nk\beta^2\left(\frac{\partial^2 \ln z}{\partial \beta^2}\right)_V .$$

5.19 Prove that a shift in the zero of energy for a set of energy levels does not affect either C_v or S. (The effect on U will be to add a constant $N \Delta \varepsilon$.)

$C_v = \left(\dfrac{\partial E}{\partial T} \right)_V$. From Eq. (5.31a), $E = \dfrac{-N\left(\dfrac{\partial z}{\partial \beta} \right)}{z}$. If we shift the zero of energy by a constant, c, then z changes as follows:

$$z = \sum_i e^{-\beta \epsilon_i} \rightarrow z' = \sum_i e^{-\beta(\epsilon_i + c)} .$$

$$\frac{\partial z'}{\partial \beta} = \frac{\partial \left[e^{-\beta c} \sum_i e^{-\beta \epsilon_i} \right]}{\partial \beta} = -c e^{-\beta c} \sum_i e^{-\beta \epsilon_i} - e^{-\beta c} \sum_i \epsilon_i e^{-\beta \epsilon_i} .$$

Thus

$$E' = \frac{-N\left(\dfrac{\partial z'}{\partial \beta} \right)}{z'} = \frac{N \left[c e^{-\beta c} \sum_i e^{-\beta \epsilon_i} - e^{-\beta c} \sum_i \epsilon_i e^{-\beta \epsilon_i} \right]}{e^{-\beta c} \sum_i e^{-\beta \epsilon_i}}$$

$$E' = Nc + \frac{N \sum_i \epsilon_i e^{-\beta \epsilon_i}}{\sum_i e^{-\beta \epsilon_i}} .$$

When we take the temperature derivative of E' , the constant term will drop. Thus C_v is independent of c. From Eq. (5.34), $S = Nk \ln z + \dfrac{E}{T}$. Proceeding as before,

$$\ln z' = -\beta c + \ln \sum_i e^{-\beta \epsilon_i} .$$

Then

$$S' = Nk \ln z' + \frac{E'}{T}$$

$$S' = Nk \ln \sum_i e^{-\beta \epsilon_i} + \frac{N \sum_i \epsilon_i e^{-\beta \epsilon_i}}{T\left(\sum_i e^{-\beta \epsilon_i} \right)} = Nk \ln z + \frac{E}{T} = S .$$

5.20 If the volume of a cell (that is, state) in phase space is h^3, estimate the number of such states for a He atom in a 1-cm^3 box having $\varepsilon < kT$ at 4 K.

The maximum value of p_x , p_y or p_z is $\sqrt{2mE}$. Thus

$$V = \int_0^{1\ \mathrm{cm}} dx \int_0^{1\ \mathrm{cm}} dy \int_0^{1\ \mathrm{cm}} dz \int_0^{\sqrt{2mE}} dp_x \int_0^{\sqrt{2mE}} dp_y \int_0^{\sqrt{2mE}} dp_z$$

$$V = (1\ \mathrm{cm})^3\left(\sqrt{2mE}\right)^3 .$$

The number of states is then $N = \dfrac{V}{h^3} = \dfrac{1\ \mathrm{cm}^3(2mE)^{3/2}}{h^3}$.

Using $E \cong kT$,

$$N = \frac{(1\ \mathrm{cm}^3)\left(2\left[\dfrac{4\ \mathrm{g}}{6.022 \times 10^{23}}\right](4\ \mathrm{K})(1.380 \times 10^{-16}\ \mathrm{erg\ K})\right)^{3/2}}{(6.626 \times 10^{-27}\ \mathrm{erg\ s})^3}$$

$$N = 2.16 \times 10^{21} .$$

5.21 Calculate the standard entropy of Ar at 298.15 K. This can be compared to the third-law value of 154.6 ± 0.8 J K^{-1}.

$$S_m^{\ominus} = \frac{3}{2}\ R\ \ln M + \frac{5}{2}\ R\ \ln T - 1.1517\ R .$$

For Argon:

$$S_m^{\ominus} = 8.31451\ \mathrm{J\ K^{-1}}\left[\tfrac{3}{2}\ln(39.95) + \tfrac{5}{2}\ln(298.15) - 1.1517\right] .$$

$$S_m^{\ominus} = 154.85\ \mathrm{J\ K^{-1}} .$$

5.22 Use Eq. (5.61) to prove that when $T \gg \theta_v$, the vibrational heat capacity will have the equipartition value, R per mole.

$$C_{vm}(\text{vib}) = \frac{Ru^2e^u}{(e^u - 1)^2} \quad \text{where} \quad u = \frac{\theta_v}{T}. \quad \text{If } \frac{\theta_v}{T} << 1 \text{ , then}$$

$$e^{\theta_v/T} \sim \left(1 + \frac{\theta_v}{T}\right) \quad \text{and} \quad C_{vm}(\text{vib}) \sim R\left(1 + \frac{\theta_v}{T}\right) \sim R \text{ .}$$

5.23 Calculate the exact rotational partition function [Eq. (5.69)] of CO gas at $T = 13.9$ K and compare the result to the approximate value given by Eq. (5.70).

From Eq. (5.69), $z_{rot} = \sum_{J=0}^{\infty} (2J + 1)\, e^{-J(J+1)\theta_r/T}$. From Table 5.2, $\theta_r = 2.78$ K , thus:

$$z_{rot} = \sum_{J=0}^{\infty} (2J + 1)\, e^{-(J^2 + J)(0.20)}$$

$$z_{rot} = 1 + 2.011 + 1.506 + 0.635 + 0.165 + 0.027 + 0.002 + \text{small terms} = 5.35 \text{ .}$$

From Eq. (5.70) $z_{rot} = \dfrac{T}{\sigma\theta_r} = 5.00$.

5.24 Calculate the rotational partition function of O_2 gas for $T = 20.8$ K; do this exactly [Eq. (5.69) with $J = 1, 3, 5, 7, \ldots$] and compare this result to the approximation of Eq. (5.70).

As in 5.23,

$$z_{rot} = \frac{1}{\sigma}\left(\sum_{J=\text{odd}}^{\infty} (2J + 1)\, e^{-J(J + 1)(0.1)}\right)$$

$$z_{rot} = \frac{1}{2}(2.546 + 2.108 + 0.548 + 0.055 + 0.002) = 5.17 \text{ .}$$

From Eq. (5.70),

$$z_{rot} = \frac{20.8 \text{ K}}{2(2.08 \text{ K})} = 5.00 \text{ .}$$

5.25 Calculate the fraction of molecules in each of the $J = 0, 3, 10$ rotational states of HCl at 304.76 K. If a computer or programmable calculator is available, do all J's and graph your results.

$$\frac{n_i}{N} = \frac{e^{-\beta\epsilon_i}}{z_{rot}} = \frac{(2J + 1)\ e^{-J(J+1)\theta_r/T}}{z_{rot}} .$$

With $z_{rot} = \frac{T}{\sigma\theta_r} = \left(\frac{304.76}{15.238}\right) = 20$ we find:

$$\frac{n_i}{N}(0) = \frac{1}{20} = 0.050$$

$$\frac{n_i}{N}(3) = \frac{3.842}{20} = 0.192$$

$$\frac{n_i}{N}(10) = \frac{0.0858}{20} = 0.004 .$$

5.26 Derive the formula for the rotational contribution to the internal energy (per mole) (a) for linear molecules, (b) for nonlinear molecules.

a) The internal energy is $U_m - U_0 = \frac{RT^2}{z}\frac{\partial z}{\partial T}$. From Eq. (5.70),

$z_{rot} = \frac{T}{\sigma\theta_r}$, thus $(U_m - U_0)_{rot} = \frac{RT^2}{T}\left(\frac{\sigma\theta_r}{\sigma\theta_r}\right) = RT$.

b) From Eq. (5.74), $z_{rot} = \frac{8\pi^2}{\sigma h^3}(2\pi kT)^{3/2}(I_xI_yI_z)^{1/2}$, thus

$$(U_m - U_0)_{rot} = \frac{RT^2\ \frac{3}{2}\left(\frac{8\pi^2}{\sigma h^3}\right)(2\pi k)^{3/2}\ T^{1/2}\ (I_xI_yI_z)^{1/2}}{\left(\frac{8\pi^2}{\sigma\ h^3}\right)\ (2\pi kT)^{3/2}\ (I_xI_yI_z)^{1/2}} = \frac{3}{2}\ RT .$$

5.27 For the rotation of a linear molecule, prove:

$$S_m^{\ominus}(\text{rot}) = R\left(\ln \frac{T}{\sigma\theta} + 1\right)$$

S_m^{θ} is given by $S_m^{\theta} = R \ln z + \frac{(U_m - U_0)}{T}$. From Eq. (5.70),

$z_{rot} = \frac{T}{\sigma\theta_r}$, and the result of problem 5.26a), we have

$$(S_m^{\theta})_{rot} = R \ \ln \frac{T}{\sigma\theta_r} + R = R\left(\ln \frac{T}{\sigma\theta_r} + 1\right) .$$

5.28 The product of the moments of inertia of SF_4 is:

$$I_x I_y I_z = 6.721 \times 10^{-114} \text{ g}^3 \text{ cm}^6$$

(a) Calculate the rotational partition function at 298.15 K ($\sigma = 2$).
(b) Calculate S(rot) for this case.

a) From Eq. (5.74),

$$z_{rot} = \frac{8\pi^2}{\sigma h^3} (2\pi kT)^{3/2} (I_x I_y I_z)^{1/2}$$

$$z_{rot} = \frac{8\pi^2 (2\pi (1.381 \times 10^{-16} \text{ erg K}^{-1})(298 \text{ K}))^{3/2}}{2(6.626 \times 10^{-27} \text{ erg s})^3} \times$$

$$(6.721 \times 10^{-114} \text{ g}^3 \text{ cm}^{-6})^{1/2}$$

$$z_{rot} = 4.62 \times 10^4 .$$

b) $(S_m^{\theta})_{rot} = R \ln z_{rot} + \frac{(U_m - U_0)_{rot}}{T}$. From problem 5.26b),

$(U_m - U_0)_{rot} = \frac{3}{2} RT$, thus $(S_m^{\theta})_{rot} = R \ln z_{rot} + \frac{3}{2} R$. Then

$$(S_m^{\theta})_{rot} = (8.3143 \text{ J K}^{-1})\left[\ln(4.62 \times 10^4) + \frac{3}{2}\right] = 1.02 \times 10^2 \text{ J K}^{-1} .$$

5.29 List the symmetry numbers of the following molecules: H—C≡N, S=C=S (both linear), H—O—H, H—O—D (both bent), CH_3Cl, CH_2Cl_2.

The symmetry number is the number of indistinguishable molecular orientations:

H - C ≡ N $\sigma = 1$

S = C = S $\sigma = 2$

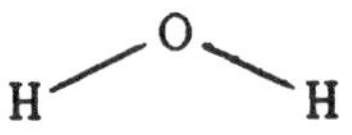

$\sigma = 2$

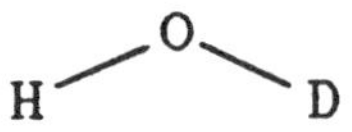

$\sigma = 1$

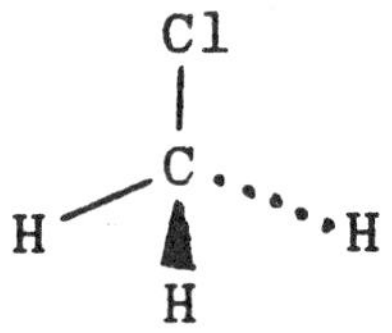

$\sigma = 3$ (rotation about C - Cl axis)

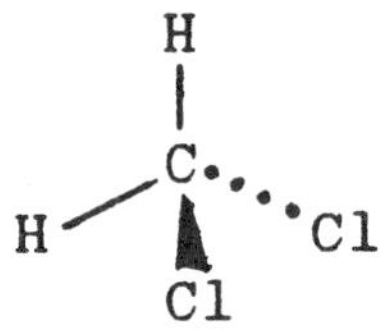

$\sigma = 2$

5.30 Give symmetry numbers for the following substituted benzene molecules:

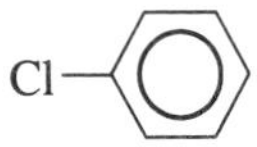

$\sigma = 2$

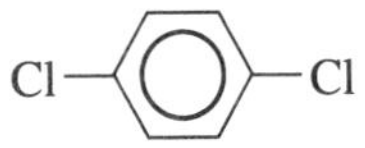

$\sigma = 4$

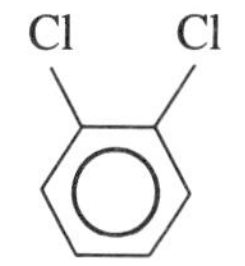

$\sigma = 2$

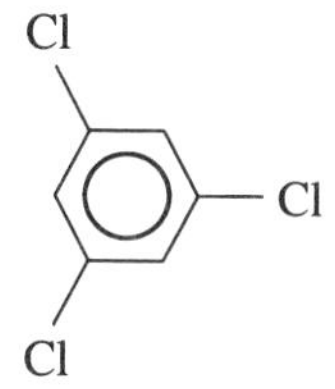

$\sigma = 6$ (1 rotation about each C - Cl bond)

5.31 (a) Show that the rotational characteristic temperature has the value:

$$\theta_r = \frac{h^2}{8\pi^2 Ik} = \frac{4.0284 \times 10^{-39}}{I}$$

(with I in g cm^2).

(b) For a nonlinear molecule, three rotational constants can be defined, one for each moment of inertia. Show that the rotational partition function [Eq. (5.74)] can be written:

$$z_{\text{rot}} = \frac{\sqrt{\pi}}{\sigma} \frac{T^{3/2}}{(\theta_x \theta_y \theta_z)^{1/2}}$$

a)
$$\theta_r = \frac{h^2}{8\pi^2 Ik} = \frac{(6.626075 \times 10^{-27} \text{ erg s})^2}{8\pi^2(1.38036 \times 10^{-16} \text{ erg K}^{-1})I}$$

$$\theta_r = \frac{4.0284 \times 10^{-39} \text{ g cm}^3 \text{ K}}{I}$$

b) From Eq. (5.74), $z_{rot} = \frac{8\pi^2}{\sigma h^3}(2\pi kT)^{3/2}(I_x I_y I_z)^{1/2}$. We define the rotational constants as $\theta_x = \frac{h^2}{8\pi^2 I_x k}$ and similarly for θ_y and θ_z. Thus $I_x = \frac{h^2}{8\pi^2 \theta_x k}$, etc., and substitution gives $z_{rot} = \frac{\sqrt{\pi}}{\sigma} \frac{T^{3/2}}{(\theta_x \theta_y \theta_z)^{1/2}}$.

5.32 It was stated that the high-temperature limit for the rotational partition function was valid for all gases above their normal boiling points, except for H_2, which has a very small moment of inertia (large θ_r) and a very low boiling point. Methane also has a very small moment of inertia (the carbon is at the center of mass):

$$I = 5.313 \times 10^{-40} \text{ g cm}^2$$

and a low boiling point (111.7 K). Calculate the rotational characteristic temperature of methane to see if it is indeed an order of magnitude smaller than the boiling temperature, as required (use the results of problem 5.31).

$I_x = I_y = I_z$. From the result of problem 5.31a) ,

$$\theta_r = \frac{4.0284 \times 10^{-39} \text{ K}}{5.313 \times 10^{-40}} = 7.58 \text{ K} .$$

Table 4.2 gives T_b = 90.18 K so $T_b \gg \theta_r$ as required.

5.33 Calculate the electronic partition function for a nitrogen atom at 10,000 K.

From Eq. (5.75), $z_{elec} = g_0 + g_1 e^{-\epsilon_1/kT} + \ldots$. From Table 5.3,

$$\epsilon_1 = 19224 \text{ cm}^{-1} = 3.8185 \times 10^{-12} \text{ erg} , \; g_1 = 6 ,$$

$$\epsilon_2 = 19233 \text{ cm}^{-1} = 3.8203 \times 10^{-12} \text{ erg} , \; g_2 = 4 ,$$

$$\epsilon_3 = 28839 \text{ cm}^{-1} = 5.7283 \times 10^{-12} \text{ erg} .$$

Thus

$$z_{elec} = 4 + 6 \exp\left(- \frac{(3.8185 \times 10^{-12})}{(1.3804 \times 10^{-16})(10^4)} \right) +$$

$$4 \exp\left(- \frac{(3.8203 \times 10^{-12})}{(1.3804 \times 10^{-16})(10^4)} \right) +$$

$$6 \exp\left(- \frac{(5.7283 \times 10^{-12})}{(1.3804 \times 10^{-16})(10^4)} \right)$$

$$z_{elec} = 4.723 .$$

5.34 Atomic sodium has a doubly degenerate ground state, and no low-lying excited electronic states. Calculate its molar entropy at 1800 K.

For atomic sodium: $S_m^\ominus = S_m^\ominus(\text{trans}) + S_m^\ominus(\text{elec})$.

$$S_m^\ominus(\text{trans}) = R\left(\frac{3}{2}\ln M + \frac{5}{2}\ln T - 1.1517\right)$$

$$= 8.31451 \text{ J K}^{-1}\left(\frac{3}{2}\ln(23.00) + \frac{5}{2}\ln(1800) - 1.1517\right)$$

$$S_m^\ominus(\text{trans}) = 185.33 \text{ J K}^{-1} .$$

Also, $S_m^\ominus(\text{elec}) = R \ln 2 = 5.76 \text{ J K}^{-1}$ so that

$$S_m^\ominus = 191.09 \text{ J K}^{-1} .$$

5.35 Starting with Eq. (5.76) prove that the contribution to C_v from a low-lying electronic state (g_1, ε_1) is:

$$C_{vm}(\text{elec}) = \frac{Rg_1g_0x^2e^{-x}}{(g_0 + g_1e^{-x})^2}$$

(where $x = \varepsilon_1/kT$). Show that this function has a maximum.

From Eq. (5.76), $U_m(\text{elec}) - U_0 = \dfrac{Rg_1\left(\frac{\epsilon_1}{k}\right)}{(g_0 e^x + g_1)}$ where $x = \dfrac{\epsilon_1}{kT}$.

$$C_{vm}(\text{elec}) = \left(\frac{\partial U_m(\text{elec})}{\partial T}\right)_V = Rg_1\left(\frac{\epsilon_1}{k}\right)\left[\frac{-g_0\left(\frac{\epsilon_1}{k}\right)\left(-\frac{1}{T^2}\right)e^x}{(g_0 e^x + g_1)^2}\right]$$

$$C_{vm}(\text{elec}) = \frac{Rg_1g_0 e^x x^2}{(g_0 e^x + g_1)^2} .$$

A maximum exists if $\dfrac{\partial C_{vm}}{\partial x} = 0$.

$$\frac{\partial C_{vm}}{\partial x} = C_{vm} + 2\frac{C_{vm}}{x} - \frac{2g_0 e^x C_{vm}}{(g_0 e^x + g_1)} = 0$$

or $x = \dfrac{g_0 e^x + g_1}{g_0 e^x - g_1}$ at $x = x_{max}$.

5.36 Atomic chlorine has a ground electronic state degeneracy of 4 and a low excited state with $\varepsilon_1 = 881\ \text{cm}^{-1}$, $g_1 = 2$. Calculate C_{vm} (total) at 300 K, 600 K, 1000 K.

From problem 5.35, $(C_v)_{elec} = \dfrac{Rg_1g_0\ e^x x^2}{(g_0\ e^x + g_1)^2}$, where $x = \dfrac{\epsilon_1}{kT}$.

Then

$$x = \frac{(881\ \text{cm}^{-1})(6.6261 \times 10^{-27}\ \text{erg s})(2.9979 \times 10^{10}\ \text{cm s}^{-1})}{(1.3804 \times 10^{-16}\ \text{erg K}^{-1})(300\ \text{K})} = 4.225,$$

and $(C_v)_{elec} = \dfrac{(8.3145\ \text{J K}^{-1})(4)(2)(4.225)^2 e^{4.225}}{(4e^{4.225} + 2)^2} = 1.070\ \text{J K}^{-1}$.

At T = 600 K, x = 2.113 and $(C_v)_{elec} = 1.995\ \text{J K}^{-1}$. For T = 1000 K, x = 1.2676 and $(C_v)_{elec} = 1.445\ \text{J K}^{-1}$. Other contributions to C_v are: $(C_v^\theta)_{trans} = \frac{3}{2}R$, $(C_v^\theta)_{rot} = (C_v^\theta)_{vib} = 0$. Thus at T = 300 K ,

$C_v^\theta = \frac{3}{2}(8.3145\ \text{J K}^{-1}) + 1.070\ \text{J K}^{-1} = 13.54\ \text{J K}^{-1}$. At T = 600 K, $C_v^\theta = 14.47\ \text{J K}^{-1}$ and at T = 1000 K, $C_v^\theta = 13.92\ \text{J K}^{-1}$.

5.37 Calculate the internal energy $U_m^\ominus - U_0$ of CO at 500 K.

From Eq. (5.60),

$$U_m^\theta(\text{vib}) - U_0 = \frac{R\theta_v}{e^u - 1} = \frac{(8.3145 \text{ J K}^{-1})(3122 \text{ K})}{\exp\left(\frac{3122}{500}\right) - 1} = 50.51 \text{ J K}^{-1} .$$

From Eq. (5.50), $U_m^\theta(\text{trans}) - U_0 = \frac{3}{2}\,RT = 6.236$ kJ . From Eq. (5.71), $U_m^\theta(\text{rot}) - U_0 = RT = 4.157$ kJ . Since $U_m^\theta(\text{elec}) - U_0 = 0$, then $U_m^\theta - U_0 = 10{,}443$ J .

5.38 Calculate $H_m^\ominus - H_0^\ominus$ at 298.15 K for H_2O (ideal gas).

From Eq. (5.87), $H_m^\theta(T) - H_0 = 4RT + \sum\frac{R\theta_v}{(e^u - 1)} + \text{electronic}$.

For an ideal gas we ignore the electronic terms. From the data in Table 5.2,

$$H_m^\theta(298.15 \text{ K}) - H_0 = 4(8.3145 \text{ J K}^{-1})(298.15 \text{ K}) + \frac{(8.3145 \text{ J K}^{-1})(5254 \text{ K})}{\exp\left(\frac{5254}{298.15}\right) - 1} + \frac{(8.3145 \text{ J K}^{-1})(2295 \text{ K})}{\exp\left(\frac{2295}{298.15}\right) - 1} + \frac{(8.3145 \text{ J K}^{-1})(5404 \text{ K})}{\exp\left(\frac{5404}{298.15}\right) - 1}$$

$$H_m^\theta(298.15 \text{ K}) - H_0 = 9924.0 \text{ J} .$$

5.39 Calculate the standard entropy of N_2 at 298.15 K and 1000 K from spectroscopic data. (Compare Table 3.2.)

$$S_m^\theta(\text{trans}) = R\left(\frac{3}{2}\ln M + \frac{5}{2}\ln T - 1.1517\right)$$

$$= 8.31451 \text{ J K}^{-1}\left(\frac{3}{2}\ln(28.01) + \frac{5}{2}\ln(298.15) - 1.1517\right)$$

$$S_m^\theta(\text{trans}) = 150.42 \text{ JK}^{-1} .$$

$$S_m^\theta(\text{rot}) = R\ln\left(\frac{T}{\sigma\theta_r}\right) + R = R\left[1 + \ln\left(\frac{298.15}{2(2.89)}\right)\right] = 41.10 \text{ J K}^{-1} .$$

$$S_m^\theta(\text{vib}) = \frac{Ru}{e^u - 1} - R\ln(1 - e^{-u}) . \quad \text{With } u = \frac{3395}{298.15} ,$$

$S_m^\theta(\text{vib}) = 9.80 \times 10^{-4} \text{ J K}^{-1}$. $S_m^\theta(\text{elec}) = 0$, so that

$S_m^\theta = \sum S_m^\theta(i) = 191.52 \text{ J K}^{-1}$. Similarly, at T = 1000 K

$$S_m^\theta(\text{trans}) = 175.54 \text{ J K}^{-1}$$

$$S_m^\theta(\text{rot}) = 51.16 \text{ J K}^{-1}$$

$$S_m^\theta(\text{vib}) = 0.67 \text{ J K}^{-1}$$

$$S_m^\theta = 227.37 \text{ J K}^{-1} .$$

5.40 Calculate the total entropy of O_2 at 298.15 K and 1000 K from its spectroscopic constants. (Compare Table 3.2.)

As in the previous problem, at 298.15 K :

$$S_m^{\theta}(\text{trans}) = 152.04 \text{ J K}^{-1}$$

$$S_m^{\theta}(\text{rot}) = 43.83 \text{ J K}^{-1}$$

$$S_m^{\theta}(\text{vib}) = 0.035 \text{ J K}^{-1}$$

$$S_m^{\theta}(\text{elec}) = R \ln 3 = 9.13 \text{ J K}^{-1}$$

so that $S_m^{\theta} = 205.04 \text{ J K}^{-1}$.

At 1000 K :

$$S_m^{\theta}(\text{trans}) = 177.20 \text{ J K}^{-1}$$

$$S_m^{\theta}(\text{rot}) = 53.89 \text{ J K}^{-1}$$

$$S_m^{\theta}(\text{vib}) = 3.07 \text{ J K}^{-1}$$

$$S_m^{\theta}(\text{elec}) = 9.13 \text{ J K}^{-1}$$

so that $S_m^{\theta} = 243.30 \text{ J K}^{-1}$.

5.41 In some texts, $C_{pm} = \frac{7}{2}R$ is stated as if it represented *truth*. For which of the following gases will this statement be reasonably accurate (5%) at 25°C?

HCl, Br_2(gas), H_2O(gas), CH_4, SiF_4

It is not necessary to calculate all these heat capacities; answer qualitatively.

From Table 5.4, $C^{\ominus}_{vm}(\text{vib}) = \dfrac{Ru^2\, e^u}{(e^u - 1)^2}$, where $u = \dfrac{\theta_v}{T}$. The Taylor expansion of e^u is $(1 + u)$, thus $\lim_{u \to 0} C^{\ominus}_{vm}(\text{vib}) = R$. Also $\lim_{u \to \infty} C^{\ominus}_{vm}(\text{vib}) = 0$. Comparing θ_v (Table 5.2) with $T = 298.15$ K :

Species	$C^{\ominus}_{vm}(\text{vib})$ [approximate]
HCl	0
Br_2	$0 < C^{\ominus}_{vm} < R$
H_2O	0
CH_4	0
SiF_4	$0 < C^{\ominus}_{vm} < R$

Using $C^{\ominus}_{vm}(\text{trans}) = 1.5\,R$ and $C^{\ominus}_{vm}(\text{rot}) \begin{cases} R & \text{linear} \\ 1.5\,R & \text{non-linear} \end{cases}$ and

$C^{\ominus}_{vm} = \sum_{r,t,v} C^{\ominus}_{vm}(i)$, then with $C^{\ominus}_{pm} = C^{\ominus}_{vm} + R$

Species	$C^{\ominus}_{pm}$
HCl	$\frac{7}{2}R$
Br_2	$\frac{7}{2}R < C^{\ominus}_{pm} < \frac{9}{2}R$
H_2O	$4\,R$
CH_4	$4\,R$
SiF_4	$4\,R < C^{\ominus}_{pm} < 6\,R$

Only HCl has $C^{\ominus}_{pm}$ of $\sim \frac{7}{2}R$.

5.42 Calculate the heat capacity (at constant P) of Cl_2 at 298.15, 500, and 1000 K. What is the equipartition value?

From Table 5.4 for Cl_2, $C^{\theta}_{vm} = 1.5\ R + R + \frac{Ru^2\ e^u}{(e^u - 1)^2}$ where

$u = \frac{\theta_v}{T} = \frac{813\ K}{T}$. We then make up the following table:

T(K)	$\frac{u^2\ e^u}{(e^u - 1)^2}$	$\frac{C_v}{R}$	$\frac{C_p}{R}$
298.15	0.55699	3.05699	4.05699
500	0.80601	3.30601	4.30601
1000	0.94699	3.44699	4.44699

The equipartition value is

$$C_p = C_v + R = 1.5\ R + R + R + R = \frac{9}{2}\ R = 4.5\ R\ .$$

5.43 Calculate C°_{vm} of HCN at 300 K.

$C^{\theta}_{vm} = C^{\theta}_{vm}(\text{trans}) + C^{\theta}_{vm}(\text{vib}) + C^{\theta}_{vm}(\text{rot})$. From Table 5.4,

$C^{\theta}_{vm}(\text{trans}) = \frac{3}{2}\ R = 12.471\ J\ K^{-1}$, $C^{\theta}_{vm}(\text{rot}) = R = 8.314\ J\ K^{-1}$,

$C^{\theta}_{vm}(\text{vib}) = \sum_u \frac{Ru^2\ e^u}{(e^u - 1)^2}$. From Table 5.2, $\theta_{v1} = 3006\ K$,

$\theta_{v2} = 4756\ K$, and $\theta_{v3} = 1024\ K$ with $g = 2$. Using $u = \frac{\theta_v}{T}$ and

plugging in, we obtain $C^{\theta}_{vm} = 27.644\ J\ K^{-1}$.

5.44 Calculate $C^{\ominus}_{pm}$ of SiF_4 at 300 K.

$C^{\theta}_{vm} = C^{\theta}_{vm}(\text{trans}) + C^{\theta}_{vm}(\text{vib}) + C^{\theta}_{vm}(\text{rot})$. Since

$C^{\theta}_{vm}(\text{trans}) = \frac{3}{2} R = 12.471 \text{ J K}^{-1}$, $C^{\theta}_{vm}(\text{rot}) = \frac{3}{2} R = 12.471 \text{ J K}^{-1}$

and $C^{\theta}_{vm}(\text{vib}) = \sum_{u} \frac{Ru^2 e^u}{(e^u - 1)^2} = 39.900 \text{ J K}^{-1}$, then

$C^{\theta}_{vm} = 64.842 \text{ J K}^{-1}$. Since $C^{\theta}_{vm} = C^{\theta}_{vm} + R$, then

$C^{\theta}_{vm} = 73.156 \text{ J K}^{-1}$.

5.45 Calculate the free-energy functions ($\phi°$ and ϕ') for O_2 at 1000 K. (The JANAF tables give $\phi' = 220.77$ J.)

$$\phi^0 = R\left\{\frac{7}{2} \ln T + \frac{3}{2} \ln M - 3.6517 - \ln(\sigma\theta_r) - \sum \ln(1 - e^{-u}) + \ln z_{elec}\right\}$$

With $T = 1000$ K , $M = 32.00$, $\sigma = 2$, $\theta_r = 2.08$,

$u = 2.274 = \frac{\theta_v}{T}$, and $g = 3$, we calculate $\phi^0 = 212.06 \text{ J K}^{-1}$.

$$\phi' = \phi^0 + \frac{H^{\theta}_m(298.15) - H_0}{T} = \phi^0 + \frac{7}{2} R + \frac{R\theta_v}{T(e^u - 1)} = 220.75 \text{ J K}^{-1} .$$

5.46 HF is a difficult substance to handle in the lab, so statistical calculations are a very attractive alternative to experimentation. For this molecule, calculate $S_m^\circ(298.15\ K)$, $H_m^\circ(298.15) - H_0$ and ϕ' at 500 K.

Using the procedure illustrated in problem 5.39 , we find:

$$S_m^\theta(\text{trans}) = 146.21\ \text{J K}^{-1}$$

$$S_m^\theta(\text{rot}) = 27.37\ \text{J K}^{-1}$$

$$S_m^\theta(\text{vib}) = 3.70 \times 10^{-7}\ \text{J K}^{-1}$$

$$S_m^\theta(\text{elec}) = 0$$

$$S_m^\theta = \sum_{r,t,v} S_m^\theta(i) = 173.59\ \text{J K}^{-1}\ .$$

$H_m^\theta(298.15) - H_0 = \frac{7}{2}\ RT + \sum\frac{R\theta_v}{(e^u - 1)}$. With $\theta_v = 5954.5$ K and $u = \frac{\theta_v}{T}$, we find $H_m^\theta(298.15) - H_0 = 8676$ J .

$$\phi^0 = R\left\{\frac{7}{2}\ \ln T + \frac{3}{2}\ \ln M - 3.6517 - \ln(\sigma\theta_r) - \sum \ln(1 - e^{-u}) + \ln z_{elec}\right\}$$

$$\phi^0 = R\left\{\frac{7}{2}\ \ln(500) + \frac{3}{2}\ \ln(20.01) - 3.6517 - \ln(30.127) - \ln(1 - e^{-5954.5/500})\right\}$$

$$\phi^0 = 159.53\ \text{J K}^{-1}\ .$$

$$\phi' = \phi^0 + \frac{H_m^\theta(298.15) - H_0}{T} = 176.88\ \text{J K}^{-1}\ .$$

5.47 Calculate the heat capacity at 300 K for a system with the following energy levels:

g	ε/k
2	0
4	100 K
2	150 K
1	200 K
5	500 K
1	1000 K
1	6000 K

Using the procedure given in the text (p. 253), with:

$$z = \sum_i g_i \exp(-u_i) = \sum_i g_i \exp\left(-\frac{\epsilon_i}{kT}\right)$$

$$z = (2 + 2.866 + 1.213 + 0.513 + 0.944 + 0.036) = 7.572 .$$

$$S_1 = \sum_i g_i u_i \exp(-u_i)$$

$$S_1 = (0.955 + 0.607 + 0.342 + 1.573 + 0.120) = 3.597 .$$

$$S_2 = \sum_i g_i u_i^2 \exp(-u_i)$$

$$S_2 = (0.318 + 0.303 + 0.228 + 2.622 + 0.40) = 3.871 .$$

From Eq. (5.82):

$$C_{vm} = R\left[\left(\frac{S_2}{z}\right) - \left(\frac{S_1}{z}\right)^2\right] = 2.374 \text{ J K}^{-1} .$$

5.48 Calculate the free-energy function (ϕ') of H_2O(liq) at 100°C from its entropy (Table 3.2) and heat capacity (C°_{pm} = 75 J K^{-1}, assumed independent of T).

From Eq. (5.94) ,

$$\Phi'(T) = S^{\theta}_m(298.15) + \int_{\ln(298.15)}^{\ln(T)} C^{\theta}_{pm}\, d(\ln T) - \frac{1}{T}\int_{298.15}^{T} C^{\theta}_{pm} dT .$$

Assuming C^θ_{pm} is independent of T ,

$$\Phi'(T) = S^\theta_m(298.15) + C^\theta_{pm}\left[\ln \frac{T}{298.15} - \frac{1}{T}(T - 298.15)\right]$$

$$\Phi'(T) = 70.00 \text{ J K}^{-1} + (75 \text{ J K}^{-1}) \times$$

$$\left[\ln \frac{373.15}{298.15} - \frac{1}{373.15}(373.15 - 298.15)\right] = 71.76 \text{ J K}^{-1} .$$

5.49 Calculate the free-energy function $\phi'(T)$ for HI at 1000 K from the thermodynamic data below.

$S^\circ_m(298.15) = 49.351 \text{ cal K}^{-1}$

T/K	C_{pm}/(cal K^{-1})	T/K	C_{pm}/(cal K^{-1})
298.15	6.969	700	7.424
400	7.010	800	7.600
500	7.107	900	7.767
600	7.253	1000	7.920

From Eq. (5.94),

$$\Phi'(T) = S^\theta_m + \int_{\ln(298.15)}^{\ln(T)} C^\theta_{pm}\, d(\ln T) - \frac{1}{T}\int_{298.15}^{T} C^\theta_{pm}\, dT .$$

To solve the two integrals above, we break the temperature range into small steps where $\int_{\ln(T_1)}^{\ln(T_2)} C^\theta_{pm} d(\ln T) = \bar{C}^\theta_{pm}(T_1, T_2) \ln \frac{T_2}{T_1}$ and $\int_{T_1}^{T_2} C^\theta_{pm}\, dT = \bar{C}^\theta_{pm}(T_1, T_2)[T_2 - T_1]$. Summing over the temperature range, integral 1 is 8.7960 cal K^{-1} and integral 2 is 5169.23 cal . Then

$$\Phi'(T) = \left(49.351 + 8.796 - \frac{5169.23}{1000}\right)\text{cal K}^{-1} = 52.978 \text{ cal K}^{-1}$$

$$\Phi'(T) = 221.85 \text{ J K}^{-1} .$$

5.50 If an atom or molecule has a low-lying excited electronic state with $\varepsilon_1 \ll kT$ at some temperature, show that the contribution of the electronic state to the free energy is $\ln(g_0 + g_1)$ and to the molar energy, $Lg_1\varepsilon_1/(g_0 + g_1)$. [Since $L\varepsilon_1 \ll RT$, this permits us to ignore the small energy and approximate the situation as a single state of degeneracy $g_0 + g_1$. In other words, very small splitting of ground state degeneracies can be ignored.]

From Eq. (5.75), $z_{elec} = g_0 + g_1 e^{-\epsilon_1/kT} + \ldots$. For a low-lying excited state, we ignore all but the first two terms. Since $\epsilon_1 \ll kT$, $e^{-\epsilon_1/kT} \cong 1$ and $z_{elec} \cong g_0 + g_1$. The electronic contribution to the free energy is $\ln z_{elec} = \ln(g_0 + g_1)$. Similarly, the electronic contribution to the molar energy is

$$U_m(\text{elec}) - U_0 = \frac{Lg_1\epsilon_1}{(g_0 e^{\epsilon_1/kT} + g_1)} \cong \frac{Lg_1\epsilon_1}{(g_0 + g_1)} .$$

5.51 The CH radical is not stable under ordinary conditions but will be an important factor in reactions at high temperatures. It has a low-lying excited state (Table 5.3), but at high temperature this will only add $R \ln 4$ to the free-energy function ($\phi°$). Calculate ϕ' at 1000 K. You will need to add the electronic contribution of $L\varepsilon/2 = 107$ J/mol to $H_m(298) - H_0$. The value listed by the JANAF tables is 197.95 J K^{-1}. (Use $\theta_v = 3932$ K, $\theta_r = 20.79$ K.)

For a linear molecule :

$$H_m^{\theta}(298.15) - H_0 = \frac{7}{2} RT + \sum \frac{R\theta_v}{(e^u - 1)} + \text{electronic contribution} .$$

Substitution gives : $H_m^{\theta}(298.15) - H_0 = 8783$ J . Similarly:

$$\phi^0 = R\left\{\frac{7}{2} \ln T + \frac{3}{2} \ln M - 3.6517 - \ln(\sigma\theta_r) - \sum \ln(1 - e^{-u}) + \ln z_{elec}\right\}$$

$$\phi^0 = 189.11 \text{ J K}^{-1} .$$

$$\phi' = \phi^0 + \frac{H_m^{\theta}(298.15) - H_0}{T} = 197.89 \text{ J K}^{-1} .$$

5.52 Gas-phase ionizations can be treated in the same fashion as other chemical reactions:

$$M \longrightarrow M^+ + e$$

To this end, one must know the thermodynamic properties of the product—an electron gas. Calculate $S_m^{\ominus}(298.15)$ for a mole of electrons. This can be compared to an early estimate by Lewis and Randall (1922), 3.28 cal K^{-1}. Note: this calculation ignores the spin-degeneracy contribution, $R \ln g_2$, due to the two degenerate states of the electron spin: spin-up and spin-down.

$$S_m^{\theta}(\text{trans}) = \frac{3}{2}R \ln M + \frac{5}{2}R \ln T - 1.1517R$$

$$M = (6.022 \times 10^{23})(9.109 \times 10^{-28} \text{ g}) = 5.486 \times 10^{-4} \text{ g}.$$

Substitution gives:

$$S_m^{\theta}(\text{trans}) = 15.22 \text{ J K}^{-1} = 3.64 \text{ cal K}^{-1} .$$

5.53 Starting with Eq. (5.82) and the appropriate partition function, show that the free-energy function of a monatomic species is:

$$\phi^\circ = R[2.5 \ln (T/\mathrm{K}) + 1.5 \ln (M/\mathrm{g}) - 3.652 + \ln z_{\mathrm{elec}}]$$

From Eq. (5.87) ,

$$\phi^0 = R \ln\left(\frac{z^\ominus}{L}\right) = R\left\{\ln \frac{z^\ominus(\mathrm{trans})}{L} + \ln z^\ominus(\mathrm{vib}) + \ln z^\ominus(\mathrm{rot}) + \ln z^\ominus(\mathrm{elec})\right\} .$$

$z^\ominus(\mathrm{trans}) = \dfrac{(2\pi mkT)^{3/2}V}{h^3}$. Using $V = \dfrac{RT}{p^\ominus}$ and $m = \dfrac{M}{L}$,

$$\ln\left(\frac{z^\ominus(\mathrm{trans})}{L}\right) = \frac{3}{2} \ln M + \frac{5}{2} \ln T + \ln \frac{(2\pi)^{3/2}R^{5/2}}{L^4h^3p^\ominus} .$$

Substituting and converting to the correct units,

$\ln\left(\dfrac{z^\ominus(\mathrm{trans})}{L}\right) = \dfrac{3}{2} \ln M + \dfrac{5}{2} \ln T - 3.652$. For a monatomic species, $z_{rot} = 1$ and $z_{vib} = 1$, thus

$$\phi^0 = R\left\{\frac{3}{2} \ln M + \frac{5}{2} \ln T - 3.652 + \ln z_{elec}\right\} .$$

5.55 From Eq. (5.97), show that the temperature (T_c), at which (and above which) the order parameter (J) will be zero, is given by:

$$T_c = 2\left[\frac{\varepsilon_{AA} + \varepsilon_{BB} - 2\varepsilon_{AB}}{k}\right]$$

Starting with Eq. (5.97):

$$T[\ln(1 + J) - \ln(1 - J)] = \frac{4J[\epsilon_{AA} + \epsilon_{BB} - 2\epsilon_{AB}]}{k} .$$

Expand the logarithms in the Taylor series:

$$T[(J + \ldots) - (-J + \ldots)] = \frac{4J[\epsilon_{AA} + \epsilon_{BB} - 2\epsilon_{AB}]}{k} .$$

Retaining only the first term of the series, valid for small J:

$$T(2J) = \frac{4J[\epsilon_{AA} + \epsilon_{BB} - 2\epsilon_{AB}]}{k}$$ thus as $J \rightarrow 0$:

$$T_c = \frac{2[\epsilon_{AA} + \epsilon_{BB} - 2\epsilon_{AB}]}{k} .$$

5.56 In a partially ordered crystal (with equal sites), $\varepsilon_{AA}/k = 100$ K, $\varepsilon_{BB}/k = 200$ K, and $\varepsilon_{AB}/k = 50$ K. At what temperature would the order parameter be equal to one half?

Rearrange Eq. (5.97) to:

$$T = \left(\ln\left[\frac{1 + J}{1 - J}\right]\right)^{-1} \frac{4J[\epsilon_{AA} + \epsilon_{BB} - 2\epsilon_{AB}]}{k}$$

$$T = \left(\ln\left[\frac{1 + \frac{1}{2}}{1 - \frac{1}{2}}\right]\right)^{-1} \frac{4}{2}\,[100 + 200 - 2(50)]\text{K}$$

$$T = \frac{2}{\ln 3}\,(200\text{ K}) = 364\text{ K} .$$

5.57 For the system of the previous problem, what would be the order parameter at 300 K?

Rearrange Eq. (5.97) to :

$$\ln\left[\frac{1 + J}{1 - J}\right] = \frac{4J[\epsilon_{AA} + \epsilon_{BB} - 2\epsilon_{AB}]k}{T}$$

$$\frac{1 + J}{1 - J} = \exp\left[\frac{800\ J}{300}\right]$$

$$J = \frac{\exp\left[\frac{8}{3} J\right] - 1}{\exp\left[\frac{8}{3} J\right] + 1} .$$

Starting with $J^{(1)} = \frac{1}{2}$, we find $J^{(2)} = 0.583$, $J^{(3)} = 0.651$, $J^{(4)} = 0.700$, $J^{(5)} = 0.732$, $J^{(6)} = 0.752$, $J^{(7)} = 0.762$, $J^{(8)} = 0.768$, $J^{(9)} = 0.772$, $J^{(10)} = 0.774$, $J^{(11)} = 0.774$.

REFERENCE: See Appendix AI.3 for methods of finding roots.

5.58 Derive formulas for the partition function, internal energy (U) and heat capacity for a system of energy levels with:

$$\varepsilon_N = N^2\theta$$

with $N = 0, 1, 2, \ldots$, for the high-temperature limit $T \gg \theta$.

In the high temperature limit, z may be considered a continuous variable, so that

$$z = \int_0^\infty \exp\left(-\frac{N^2\theta}{kT}\right)dN = \frac{1}{2}\sqrt{\frac{\pi kT}{\theta}} .$$

$$U - U_0 = \frac{RT^2}{z}\left(\frac{\partial z}{\partial T}\right) = \frac{RT}{2}$$

$$C_v = \frac{\partial U}{\partial T} = \frac{R}{2} .$$

6

Chemical Reactions

6.1 Give the formation reactions for the following:

$C_{12}H_{22}O_{11}(s)$, $PbSO_4(s)$, $NaIO_3(s)$, $C_2H_5OH(liq)$, $C_2H_5OH(g)$

$$12\ C\ (s)\ (graphite) + 11\ H_2\ (g) + \frac{11}{2}\ O_2\ (g) = C_{12}H_{22}O_{11}\ (s)$$

$$Pb\ (s) + S\ (s, rh) + 2\ O_2\ (g) = PbSO_4\ (s)$$

$$Na\ (s) + \frac{1}{2}\ I_2\ (s) + \frac{3}{2}\ O_2\ (g) = NaIO_3\ (s)$$

$$2\ C\ (s)\ (graphite) + 3\ H_2\ (g) + \frac{1}{2}\ O_2\ (g) = C_2H_5OH\ (l)\ .$$

6.2 The heat of combustion of acetic acid, $CH_3COOH(l)$, (at 25°C and constant pressure) is $\Delta_c H^\circ = -871.7$ kJ/mol. Use this to determine its heat of formation.

The combustion reaction is

$$CH_3COOH\ (l) + 2\ O_2\ (g) = 2\ CO_2\ (g) + 2\ H_2O\ (l)\ .$$

The heat of formation of CH_3COOH is

$$\Delta_f H^\ominus(CH_3COOH(l)) = 2\Delta_f H^\ominus(H_2O(l)) + 2\Delta_f H^\ominus(CO_2(g)) - \Delta_c H^\ominus$$

$$\Delta_f H^\ominus(CH_3COOH(l)) = 2(-285.83\ kJ) + 2(-393.509\ kJ) + 871.7\ kJ$$

$$\Delta_f H^\ominus(CH_3COOH(l)) = -486.98\ kJ\ .$$

6.3 Calculate the heat of formation of thiophene from its heat of combustion, Table 6.2.

The combustion reaction of thiophene is

$$C_4H_4S\ (l) + 7\ O_2\ (g) = 4\ CO_2\ (g) + 2\ H_2O\ (l) + SO_2\ (g)$$

The heat of formation of C_4H_4S is then

$$\Delta_f H^\theta(C_4H_4S) = 4\Delta_f H^\theta(CO_2(g)) + 2\Delta_f H^\theta(H_2O)(l)) + \Delta_f H^\theta(SO_2(g)) - \Delta_c H^\theta$$

$$\Delta_f H^\theta(C_4H_4S) = 4(-393.509\ kJ) + 2(-285.830\ kJ) + (-296.83\ kJ) + 2805\ kJ$$

$$\Delta_f H^\theta(C_4H_4S) = 362.47\ kJ\ .$$

6.4 Calculate the heat of formation of TiN from the data (T = 298.15 K):

$$Ti(s) + O_2(g) = TiO_2(s, \text{rutile}), \qquad \Delta H = -939.7\ kJ$$

$$TiN(s) + O_2(g) = TiO_2(s, \text{rutile}) + \tfrac{1}{2}N_2(g), \qquad \Delta H = -606.7\ kJ$$

Subtracting the second reaction from the first gives the formation reaction:

$$Ti\ (s) + \frac{1}{2}\ N_2\ (g) = TiN\ (s)\ .$$

Then $\Delta_f H^\theta(TiN) = -939.7\ kJ + 606.7\ kJ = -333.0\ kJ$.

6.5 The reactions:

(1) $H_2S(g) + \frac{3}{2}\ O_2(g) = SO_2(g) + H_2O(g)$

(2) $SO_2(g) + 2\ H_2S(g) = 3\ S(s) + 2\ H_2O(g)$

are important in a process for removing H_2S from gas streams. Calculate the heats of these reactions at 298 K.

$$\Delta H^\theta_{(1)} = \Delta_f H^\theta(SO_2(g)) + \Delta_f H^\theta(H_2O(g)) - \Delta_f H^\theta(H_2S(g))$$

$$\Delta H^\theta_{(1)} = -296.83\ kJ - 241.818\ kJ + 20.63\ kJ = -518.02\ kJ\ .$$

Similarly,

$$\Delta H^\theta_{(2)} = 2\Delta_f H^\theta(H_2O(g)) - 2\Delta_f H^\theta(H_2S(g)) - \Delta_f H^\theta(SO_2(g))$$

$$\Delta H^\theta_{(2)} = -145.55\ kJ\ .$$

6.6 Calculate the heat of combustion per kilogram of water gas, which consists of 40% (weight) CO, 3% CO_2, 52% H_2, and 5% N_2.

The combustion reactions are:

$$CO\ (g) + \frac{1}{2}\ O_2\ (g) = CO_2\ (g) \qquad (1)$$

$$H_2\ (g) + \frac{1}{2}\ O_2\ (g) = H_2O\ (l) \qquad (2)$$

with $\Delta H^{\ominus}_{(1)} = -282.99$ kJ mol^{-1} and $\Delta H^{\ominus}_{(2)} = -285.83$ kJ mol^{-1} .

Each kilogram of water gas contains

$\left(\frac{400\ g}{28\ g\ mol^{-1}}\right) = 14.3$ moles CO kg^{-1} and

$\left(\frac{520\ g}{2\ g\ mol^{-1}}\right) = 260$ moles H_2 kg^{-1} so that

$$\Delta_c H^{\ominus} = 14.3(\Delta H^{\ominus}_{(1)}) + 260(\Delta H^{\ominus}_{(2)}) = 78\ MJ\ kg^{-1}\ .$$

6.7 The heat of vaporization of Hg at 25°C is 31.76 kJ/mole. Calculate ΔH° of the reaction:

$$HgO(s, red) = Hg(g) + \tfrac{1}{2}O_2(g)$$

at 25°C from the heat of formation.

$$\Delta H^{\ominus} = -\Delta_f H^{\ominus}(HgO(s,\ red)) + \Delta_v H^{\ominus}(Hg(l))$$

$$\Delta H^{\ominus} = 90.83\ kJ + 31.76\ kJ = 122.59\ kJ\ .$$

6.8 Estimate the heat of the reaction:

$$H_2O(g) + CO(g) = H_2(g) + CO_2(g)$$

at 425°C. Assume constant C_p.

From Eq. (6.8), $\Delta_{rxn}H(T_2) = \Delta_{rxn}H(T_1) + \int_{T_1}^{T_2} \Delta C_p \, dT$.

$\Delta_{rxn}H^\theta(25°C) = \Delta_f H^\theta(CO_2(g)) - \Delta_f H^\theta(H_2O(g)) - \Delta_f H^\theta(CO(g))$.

$\Delta_{rxn}H^\theta(25°C) = -393.509 \text{ kJ} + 241.818 \text{ kJ} + 110.525 \text{ kJ} = -41.17 \text{ kJ}$.

From Eq. (6.6), $\Delta C_p = \sum_i \nu_i \, C_{pm}(i)$. Using data from Tables 6.1 and 2.1 at 25°C, $\Delta C_p = 2.990 \text{ J K}^{-1}$. Assuming constant heat capacities,

$$\Delta_{rxn}H^\theta(425°C) = \Delta_{rxn}H^\theta(25°C) + \Delta C_p \,(425°C - 25°C)$$

$$\Delta_{rxn}H^\theta(425°C) = -39.97 \text{ kJ}$$

6.9 Estimate the heat of reaction at 800 K for

$$Si(s) + 2\, Cl_2(g) = SiCl_4(g)$$

Assume constant C_p.

For temperature independent heat capacities:

$$\Delta_{rxn}H(T_2) = \Delta_{rxn}H(T_1) + \Delta_{rxn}C_p(T_2 - T_1) \, .$$

Using the data of Table 6.1:

$\Delta_{rxn}H(298.15 \text{ K}) = -657.01 \text{ kJ}$, $\Delta_{rxn}C_p = 2.44 \text{ J K}^{-1}$, $T_2 = 800 \text{ K}$

so that $\Delta_{rxn}H(800 \text{ K}) = -655.79 \text{ kJ}$.

6.10 The reaction:

$$4\,H_2(g) + 2\,CO(g) = C_2H_4(g) + 2\,H_2O(g)$$

is one of those in the Fischer-Tropsch synthesis of hydrocarbons. Derive a formula for the ΔH of this reaction as a function of T, assuming constant heat capacities (Tables 2.1 and 6.1). Calculate ΔH at 600 K.

For the reaction ,

$$4\ H_2\ (g) + 2\ CO\ (g) = C_2H_4\ (g) + 2\ H_2O\ (g)$$

we use Eq. (6.4) , $\Delta_{rxn}H(25°C) = \sum_i \nu_i \Delta_f H_i^\theta$, to find

$\Delta_{rxn}H(25°C) = -210.33$ kJ . From Eq. (6.6) ,

$\Delta C_p = \sum_i \nu_i\ C_{pm}(i) = -61.88\ J\ K^{-1}$. With ΔC_p considered constant,

Eq. (6.8) becomes $\Delta_{rxn}H(T_2) = \Delta_{rxn}H(T_1) + \Delta C_p(T_2 - T_1)$.

With $T_1 = 25°C$, $\Delta_{rxn}H(T) = -210.33\ kJ - \dfrac{61.88(T - 298.15)}{1000}\ kJ$.

For T = 600 K , $\Delta_{rxn}H = -229$ kJ .

6.11 Derive a formula for the heat of the reaction:

$$C(graphite) + 2\,H_2(g) = CH_4(g)$$

as a function of T. (Use data from Tables 6.1 and 2.1 and assume constant heat capacity.) Calculate ΔH at 500 and 1000 K.

At constant C_p , $\Delta_{rxn}H(T_2) = \Delta_{rxn}H(T_1) + \Delta C_p(T_2 - T_1)$.

The reaction is

$$C\ (graphite) + 2\ H_2\ (g) = CH_4\ (g)\ .$$

From Eq. (6.4) , $\Delta_{rxn}H(25°C) = \sum_i \nu_i \Delta_f H_i^\theta$ and using data from

Tables 2.1 and 6.1 , $\Delta_{rxn}H(25°C) = -74.81$ kJ . From Eq. (6.6),

$\Delta C_p = \sum_i \nu_i\ C_{pm(i)} = -30.090\ J\ K^{-1}$. Then

$\Delta_{rxn}H(T) = -74.81\ kJ - \dfrac{30.090(T - 298.15)}{1000}\ kJ$. For T = 500 K,

$\Delta_{rxn}H(500\ K) = -80.88\ kJ$. For T = 1000 K, $\Delta_{rxn}H(1000\ K)$,

$\Delta_{rxn}H(1000\ K) = -95.93\ kJ$.

6.12 Calculate the heat of vaporization of CCl_4 at 25°C with data from Table 6.1. Then estimate the heat of vaporization at the normal boiling point (349.9 K) assuming constant heat capacity; compare your result with the value given by Table 4.2.

From Table 6.1, for CCl_4 at 25°C:

$$\Delta_{vap}H(298.15\ K) = (-102.9\ kJ) - (-135.44\ kJ) = 32.54\ kJ\ .$$

Assuming constant heat capacities :

$$\Delta_{vap}H(349.9\ K) = \Delta_{vap}H(298.15\ K) + \Delta C_p \Delta T\ .$$

With $\Delta C_p = 83.3\ J\ K^{-1} - 131.75\ J\ K^{-1} = -48.45\ J\ K^{-1}$ and

$\Delta T = 51.75$ K, we find:

$$\Delta_{vap}H(349.9\ K) = 30.03\ kJ\ .$$

6.13 Estimate the adiabatic flame temperature of CS_2 burning in air, starting at 25°C. Assume constant heat capacity for the products.

The reaction is:

$$CS_2\ (l) + 3\ O_2\ (g) + 12\ N_2\ (g) = CO_2\ (g) + 2\ SO_2\ (g) + 12\ N_2\ (g)\ .$$

Assuming constant product heat capacities:

$$C_p(prod) = 465.3\ J\ K^{-1}\ .$$

The enthalpy of reaction is : $\Delta_{rxn}H(298.15\ K) = -1076.9\ kJ$.

Thus $\Delta T = -\dfrac{\Delta_{rxn}H}{C_p} = 2314$ K and $T_2 = T_{ad} = 2612$ K .

6.14 Estimate the adiabatic flame temperature for ethanol burning in air, starting at 25°C.

The reaction is:

$$C_2H_5OH\ (l) + 3\ O_2\ (g) + 12\ N_2\ (g) = 2\ CO_2\ (g) + 3\ H_2O\ (g) + 12\ N_2\ (g)$$

The heat capacity of the product mixture is (Table 2.2):

$C_p(\text{prod}) = 523 + (9.37 \times 10^{-2})T - \dfrac{2.324 \times 10^6}{T^2}$. Guess a mean T of 1000 K to find: $\bar{C}_p(1000\ \text{K}) = 614.4\ \text{J K}^{-1}$. The enthalpy of reaction is: $\Delta_{rxn}H(298.15\ \text{K}) = -1234\ \text{kJ}$. Using $\Delta T = -\dfrac{\Delta_{rxn}H}{\bar{C}_p}$, we draw up the following table:

	T (K)	$\bar{C}_p$ (J K^{-1})	T_2 (K)
(guess)	1000	614.4	2307
	1303	643.7	2216
	1257	639.3	2229
	1263	640.0	2227

6.15 *n*-Octane is typical of the hydrocarbons found in gasoline. In a gasoline engine, the air/fuel mixture is heated by adiabatic compression before ignition. Assuming a starting temperature of 700 K, estimate the temperature of the gases in the cylinder after ignition. Use the heat of combustion from Table 6.2 (for 25°C, assumed to be the same at 700 K) and *T*-dependent heat capacities for the products.

The chemical reaction is:

$$C_8H_{18}\ (l) + \frac{25}{2}\ O_2\ (g) + 50\ N_2\ (g) = 8\ CO_2\ (g) + 9\ H_2O\ (g) + 50\ N_2\ (g)$$

The enthalpy of reaction is : $\Delta_{rxn}H^\theta = -5055.9\ \text{kJ mol}^{-1}$.

The temperature dependent heat capacity is:

$C_p(\text{prod}) = 2057.78 + 0.3514\ T - \dfrac{1.120 \times 10^7}{T^2}$. Guess a mean temperature of 1000 K and draw up the following table:

T (K)	$\bar{C}_p$ (J K^{-1})	T_2 (K)
1000	2400	2403
1351	2528	2298
1298	2508	2313
1306	2511	2311
1305	2511	2311

6.16 The heat from chemical reactions cannot be dissipated immediately, so the products of an exothermic reaction can become quite hot; the maximum temperature can be estimated by assuming an adiabatic reaction. Estimate the maximum temperature for the lead-chamber process:

$$NO_2 + SO_2 = NO + SO_3$$

if it is carried out starting at $T_1 = 373$ K. Assume $\Delta_{rxn}H$ and C_p's independent of temperature.

$\Delta_{rxn}H(T) = \Delta_{rxn}H(298.15\text{ K}) + \Delta_{rxn}C_p(T - 298.15\text{ K})$. With $\Delta_{rxn}H(298.15\text{ K}) = -41.82$ kJ and $\Delta_{rxn}C_p = 3.44$ J K^{-1} we find $\Delta_{rxn}H(373\text{ K}) = 41.47$ kJ . $\Delta T = -\dfrac{\Delta_{rxn}H}{C_p(\text{products})}$, $C_p(\text{products}) = 80.51$ J K^{-1} . Thus $\Delta T = 515.1$ K and $T_{ad} = 888$ K .

6.17 The reaction:

$$C(s) + S_2(g) = CS_2(g)$$

was equilibrated at 1282 K; the product mixture was found to be 85% CS_2. Calculate K_p.

$X_{CS_2} = 0.85$, $X_{S_2} = 0.15$. $K_p = \dfrac{P_{CS_2}}{P_{S_2}} = \dfrac{X_{CS_2}P}{X_{S_2}P}$ or

$$K_p = \frac{0.85}{0.15} = 5.67 .$$

6.18 The dimerization of acetic acid (M = 60.05 g/mole):

$$2\ HAc(g) = (HAc)_2(g)$$

was studied by determining the apparent molecular weight (M_a) from vapor-density measurements. At 132°C, P = 0.4862 atm, M_a = 78.13 g. Calculate K_p.

If "d" denotes dimer and "m" denotes monomer, then:

$$K_p = \frac{P_d}{P_m^2} = \frac{X_d}{PX_m^2} .$$

Also: $M_a = X_dM_d + X_mM_m$, $M_a = 2M_m(1 - X_m) + M_mX_m$. Solving for X_m: $X_m = 2 - \frac{M_a}{M_m} = 2 - \frac{78.13}{60.05} = 0.699$. Thus $X_d = 0.301$ and

$$K_p = \frac{(0.301)}{(0.4862\ \text{atm})(0.699)^2} = 1.267\ \text{atm}^{-1} .$$

6.19 The reaction:

$$2\ NaHCO_3(s) = Na_2CO_3(s) + H_2O(g) + CO_2(g)$$

has a total P = 0.5451 atm at 90°C.

(a) Calculate K_p from this pressure.

(b) Calculate the total pressure if the $NaHCO_3$ is placed into a container with 1 atm of CO_2 (before reaction) at 90°C.

a) From Eq. (6.20) , $K_p = P_{H_2O}P_{CO_2}$. If the container was initially evacuated, $P_{H_2O} = P_{CO_2} = \frac{1}{2}P$ and

$$K_p = \frac{1}{4}P^2 = 7.43 \times 10^{-2}\ \text{atm}^2 .$$

b) Define an extent of reaction x, so that $P_{H_2O} = x$, $P_{CO_2} = 1 + x$ and $P_{total} = 1 + 2x$. From part a), $K_p = 7.43 \times 10^{-2}\ \text{atm}^2 = P_{H_2O}\ P_{CO_2} = x(1 + x)$ or $x = 6.95 \times 10^{-2}$ atm . Thus $P_{total} = 1 + 2x = 1.14$ atm .

6.20 (a) Show that the dissociation pressure (P) of ammonium carbamate:

$$NH_2COONH_4(s) = 2\ NH_3(g) + CO_2(g)$$

is related to the equilibrium constant as $K_p = \frac{4}{27}P^3$.
(b) At 25°C, the total pressure of the above reaction is 0.117 atm. Calculate $\Delta_f G^\circ$ of ammonium carbamate.

a) $K_p = P_{CO_2} P_{NH_3}{}^2$ and $P_{CO_2} + P_{NH_3} = P$. From the stoichiometry for the reaction, $P_{NH_3} = 2P_{CO_2}$, so that $P_{CO_2} = \frac{P}{3}$ and $P_{NH_3} = \frac{2P}{3}$. Substituting, $K_p = \frac{4}{27} P^3$.

b) Assuming ideal gas behavior,

$$\Delta_{rxn}G^\ominus = -RT\ \ln K_a$$

$$\Delta_{rxn}G^\ominus = -RT\ \ln K_p = -(8.3143\ J\ K^{-1})(298.15\ K)\ln\left[(0.117)^3\left(\frac{4}{27}\right)\right]$$

$$\Delta_{rxn}G^\ominus = 20.69\ kJ\ .$$

Also $\Delta_f G^\ominus(NH_2COONH_4) = 2\Delta_f G^\ominus(NH_3(g)) + \Delta_f G^\ominus(CO_2(g)) - \Delta_{rxn}G^\ominus$.

Using data from Table 6.1,

$$\Delta_f G^\ominus(NH_2COONH_4) = 2(-16.45\ kJ) - 394.359\ kJ - 20.69\ kJ$$

$$\Delta_f G^\ominus(NH_2COONH_4) = -447.97\ kJ\ .$$

6.21 Calculate $\Delta_f G^\circ$ at 298.15 K for C_2H_5OH(liq) from its heat of combustion (Table 6.2) and its standard entropy (Table 3.2). (Compare Table 6.1).

The combustion reaction is

$$C_2H_5OH\ (l) + 3\ O_2\ (g) = 2\ CO_2\ (g) + 3\ H_2O\ (l)$$

Thus

$$\Delta_f H^\ominus(C_2H_5OH(l)) = 2\Delta_f H^\ominus(CO_2(g)) + 3\Delta_f H^\ominus(H_2O(l)) - \Delta_c H$$

$$\Delta_f H^\ominus(C_2H_5OH(l)) = 2(-393.509\ kJ) + 3(-285.830\ kJ) + 1367\ kJ$$

$$\Delta_f H^\ominus(C_2H_5OH(l)) = -277.508\ kJ\ .$$

From Eq. (6.23), $\Delta_f G^\theta = \Delta_f H^\theta - T\,\Delta_f S^\theta$. The formation reaction for C_2H_5OH (l) is

$$2\ C\ (s) + 3\ H_2\ (g) + \tfrac{1}{2}\ O_2\ (g) = C_2H_5OH\ (l)\ .$$

With $\Delta_f S^\theta = \sum \nu_i S_m^\theta(i)$ and data from Table 3.2,

$\Delta_f S^\theta = -344.7\ J\ K^{-1}$ so that $\Delta_f G^\theta(298.15) = -175\ kJ$.

6.22 A standard reaction for coal gasification is:

$$H_2O(g) + \text{coal} = H_2(g) + CO(g)$$

(a) Treating coal as (approximately) graphite, calculate the equilibrium constant of this reaction at 1000 K (use free-energy functions).
(b) Calculate the percent H_2O reacted if the initial H_2O pressure is 10 atm (assume ideal gas).

a) From Eq. (6.25) , $K_a = \exp\left[\frac{\Delta\phi^0}{R} - \frac{\Delta H_0^\theta}{RT}\right]$. Using

$$H_2O\ (g) + C\ (\text{graphite}) = H_2\ (g) + CO\ (g)$$

and data from Table 6.4 , $\Delta\phi^0(1000\ K) = 132.8\ J\ K^{-1}$ and $\Delta H_0^\theta = 125.13\ kJ$. Thus $K_a(1000\ K) = 2.52$.

b) Assuming ideal gas behavior, $K_a = K_p = \frac{P_{CO}P_{H_2}}{P_{H_2O}}$. From the stoichiometry, $P_{CO} = P_{H_2}$ and $P_{H_2} = 10\ atm - P_{CO}$ and $P = P_{CO} + P_{H_2} + P_{H_2O} = 10 + P_{CO}$. Letting $x = P_{CO}$, $K_p = \frac{x^2}{10 - x}$.

With $K_p = 2.516$, $x^2 + 2.516x - 25.16 = 0$ or $x = 3.913$.

The % decomposition is then $100\left(\frac{x}{10}\right) = 39.13\%$.

6.23 (a) Estimate the vapor pressure of CCl_4 at 25°C with data from Table 6.1. (Remember that the data on this table are referenced to 1 bar = 750 torr.)
(b) Using the methods of Chapter 4 and data from Table 4.2 (assuming the enthalpy of vaporization is constant), estimate the same quantity and compare to the answer of (a). Which answer should be the more accurate? Why?
(c) In problem 6.12 the heat of vaporization was calculated for 298 K and the normal boiling point (349.9 K). Repeat the calculation of part (b) using the mean value of the heat of vaporization.

a) For the vaporization reaction: $CCl_4\ (l) = CCl_4\ (g)$.

$\Delta_{vap}G^{\ominus} = -RT \ln K_p = -RT \ln P(CCl_4) = 4.62$ kJ . $T = 298.15$ K so that $P(CCl_4) = 0.155$ bar $= 116$ torr .

b) From chapter 4, if $\Delta_v H^{\ominus}$ is constant:

$$\ln\left(\frac{P_2^0}{P_1^0}\right) = -\frac{\Delta_v H^{\ominus}}{R}\left(\frac{1}{T_2} - \frac{1}{T_1}\right) .$$

If we let $T_1 = T_b = 349.9$ K for CCl_4 , then with $P_1^0 = 1$ atm , $\Delta_v H^{\ominus} = 30$ kJ mol^{-1} and $T_2 = 298$ K, we calculate:

$$P_2^0(25°C) = 0.166 \text{ atm} = 126 \text{ torr} .$$

c) With $\Delta_v H^{\ominus} = 31.285$ kJ mol^{-1} , we find:

$$P_2^0 = 0.155 \text{ atm} = 118 \text{ torr} .$$

6.24 Carbon tetrachloride is generally considered to be noncombustible; in fact, it has been used in fire extinguishers and as a nonflammable spot-remover. (However, such uses have been abandoned because of concerns about its toxicity.) Calculate the equilibrium constant and heat of reaction at 1000 K for the combustion of carbon tetrachloride:

$$CCl_4(g) + 3O_2(g) = 4\ ClO(g) + CO_2(g)$$

(Use data from Table 6.1 and assume constant C_p.) You should find that the reaction is spontaneous at this temperature; however, since it is endothermic, it cannot sustain a flame. ClO, presumably produced by the decomposition of chlorofluorocarbons (CFC) has been a prime suspect as a catalyst for the decomposition of ozone in the stratosphere.

Assuming constant heat capacitites:

$$\ln K_a = \ln K_a(298.15) - \left[\frac{\Delta_{rxn}H(298.15) - (298.15\ K)\Delta_{rxn}C_p}{R}\right]\left(\frac{1}{T} - \frac{1}{298.15\ K}\right) + \left(\frac{\Delta_{rxn}C_p}{R}\right)\ln\left(\frac{T}{298.15\ K}\right).$$

For the reaction

$$CCl_4\ (g) + 3\ O_2\ (g) = 4\ ClO\ (g) + CO_2\ (g)$$

$\Delta_{rxn}G^\theta = 58.671$ kJ , $\ln K_a(298.15) = -\dfrac{\Delta_{rxn}G^\theta}{RT} = -23.67$,

$\Delta_{rxn}H(298.15) = 116.751$ kJ , $\Delta_{rxn}C_p = -8.415$. With $T = 1000$ K

we calculate: $\ln K_a(1000\ K) = 8.871$, $K_a(1000\ K) = 7.1 \times 10^3$.

Also, $\Delta_{rxn}H = \Delta_{rxn}H(298.15) - \Delta_{rxn}C_p(298.15\ K - T)$ so that:

$$\Delta_{rxn}H(1000\ K) = 111\ kJ .$$

6.25 Estimate the equilibrium constant at 900 K for:

$$COCl_2(g) = CO(g) + Cl_2(g)$$

assuming (a) constant H, (b) constant C_p.

a) If the enthalpy is assumed to be constant, then:

$$\ln K_a(T_2) = \ln K_a(T_1) - \frac{\Delta_{rxn}H^\theta}{R}\left(\frac{1}{T_2} - \frac{1}{T_1}\right)$$

At T_1 = 298.15 K: $K_a(298.15) = 1.535 \times 10^{-12}$,

$\Delta_{rxn}G^\theta$ = 67.432 kJ , $\Delta_{rxn}H^\theta$ = 108.275 kJ so that

$$K_a(900\ K) = 7.44\ .$$

b) If the heat capacity is assumed to be constant, then:

$$\ln K_a(T_2) = \ln K_a(T_1) -$$

$$\left(\frac{\Delta_{rxn}H(T_1) - T_1\Delta_{rxn}C_p}{R}\right)\left(\frac{1}{T_2} - \frac{1}{T_1}\right) + \left(\frac{\Delta_{rxn}C_p}{R}\right)\ln\left(\frac{T_2}{T_1}\right).$$

With $\Delta_{rxn}C_p = 5.389\ J\ K^{-1}$ and other parameters as in part a),

we find: $K_a(900\ K) = 9.87$.

6.26 Calculate the equilibrium constant for the reaction:

$$Ti(s) + \tfrac{1}{2}N_2(g) = TiN(s)$$

at 1500 K. Will this reaction be spontaneous if P_{N_2} = 1 torr?

$$Ti\ (s) + \frac{1}{2} N_2\ (g) = TiN\ (s)$$

$$\ln K_a = \frac{\Delta\Phi'}{R} - \frac{\Delta H^\theta(298.15)}{RT}\ .$$

For this reaction, $\Delta\Phi' = -94.0\ J\ K^{-1}$ and $\Delta H^\theta(298.15)$ = -338 kJ,

so that $K_a(1500\ K) = 7.2 \times 10^6$. If $K_p = K_a = \dfrac{1}{(P_{N_2})^{1/2}}$ (ideal gas behavior), then $\frac{1}{(P_{N_2})^{1/2}} = (760\ \text{atm}^{-1})^{1/2} = 27.6\ \text{atm}^{-1/2}$.

The reaction will proceed as written until

$$P_{N_2} = \frac{1}{(K_p)^2} = 1.9 \times 10^{-14}\ \text{atm} .$$

6.27 Oxygen as an impurity in a gas stream can be removed by passing the gas over hot copper turnings and permitting the reaction:

$$2\ Cu(s) + \tfrac{1}{2}\ O_2(g) = Cu_2O(s)$$

What would be the concentration of O_2 (per cm^3) in the gas stream following this reaction at 500 K? (Use data from Table 6.5.)

$$K_p = K_a = \exp\left[\frac{\Delta\Phi'}{R} - \frac{\Delta H^\ominus(298.15)}{RT}\right] .$$

For this reaction, $K_p = \frac{1}{(P_{O_2})^{1/2}}$ so that

$$P_{O_2} = \exp\left\{-2\left(\frac{\Delta\Phi'}{R} - \frac{\Delta H^\ominus(298.15)}{RT}\right)\right\} .$$

Also, $\Delta\Phi'(500\ K) = -75.95\ J\ K^{-1}$ and $\Delta H^\ominus(298.15\ K) = -170\ kJ$ so that $P_{O_2} = 2.60 \times 10^{-28}$ atm, which corresponds to a concentration of: $[O_2] = \frac{N_{O_2}}{V} = \frac{PL}{RT} = 3.82 \times 10^{-9}$ molecules cm^{-3} or one molecule in 260 m^3 .

6.28 Calculate the equilibrium constant K_a for the formation of ammonia at 773 K. Use $\Delta_f H^\circ(298) = -10.97 \pm 0.1$ kcal. The free energy functions (298 based) from the JANAF tables are given below (in cal K^{-1}).

	H_2	N_2	NH_3
$\phi'(700)$	33.153	47.731	48.647
$\phi'(800)$	33.715	48.303	49.467

Check the effect of the error in ΔH by repeating the calculation with $\Delta_f H = -10.90$ kcal. Compare your answer to Table 6.8.

From Eq. (6.28), $K_a = \exp\left[\frac{\Delta\Phi'}{R} - \frac{\Delta H^\ominus(298.15)}{RT}\right]$. Interpolate the data to 773 K to find $\Phi'(H_2) = 33.563$ cal K^{-1}, $\Phi'(N_2) = 48.149$ cal K^{-1} and $\Phi'(NH_3) = 49.246$ cal K^{-1}. The formation reaction is

$$\frac{3}{2}\,H_2\ (g) + \frac{1}{2}\,N_2\ (g) = NH_3\ (g)\ ,$$

thus $\Delta\Phi' = \sum_i \nu_i \Phi'(i) = -25.173$ cal K^{-1} and $K_a = 3.98 \times 10^{-3}$.

With $\Delta_f H^\ominus = -10.90$ kcal, $K_a = 3.80 \times 10^{-3}$.

6.29 One of the oldest reactions studied in a laboratory is the conversion of mercuric oxide to mercury by heat:

$$2\,HgO(s, red) = 2\,Hg(g) + O_2$$

Estimate the temperature at which this conversion will occur if HgO is heated in air. For this reaction at 25°C, $\Delta H = 303.67$ kJ, $\Delta G^\circ = 180.60$ kJ. (You may assume ΔH is constant.) (When the vapor is condensed, shining droplets of mercury appear. This seemingly magical transformation of a red powder to a silvery liquid was used by alchemists to impress their research sponsors.)

$$K_p(298.15\ K) = \exp\left(-\frac{\Delta_{rxn}G^\ominus}{RT}\right) = \exp\left(\frac{-180.6 \times 10^3\ J}{(8.3143\ J\ K^{-1})(298.15\ K)}\right)$$

$K_p(298.15\ K) = 2.28 \times 10^{-32}$ atm $= P_{O_2}$.

Rearranging Eq. (6.31), $T = \left\{\frac{1}{298.15} - \frac{R}{\Delta H^\ominus}\ln\left(\frac{K_p(T)}{K_p(298.15)}\right)\right\}^{-1}$.

With $K_p(T) = P_{O_2}(air) = 0.21$ atm and $\Delta_r H^\ominus = 303.67 \times 10^3$ J,

$T = 713$ K.

6.30 The heat-capacity change for a reaction can be expressed (as in Table 2.1):

$$\Delta C_p = \Delta a + \Delta b T + \frac{\Delta c}{T^2}$$

(a) Derive an expression for ln K in terms of Δa, Δb, Δc, the enthalpy of reaction at 298.15 K, and two constants of integration (I and J) which can be determined if K and ΔH are known at any one temperature.
(b) Derive such a formula for the Haber synthesis and compare its results to Table 6.8.

a) $\Delta_{rxn}H(T) = \Delta_{rxn}H(T_0) + \int_{T_0}^{T} \Delta C_p \, dT$ so that, with

$\Delta C_p = \Delta a + \Delta bT + \frac{\Delta c}{T^2}$, $\Delta_{rxn}H(T) = \Delta aT + \frac{1}{2}\Delta bT^2 - \frac{\Delta c}{T} + J$ where

J is a constant: $J = \Delta H(T_0) - \Delta aT_0 - \frac{1}{2}\Delta bT_0{}^2 + \frac{\Delta c}{T_0}$.

Plugging this into Eq. (6.30) and integrating

$$R \ln K_p = \int_{T_1}^{T} \frac{\Delta aT + \frac{1}{2}\Delta bT^2 - \frac{\Delta c}{T} + J}{T^2} \, dT$$

$$R \ln K_p = \Delta a \ln T + \frac{1}{2}\Delta bT + \frac{1}{2}\frac{\Delta c}{T^2} - \frac{J}{T} + I \ ,$$

where I is a constant,

$$I = -\Delta a \ln T_1 + \frac{1}{2}\Delta bT_1 - \frac{1}{2}\frac{\Delta c}{T_1{}^2} + \frac{J}{T_1} + R \ln K_p(T_1) \ .$$

b) The Haber synthesis is

$$\frac{1}{2} N_2\ (g) + \frac{3}{2} H_2\ (g) = NH_3\ (g)$$

Using data from Table 2.21, $\Delta a = -25.46$, $\Delta b = 18.325 \times 10^{-3}$ and $\Delta c = -2.050 \times 10^5$. As a reference temperature use $T_0 = T_1 = 298.15$ K . Using data from Table 6.1,

$\Delta_{rxn}H^\theta(298.15) = -46.19$ kJ and $\Delta_{rxn}G^\theta(298.15) = -16.64$ kJ .

$\ln K_p(298.15) = 6.7129$, so that

$$\ln K_p = 7.7929 + \frac{4823}{T} - 3.062 \ln T + 1.102 \times 10^{-3} T - \frac{1.233 \times 10^4}{T^2} .$$

6.31 (a) Use the results for $\Delta H(T)$ obtained in Problem 6.11 to derive a formula for ln K as a function of T for the reaction:

$$C(\text{graphite}) + 2 H_2(g) = CH_4(g)$$

(b) Compare your calculation at 1000 K to that obtained from the free-energy functions, Table 6.4.

a) Using data from Table 6.1, $\ln K_0 = -\frac{\Delta_f G^\theta(CH_4)}{RT} = 20.49$ with $T_0 = 298.15$ K . Then $\ln K = 14.54 + \frac{7923}{T} - 3.619 \ln T$.

b) Using data from Table 6.4, ln K(1000 K) = -2.321 or $K = 9.814 \times 10^{-2}$. From part a), ln K(1000 K) = -2.536 or

$$K = 7.917 \times 10^{-2} .$$

6.32 Estimate ΔH° of the reaction:

$$H_2(g) + \tfrac{1}{2} S_2(g) = H_2S(g)$$

given $K_p = 106$ at 1023 K, $K_p = 20.2$ at 1218 K.

From Eq. (6.31) , $\Delta_{rxn}H^\theta = -R\ln\left(\frac{K(T_2)}{K(T_1)}\right)\left[\frac{1}{T_2} - \frac{1}{T_1}\right]^{-1}$. With the data of the problem we find $\Delta_{rxn}H^\theta = -88.07$ kJ .

6.33 Estimate the equilibrium constant at 500 K for:

$$SO_2(g) + 2\,H_2S(g) = 3\,S(s) + 2\,H_2O(g)$$

Assume ΔH is independent of T.

Using data from Table 6.1, $\Delta_{rxn}H^{\ominus}(298.15) = -145.55$ kJ and $\Delta_{rxn}G^{\ominus} = -89.830$ kJ . From Eq. (6.31),

$$\ln K = \ln K(298.15) - \frac{\Delta_{rxn}H^{\ominus}}{R}\left(\frac{1}{T} - \frac{1}{298.15}\right)$$

. From Eq. (6.17),

$$\ln K(298.15) = -\frac{\Delta_{rxn}G^{\ominus}(298.15)}{R(298.15\ K)} = 36.24$$

. Thus at T = 500 K

$$\ln K = 36.24 + 17\ ,\ 505\left(\frac{1}{500} - \frac{1}{298.15}\right) = 12.54$$

and

$$K(500\ K) = 2.78 \times 10^5 .$$

6.34 From the equilibrium constants below for the reaction:

$$V_2O_5(s) + SO_2(g) = V_2O_4(s) + SO_3(g)$$

calculate (a) $\Delta_{rxn}H^{\ominus}$, (b) $\Delta_{rxn}G^{\ominus}$, (c) the percent of the SO_2 converted to SO_3 at 878 K.

T	K_p
831	0.0154
857	0.0170
878	0.0182
906	0.0202
918	0.0215

a) From Eq. (6.29), a plot of $\ln K_p$ vs. $\frac{1}{T}$ should be a straight line with slope $= -\frac{\Delta_{rxn}H^{\ominus}}{R}$. We find by linear regression

$\frac{\Delta H^\theta}{R} = 2.89 \times 10^3$ with $\sigma = 0.12 \times 10^3$ and $\Delta_{rxn}H^\theta = 24$ kJ with $\sigma = 1$ kJ .

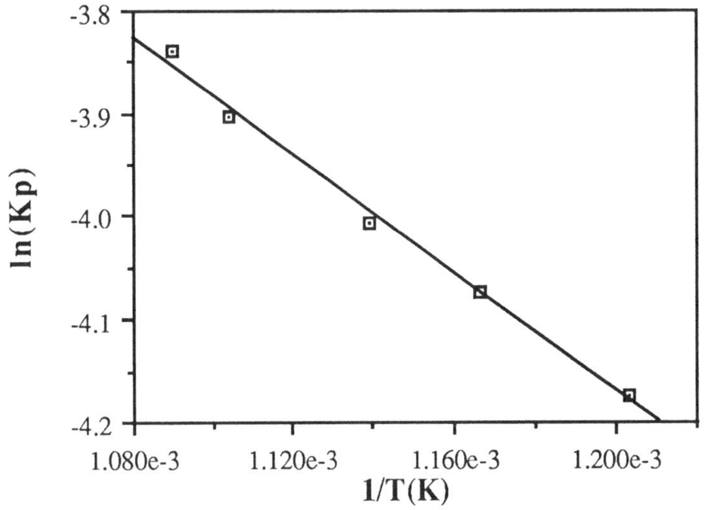

b) $\Delta_{rxn}G^\theta = -RT \ln K_p = -(8.3143 \text{ J K}^{-1})(878 \text{ K}) \ln(0.0182)$

$\Delta_{rxn}G^\theta = 29.2$ kJ .

c) $K_p = \frac{P_{SO_3}}{P_{SO_2}}$. Assuming the equilibrium occurs in a container initially filled with SO_2 (g) at P_0 , then $P_0 = P_{SO_2} + P_{SO_3}$ and $P_{SO_2} = \frac{P_0}{(1 + K_p)}$. The % decomposed is

$$\left(\frac{P_{SO_3}}{P_0}\right) 100 = \frac{100\ K_p}{(1 + K_p)} = 1.8\% \text{ at } T = 878 \text{ K} .$$

6.35 The dissociation pressures of:

$$CaCO_3(s) = CaO(s) + CO_2(g)$$

are given below. Calculate the heat of this reaction. Use either linear regression (Appendix I) or a graphical method.

T	P/atm	T	P/atm
1115.4	0.4513	1177.4	1.157
1126.0	0.5245	1179.6	1.151
1127.6	0.5317	1210.1	1.770
1142.0	0.6722		

From Eq. (6.29), a plot of $\ln K_p$ vs. $\frac{1}{T}$ is a straight line of slope $= -\frac{\Delta_{rxn}H^{\theta}}{R}$. For the given reaction, $K_p = P_{CO_2}$, thus

$\Delta_{rxn}H^{\theta} = 163.9$ kJ with $\sigma = 1.9$ kJ .

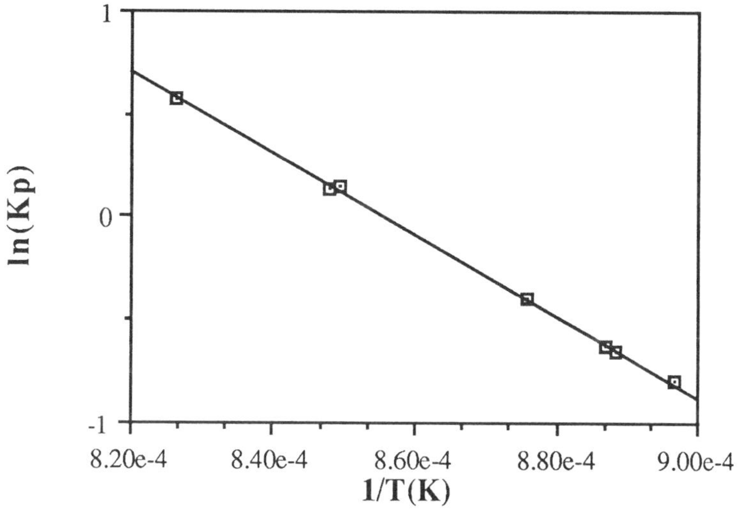

6.36 In Problem 6.10 the heat of reaction for:

$$4\ H_2(g) + 2\ CO(g) = C_2H_4(g) + 2\ H_2O(g)$$

was estimated as:

$$\Delta H = -191{,}844 - 61.98T$$

Derive a formula for ln K as a function of T and estimate K at 600 K.

From problem 6.10, $\Delta_{rxn}H^{\theta}(T) = -191{,}873 - 61.88\ T$. Using

$\dfrac{d\ \ln K_p}{dT} = \dfrac{\Delta_{rxn}H^{\theta}}{RT^2}$ and $R = 8.3143\ J\ K^{-1}$, $\dfrac{d\ \ln K_p}{dT} = \dfrac{-23{,}078}{T^2} - \dfrac{7.45}{T}$.

Integrating from T = 298.15 to T,

$$\ln\left(\frac{K_p(T)}{K_p(298.15)}\right) = \frac{23{,}078}{T} - 7.45\ \ln T - 34.96\ .$$

For the given reaction, we calculate $K_p(298.15)$ from the data of Table 6.1:

$$\ln K_p(298.15) = -\frac{\Delta_{rxn}G^{\theta}(298.15)}{RT} = \frac{114.658 \times 10^3\ J}{(8.3143\ J\ K^{-1})(298.15\ K)}$$

$$\ln K_p(298.15) = 46.2\ .$$

Then $\ln K_p(T) = \dfrac{23{,}078}{T} - 7.45\ \ln T + 11.24$ and at T = 600 K ,

$$K_p = 7.77\ .$$

6.37 The equation of state:

$$PV_m = RT(1 + 6.4 \times 10^{-4}\, P/\text{atm})$$

works for hydrogen gas at 25° up to 1500 atm with a maximum of 0.5% error. Use it to calculate the fugacity of hydrogen at 500 and 1000 atm.

From Eq. (6.37), $\ln \gamma = \frac{1}{RT}\int_0^P \left(V_m - \frac{RT}{P}\right) dP$. Substituting $V_m = \frac{RT}{P} + RT(6.4 \times 10^{-4})$ and integrating the above, $\ln \gamma = 6.4 \times 10^{-4}P$ or $\gamma = \exp(6.4 \times 10^{-4}P)$. At P = 500 atm, $\gamma = 1.377$ and at P = 1000 atm, $\gamma = 1.896$. From Eq. (6.36), $f = \gamma P$, so that f(500 atm) = 688.6 atm and

$$f(1000\ \text{atm}) = 1896\ \text{atm}.$$

6.38 Show that the fugacity of a van der Waals gas is given by:

$$f = \left(\frac{RT}{V_m - b}\right) \exp\left(\frac{b}{V_m - b} - \frac{2a}{RTV_m}\right)$$

This is best done by integrating Eq. (6.35) by parts from a low-pressure point (P^*, V^*) at which the ideal gas law is valid $(P^*V^* = RT, f^* = P^*)$; then find the limit $P^* \to 0$, $V^* \to \infty$.

$RT\, d(\ln f) = V_m\, dP$. For a van der Waals gas,

$RT\, d(\ln f) = -\dfrac{RTV_m\, dV_m}{(V_m - b)^2} + \dfrac{2a}{V_m^2}\, dV_m$. Dividing by RT and integrating from $V^* = \dfrac{RT}{P^*}$ at $f^* = P^*$ to V_m at f(ideal gas limit at $f^* = P^*$): $\ln\left(\dfrac{f}{f^*}\right) = \displaystyle\int_{\frac{RT}{P^*}}^{V_m} \left(\frac{2a}{RTV_m^2} - \frac{V_m}{(V_m - b)^2}\right) dV_m$. The first integral is $\displaystyle\int_{\frac{RT}{P^*}}^{V_m} \frac{2a}{RTV_m^2}\, dV_m = \frac{2aP^*}{(RT)^2} - \frac{2a}{RTV_m}$. We do the second integral by parts

$$-\int_{\frac{RT}{P^*}}^{V_m} \frac{V_m\, dV_m}{(V_m - b)^2} = \frac{V_m}{V_m - b} - \frac{\frac{RT}{P^*}}{\left(\frac{RT}{P^*} - b\right)} - \ln\left[\frac{(V_m - b)}{\left(\frac{RT}{P^*} - b\right)}\right] .$$

Collecting terms,

$$\ln\left(\frac{f}{f^*}\right) = \frac{2aP^*}{(RT)^2} - \frac{2a}{RTV_m} + \frac{V_m}{V_m - b} - \frac{1}{\left(1 - \frac{bP^*}{RT}\right)} - \ln\left[\frac{P^*(V_m - b)}{(RT - P^*b)}\right] .$$

By definition, $f^* = P^*$ so the $\ln P^*$ terms cancel. Taking the limit as $P^* \to 0$ (ideal gas limit):

$$\ln f = \ln\left(\frac{RT}{V_m - b}\right) + \frac{b}{(V_m - b)} - \frac{2a}{RTV_m}$$

$$f = \frac{RT}{(V_m - b)} \exp\left\{\frac{b}{(V_m - b)} - \frac{2a}{RTV_m}\right\} .$$

6.39 Calculate the fugacity coefficients of methane between 100, 500, and 1000 atm from the data below (T = 203 K).

P/atm	z	P/atm	z
1	0.9940	160	0.5252
10	0.9370	180	0.5752
20	0.8683	200	0.6246
30	0.7928	250	0.7468
40	0.7034	300	0.8663
50	0.5936	400	1.0980
60	0.4515	500	1.3236
80	0.3429	600	1.5409
100	0.3767	800	1.9626
120	0.4259	1000	2.3684
140	0.4753		

We begin by estimating the second virial coefficient of CH_4. Using Eq. (1.16) and data from Table 1.2, $B(203\text{ K}) = -0.0962\text{ dm}^3$. Using Eq. (6.39), $\ln \gamma = \int_0^P \frac{z-1}{P}\,dP$, and the trapezoidal rule (AI.4) to numerically integrate the data, we draw up the following table: (Note that from Eq. (6.40), $\lim_{P\to 0}\left[\frac{z-1}{P}\right] = \frac{B}{RT} = -0.0058\text{ atm}^{-1}$.)

P	$\frac{(z-1)}{P}$ (atm^{-1})	ΔP (atm)	$\int_0^P \frac{z-1}{P}\,dP$	γ
0	-0.0058			
1	-0.0060	1	-0.0059	0.99
10	-0.0063	9	-0.0613	0.94
20	-0.0066	10	-0.1258	0.88
30	-0.0069	10	-0.1933	0.82
40	-0.0074	10	-0.2648	0.77
⋮	⋮	⋮	⋮	⋮
100	-0.0062	20	-0.7453	0.47
⋮	⋮	⋮	⋮	⋮
500	0.0006	100	-1.1343	0.32
⋮	⋮	⋮	⋮	⋮
1000	0.0014	200	-0.5893	0.55

6.40 Calculate the fugacity coefficients of ammonia between 100 and 1000 atm from the data below (T = 473 K).

P/atm	z	P/atm	z
10	0.9805	200	0.5505
20	0.9611	300	0.4615
30	0.9418	400	0.4948
40	0.9219	500	0.5567
60	0.8821	600	0.6212
80	0.8411	800	0.7545
100	0.8008	1000	0.8914

Proceed as in problem 6.39, using Eq. (6.39) and the trapezoidal rule (AI.4) to integrate the data. To find the integrand at P = 0, use Eq. (6.40), $\lim_{P\to 0}\left[\frac{z-1}{P}\right] = \frac{B}{RT}$. From Eq. (1.17) and the data in Table 1.1, B(473 K) = -0.0715 and

$\lim_{P\to 0}\left[\frac{z-1}{P}\right]$ = -0.0018 . We then have the following table:

P	$\frac{(z-1)}{P}$ (atm^{-1})	ΔP (atm)	$\int_0^P \frac{z-1}{P}\,dP$	γ
0	-0.0018			
10	-0.0020	10	-0.0190	0.98
20	-0.0019	10	-0.0385	0.96
.	.	.	.	.
.	.	.	.	.
100	-0.0020	20	-0.1970	0.82
.	.	.	.	.
.	.	.	.	.
500	-0.0009	100	-0.8720	0.42
.	.	.	.	.
.	.	.	.	.
1000	-0.0001	200	-1.0770	0.34

6.41 (a) Derive a formula for the fugacity of a gas from the equation of state:

$$PV_m = RT + \beta P + \gamma P^2 + \delta P^3 + \varepsilon P^4$$

(b) For hydrogen at 0°C, $\beta = 1.3638 \times 10^{-2}$, $\gamma = 7.851 \times 10^{-6}$, $\delta = -1.206 \times 10^{-8}$, $\varepsilon = 7.354 \times 10^{-12}$ (P in atm, V in dm^3). Calculate the fugacity of hydrogen at $P = 500$ atm, 0°C.

a) From Eq. (6.37) ,

$$\ln \gamma = \frac{1}{RT}\int_0^P \left[V_m - \frac{RT}{P}\right]dP = \ln \gamma = \frac{1}{RT}\int_0^P [\beta + \gamma P + \delta P^2 + \xi P^3]dP ,$$

so that $\ln \gamma = \frac{1}{RT}\left(\beta P + \frac{\gamma P^2}{2} + \frac{\delta P^3}{3} + \frac{\xi P^4}{4}\right)$ and

$$\gamma = \exp\left(\left[\beta P + \frac{\gamma P^2}{2} + \frac{\delta P^3}{3} + \frac{\xi P^4}{4}\right]\frac{1}{RT}\right) .$$

b) Plugging in the given values at P = 500 atm and T = 273.15 K, $\gamma = 1.392$ and $f = \gamma P = 696$ atm .

6.42 Zinc has $V_m = 7.1$ cm^3 (20°C) and (Table 1.8):

$$\kappa_T = 1.5 \times 10^{-7} \text{ atm}^{-1}$$

Estimate the activity of zinc at 298 K and $P = 1000$ atm, assuming: (a) it is incompressible; (b) using Eq. (1.62).

a) $\Gamma = \exp\left[\frac{(P - P^\theta)V_m}{RT}\right] = \exp\left[\frac{((999)(7.1 \times 10^{-3})}{(0.08206)(298.15)}\right] = 1.336$.

b) $V_m(P) = V_m^\theta\left[1 - \kappa_T(P - P^\theta)\right]$ and $\ln \Gamma = \frac{1}{RT}\int_{P^\theta}^P V_m\, dP$.

Substituting $P_0 = P^\theta \sim 1$ atm:

$$\ln \Gamma = \frac{V_m^\theta}{RT}\left[P - \frac{\kappa P^2}{2} + \kappa_T P^\theta P\right]_{1\text{ atm}}^{1000\text{ atm}} .$$

Evaluating the r.h.s., we find $\ln \Gamma = 0.2899$ and $\Gamma = 1.336$.

6.43 A mixture containing 200 atm methane and 400 atm carbon dioxide is heated to 900 K. Use Newton's graphs (Figure 6.9) to calculate the fugacity of each gas.

Reduced temperatures and pressures are:

Species	T_R	P_R
CH_4	4.72	13.10
CO_2	2.96	8.22

From Figure 6.9, $\gamma(CH_4) = 1.25$ and $\gamma(CO_2) = 1.12$ so that

$$f(CH_4) = (1.25)(200) = 250 \text{ atm}$$
$$f(CO_2) = (1.12)(400) = 448 \text{ atm} .$$

6.44 The reaction:

$$C(s) + 2\,H_2(g) = CH_4(g)$$

has $K_a = 0.46$ at 873 K. Estimate K_p and the percent methane in the equilibrium mixture when the equilibrium total pressure is 1000 atm. You may assume that graphite is incompressible with density 2.26 g/cm^3.

$K_p = \frac{K_a}{K_\gamma}$. Using data from Table 1.1,

Species	T_R	P_R
CH_4	4.58	21.8
H_2	26.3	78.1

From Figure 6.9 , $\gamma(CH_4) = 1.43$ and $\gamma(H_2) = 1.36$. The activity coefficient for C(s) is given by $\Gamma = \exp\left(\frac{PV_m}{RT}\right)$. Since

$$V_m = \frac{M}{\rho} = \frac{12.011 \text{ g}}{2.26 \times 10^3 \text{ g dm}^{-3}} = 5.315 \times 10^{-3} \text{ dm}^3 \text{ , then } \Gamma = 1.077 .$$

From Eq. (6.42), $K_\gamma = \frac{\gamma(CH_4)}{(\gamma(H_2))^2\,\Gamma} = \frac{1.43}{(1.36)^2(1.077)} = 0.7179$.

Thus $K_p = \frac{0.46}{0.718} = 0.64$. Since,

$$K_p = \frac{X_{CH_4}}{(X_{H_2})^2}\left(\frac{1}{P}\right) = \frac{X_{CH_4}}{(1 - X_{CH_4})^2}\left(\frac{1}{P}\right)$$, then

$$(X_{CH_4})^2 - \left(2 + \frac{1}{PK_p}\right)X_{CH_4} + 1 = 0$$ and the solution is

$X_{CH_4} = 0.961$. Thus there is 96% CH_4 at equilibrium .

6.45 The equilibrium:

$$N_2O_4(g) = 2\ NO_2(g)$$

was studied by equilibrating the gas at 37.0°C in a container with $V = 2042$ cm³. The pressure was adjusted to 750 torr (by allowing gas to escape) and the container weighed; it contained 5.80 g of gas. Calculate the degree of dissociation and K_p at this temperature.

Draw up the folowing table, in which α is the degree of dissociation:

Species	Initial Moles	Final Moles	Final Mole Fraction
N_2O_4	n_0	$n_0(1 - \alpha)$	$\frac{(1 - \alpha)}{(1 + \alpha)}$
NO_2	0	$2\alpha n_0$	$\frac{2\alpha}{(1 + \alpha)}$

The mass of gas in the container is

$$W = W_{NO_2} + W_{N_2O_4} = n_{NO_2}M_{NO_2} + n_{N_2O_4}M_{N_2O_4} = n_T\ M_{NO_2}(X_{NO_2} + 2(1 - X_{NO_2}))$$

where n_T = total moles. Using the ideal gas law for n_T,

$$X_{NO_2} = 2 - \frac{WRT}{PVM_{NO_2}}$$

$$X_{NO_2} = 2 - \frac{(5.80)(0.08206\ dm^3\ atm\ K^{-1})(310.15\ K)}{(0.987\ atm)(2.042\ dm^3)(46.0)} = 0.408\ .$$

$$\alpha = \frac{X_{NO_2}}{2 - X_{NO_2}} = 0.256$$ so that, with $K_p = \frac{4\alpha^2 P}{(1 - \alpha)\ (1 + \alpha)}$,

$$K_p = 0.277\ .$$

6.46 Calculate the degree of dissociation for:

$$N_2O_4 = 2\ NO_2$$

using data from Table 6.1 at $P = 1$ atm, $T = 298.15$ K.

Using data from Table 6.1,

$$\Delta_{rxn}G^{\theta} = 2\Delta_f G^{\theta}(NO_2) - \Delta_f G^{\theta}(N_2O_4) = 5.394 \text{ kJ} .$$

$K_p = \exp\left(-\dfrac{\Delta_{rxn}G^{\theta}}{RT}\right) = 0.113$ atm . If α = degree of dissociation,

then $X_{NO_2} = \dfrac{2\alpha}{(1 + \alpha)}$, $X_{N_2O_4} = \dfrac{(1 - \alpha)}{(1 + \alpha)}$ and $K_p = \dfrac{P(X_{NO_2})^2}{X_{N_2O_4}} = \dfrac{4\alpha^2 P}{1 - \alpha^2}$

or $\alpha = \left[\dfrac{K_p}{4P + K_p}\right]^{1/2}$. Thus $\alpha = 0.166$ or 16.6% dissociation .

6.47 The equilibrium constant for the dissociation of phosgene:

$$COCl_2(g) = CO(g) + Cl_2(g)$$

is 22.5 atm at 668 K. Calculate the degree of dissociation at $P = 2$ atm.

The equilibrium constant is $K_p = \dfrac{PX_{Cl_2}X_{CO}}{X_{COCl_2}} = PK_x$. With degree of dissociation = α , then from Eq. (6.49), $K_x = \dfrac{\alpha^2}{(1 - \alpha^2)}$ or

$$\alpha = \left(\frac{K_p}{P + K_p}\right)^{1/2} = \left(\frac{22.5}{2 + 22.5}\right)^{1/2} = 0.958 \text{ or } 95.8\% \text{ dissociated} .$$

6.48 Calculate the equilibrium constant and degree of dissociation for:

$$SO_2Cl_2(g) = SO_2(g) + Cl_2(g)$$

at 25°C and P = .001 bar.

For the reaction: $SO_2Cl_2\ (g) = SO_2\ (g) + Cl_2\ (g)$

$\Delta_{rxn}G^{\ominus}$ = 19.806 kJ and $K_a(298.15) = 3.389 \times 10^{-4}$.

$K_a \sim \left(\dfrac{\alpha^2}{1 - \alpha^2}\right)P$. With P = 0.001 bar, we find α = 0.503 .

6.49 The equilibrium constant for the dissociation of ethanol into ethylene and water:

$$C_2H_5OH(g) = C_2H_4(g) + H_2O(g)$$

is 0.6246 atm at 351 K (the normal boiling point of ethanol). Calculate the degree of dissociation at this temperature. This reaction does not normally occur (in the absence of a catalyst) because it is too slow. If it did, it would be a major problem for the distillers of alcoholic beverages.

If we define a degree of dissociation α, then at constant P:

$K_p = \dfrac{\alpha^2 P}{1 - \alpha^2}$. Solving for α: $\alpha = \sqrt{\dfrac{K_p}{P + K_p}}$. With

K_p = 0.6426 bar and P = 1 bar , we find α = 0.625 .

6.50 Use the calculated equilibrium constants (Table 6.6) for Br_2 = 2 Br to calculate the degree of dissociation at 2000 K, 1 atm, for each of the estimated values.

From Eq. (6.48), $\alpha = \left(\dfrac{K_p}{4P + K_p}\right)^{1/2}$. With P = 1 atm, we may

use Table 6.6 we may use Table 6.6 to draw up the following

table:

K_p	α
2.77	0.64
5.54	0.76
4.83	0.74
4.94	0.74
5.10	0.75

6.51 The lead-chamber process for making sulfuric acid uses the reaction:

$$NO_2(g) + SO_2(g) = NO(g) + SO_3(g)$$

At 373 K, $K_p = 15.8 \times 10^3$. Calculate the percent conversion of SO_2 to SO_3 if the NO_2 and SO_2 are mixed in equal proportions.

$K_p' = K_x = \dfrac{X_{NO}X_{SO_3}}{X_{NO_2}X_{SO_2}}$. $X_{NO} = X_{SO_3}$, $X_{NO_2} = X_{SO_2}$ and

$X_{NO} + X_{NO_2} = X_{SO_2} + X_{SO_3} = 0.5$. Defining $X_{SO_3} = X$, then

$K_p = \dfrac{X^2}{(0.5 - X)^2}$ or $X^2 + \dfrac{K_p}{1 - K_p} X - \dfrac{0.25\ K_p}{1 - K_p} = 0$. With

$K_p = 15.8 \times 10^3$, $X = 0.4961 = X_{SO_3}$. The percent conversion

is thus $\left(\dfrac{X_{SO_3}}{0.5}\right) 100\% = 99.2\%$.

6.52 Urea can react with water vapor to form ammonia:

$$CO(NH_2)_2(s) + H_2O(g) = CO_2(g) + 2\ NH_3(g)$$

with $K_p = 1.63$ atm^2 at 25°C. If urea is stored in a closed container under moist air with an initial water pressure at 20 torr, what will be the pressure of ammonia at equilibrium?

$K_p = \dfrac{(P_{NH_3})^2 P_{CO_2}}{P_{H_2O}}$. If we define ϵ = extent of reaction , then

$P_{NH_3} = 2\epsilon$, $P_{CO_2} = \epsilon$ and $P_{H_2O} = P_0 - \epsilon$ where

P_0 = initial H_2O pressure. Thus $K_p = \dfrac{4\epsilon^3}{(P_0 - \epsilon)}$. Rearranging,

$\epsilon^3 + \left(\dfrac{K_p}{4}\right)\epsilon - \left(\dfrac{K_p}{4}\right)P_0 = 0$. With $P_0 = 2.632 \times 10^{-2}$ atm, then

$\epsilon = 0.0263$ atm and $P_{NH_3} = 2\epsilon = 0.0526$ atm $= 39.9$ torr .

6.53 The reaction:

$$CO(g) + H_2O(g) = CO_2(g) + H_2(g)$$

has $K_p = 1.374$ at 1000 K. If a mixture of CO (40%) and H_2O (60%) at 10 atm pressure is reacted at 1000 K, what will be the percent H_2 in the equilibrium mixture?

$K_p = \left(\frac{P_{H_2}P_{CO_2}}{P_{CO}P_{H_2O}}\right)$. Defining ϵ = extent of reaction,

$P_{H_2} = P_{CO_2} = \epsilon$, $P_{CO} = P_0(CO) - \epsilon = 4 - \epsilon$ and

$P_{H_2O} = P_0(H_2O) - \epsilon = 6 - \epsilon$. Then $K_p = \frac{\epsilon^2}{(6 - \epsilon)(4 - \epsilon)}$ or

$\epsilon^2 + \frac{10\ K_p}{(1 - K_p)}\epsilon - \frac{24\ K_p}{(1 - K_p)} = 0$. With $K_p = 1.374$, $\epsilon = 2.581$ atm .

The total pressure = 10 atm , so the percent $H_2 = \left(\frac{\epsilon}{10}\right) = 25.8\%$.

6.54 For the reaction

$$4\ HCl(g) + O_2(g) = 2\ Cl_2(g) + 2\ H_2O(g)$$

$K_p = 23.14\ atm^{-1}$ at 723 K. If a 4:1 (moles) mixture of HCl and oxygen is reacted at constant $P = 5$ atm, what will be the partial pressure of chlorine at equilibrium? This is the *Deacon process,* which was once used for the commercial production of chlorine.

$K_p = \frac{P_{Cl_2}{}^2 P_{H_2O}{}^2}{P_{HCl}{}^4 P_{O_2}} = 23.14\ atm^{-1}$. With extent of reaction y,

equilibrium mole fractions are: $X_{Cl_2} = X_{H_2O} = \frac{2y}{5 - y}$,

$X_{HCl} = \frac{4 - 4y}{5 - y}$, $X_{O_2} = \frac{1 - y}{5 - y}$ so that

$K_p = \left(\frac{1}{P}\right)\frac{(2y)^4(5 - y)}{(4 - 4y)^4(1 - y)} = \frac{y^4(5 - y)}{16(1 - y)^5}\left(\frac{1}{P}\right)$. With P = 5 atm,

we find y = 0.7616 so that $P_{Cl_2} = \frac{(5\ atm)(2y)}{5 - y} = 1.797$ atm .

6.55 Estimate the equilibrium constant at 800 K for the reaction:

$$Br_2(g) + Cl_2(g) = 2\ BrCl(g)$$

You may assume constant enthalpy for this calculation. This assumption is remarkably accurate in this case because the $\Delta_{rxn} C_p$ is so small (0.037 J/K). Why, based on what you learned in Chapter 5, might you have expected this?

For the reaction Br_2 (g) + Cl_2 (g) = 2 BrCl (g) , if the enthalpy of reaction is constant, then

$$\ln K_a(T_2) = \ln K_a(T_1) - \frac{\Delta_{rxn}H}{R}\left(\frac{1}{T_2} - \frac{1}{T_1}\right) .$$

$\Delta_{rxn}G(298.15) = -1.96$ kJ , $K_a(298.15) = 2.205$,

$\Delta_{rxn}H(298.15) = 29.28$ kJ and $K_a(800) = 3642$.

6.56 If hydrogen is equilibrated over solid iodine:

$$I_2(s) + H_2(g) = 2\ HI(g)$$

at 25°C and a total (constant) pressure of 3 atm, what will be the mole fraction of HI in the vapor phase?

$$K_p = \frac{(P_{HI})^2}{P_{H_2}} = \frac{P(X_{HI})^2}{X_{H_2}} .$$

Since $\Delta_{rxn}G^{\ominus} = 2\Delta_f G^{\ominus}(HI(g)) = 2.6$ kJ , then

$$K_a = \exp\left(-\frac{\Delta_{rxn}G^{\ominus}}{RT}\right) = \exp\left(-\frac{2.6 \times 10^3}{(8.3143)(298.15)}\right) = 0.35 \text{ atm} .$$

Defining ϵ = extent of reaction:

Species	Initial Moles	Final Moles	Mole Fraction
H_2	n_0	$n_0(1 - \epsilon)$	$\frac{(1 - \epsilon)}{(1 + \epsilon)}$
HI	0	$n_0 2\epsilon$	$\frac{2\epsilon}{(1 + \epsilon)}$

Then $\frac{K_p}{P} = \frac{4\epsilon^2}{1 - \epsilon^2}$. Using the approximation that $K_p = K_a$,

$0.117 = \frac{4\epsilon^2}{1 - \epsilon^2}$. The solution is $\epsilon = 0.169$ and the mole

fraction of HI in the vapor phase is $X_{HI} = \frac{2\epsilon}{(1 + \epsilon)} = 0.288$.

6.57 The reaction:

$$C(s) + 2\ H_2(g) = CH_4(g)$$

has $K_a = 1.38\ \text{atm}^{-1}$ at 800 K. Calculate the percent methane in the equilibrium mixture for final (equilibrium) pressures of 50 and 500 atm (assume ideal gas).

$$K_p = \frac{P_{CH_4}}{(P_{H_2})^2} = \frac{X_{CH_4}}{P(X_{H_2})^2} \ . \quad X_{H_2} = 1 - X_{CH_4} \text{ , so that}$$

$$K_p = \frac{X_{CH_4}}{P(1 - X_{CH_4})^2} \text{ or } X_{CH_4}{}^2 - \left(2 + \frac{1}{PK_p}\right)X_{CH_4} + 1 = 0 \ .$$

With $K_a = K_p = 1.38$ and $P = 50$ atm, $X_{CH_4} = 0.887$ or 88.7% CH_4 .

With $P = 500$ atm, $X_{CH_4} = 0.963$ or 96.3% CH_4 .

6.58 Sulfur exists in the vapor phase as either S_2 or S_8. Calculate the mole fraction of S_8 in sulfur vapor at 1000 and 1500 K when the total pressure is 3 atm.

$4\ S_2\ (g) = S_8\ (g)$ and $K_p = \frac{P_{S_8}}{(P_{S_2})^4}$. Using data from Table 6.5,

$\Delta\Phi'(1000\ K) = -466.7\ J\ K^{-1}$, $\Delta\Phi'(1500\ K) = -457.0\ J\ K^{-1}$, and

$\Delta_{rxn}H^\theta = -414.7\ kJ$. From Eq. (6.28), $K_a = \exp\left[\frac{\Delta\Phi'}{R} - \frac{\Delta_{rxn}H^\theta}{RT}\right]$, then $K_a(1000\ K) = 1.922 \times 10^{-3}$ and $K_a(1500\ K) = 3.712 \times 10^{-10}$.

Assuming ideal behavior, $K_p = K_a = \frac{X_{S_8}}{P^3(X_{S_2})^4}$. $X_{S_2} = 1 - X_{S_8}$,

so that $K_p = \frac{X_{S_8}}{P^3(1 - X_{S_8})^4}$ or $X_{S_8} = K_p P^3(1 - X_{S_8})^4$ where P = 3 atm.

Solving this by iteration, we guess $X_{S_8}^{(0)} = 0.1$, plug this into the r.h.s. and solve for $X_{S_8}^{(1)}$, etc . This gives

$X_{S_8}(1000\ K) = 4.34 \times 10^{-2} = 4.34\%$ and

$X_{S_8}(1500\ K) = 10^{-8} = 10^{-6}\ \%$.

6.59 The reaction:

$$2\ SO_2(g) + O_2(g) = 2\ SO_3(g)$$

has $K_p = 3.46\ atm^{-1}$ at 1000 K. A mixture of 10% SO_2 in air (which is initially 21% oxygen) is reacted (at constant V) with an initial total pressure of 1 atm. What percent of the SO_2 will be converted to SO_3?

$K_p = \frac{P_{SO_3}{}^2}{P_{SO_2}P_{O_2}}$. Defining ϵ = extent of reaction, $P_{SO_3} = 2\epsilon$,

$P_{O_2} = P_0(O_2) - \epsilon$ and $P_{SO_2} = P_0(SO_2) - 2\epsilon$. Since

$P_0(SO_2) = 0.10$ atm and $P_0(O_2) = 0.9(0.21) = 0.189$ atm, then

$$K_p = \frac{4\epsilon^2}{(P_0(O_2) - \epsilon)(P_0(SO_2) - 2\epsilon)^2} = \frac{4\epsilon^2}{(0.189 - \epsilon)(0.10 - 2\epsilon)^2}$$ or

$\epsilon = 2.161 \times 10^{-2}$ atm . The % conversion is then

$100\%\left(\frac{2\epsilon}{0.1\ atm}\right) = 43.2\%$.

6.60 The reaction (A = cyclopentene, B = cyclopentadiene):

$$A(g) + I_2(g) = 2\ HI(g) + B(g)$$

has $K_p = 0.30$ atm at 600 K. If an equimolar mixture of A and I_2 is reacted, and the equilibrium pressure is 2 atm, what will be the percent conversion of A to B?

$$K_p = \frac{P_{HI}{}^2 P_B}{P_A P_{I_2}} = \frac{P(X_{HI})^2 X_B}{X_A X_{I_2}}$$. Defining ϵ = extent of reaction:

Species	Moles	Mole Fraction
A	$n_0(1 - \epsilon)$	$\frac{(1 - \epsilon)}{(1 + \epsilon)}$
I_2	$n_0(1 - \epsilon)$	$\frac{(1 - \epsilon)}{(1 + \epsilon)}$
HI	$n_0 2\epsilon$	$\frac{2\epsilon}{(1 + \epsilon)}$
B	$n_0\epsilon$	$\frac{\epsilon}{(1 + \epsilon)}$

Thus $K_p = \dfrac{P4\epsilon^3}{(1 - \epsilon)^2(1 + \epsilon)}$. With P = 2 atm and $K_p = 0.30$,

$\epsilon = 0.290$ and the % conversion is 29.0% .

6.61 For the reaction of Problem 6.36, $K_p = 7.79\ \text{atm}^{-3}$ at 600 K. If a mixture of hydrogen and carbon monoxide with (initial) pressures $P_{H_2} = 4$ atm, $P_{CO} = 2$ atm, is reacted at constant V, T, calculate the partial pressure of ethylene and the total pressure in the final equilibrium mixture.

$4\ H_2\ (g) + 2\ CO\ (g) = C_2H_4\ (g) + 2\ H_2O\ (g)$. $K_p = \dfrac{P_{H_2O}{}^2 P_{C_2H_4}}{P_{H_2}{}^4 P_{CO}{}^2}$.

Draw up the following table, with ϵ = extent of reaction in atmospheres:

	H_2	CO	C_2H_4	H_2O	total
$P_{initial}$	4	2	0	0	6
P_{final}	$4 - 4\epsilon$	$2 - 2\epsilon$	ϵ	2ϵ	$6 - 3\epsilon$

$$K_p = 7.79 = \frac{4\epsilon^3}{(4 - 4\epsilon)^4(2 - 2\epsilon)^2}$$. The solution is

$\epsilon = 0.755 = P_{C_2H_4}$ corresponding to a total pressure of 3.73 atm.

6.62 The reaction:

$$2\ H_2(g) + S_2(g) = 2\ H_2S(g)$$

has $K_p = 408\ atm^{-1}$ at 1218 K. A reaction mixture with initial pressures of 2 atm for H_2 and 1 atm for S_2 is reacted at constant V. Calculate the final partial pressure of H_2S.

$$K_p = \frac{P_{H_2S}{}^2}{P_{H_2}{}^2\ P_{S_2}}$$. Defining ϵ = extent of reaction, $P_{H_2S} = 2\epsilon$,

$P_{S_2} = 1 - \epsilon$ and $P_{H_2} = 2 - 2\epsilon$. Then

$$K_p = \frac{4\epsilon^2}{(2 - 2\epsilon)^2(1 - \epsilon)} = \frac{\epsilon^2}{(1 - \epsilon)^3}$$. With $K_p = 408$, $\epsilon = 0.877$ atm

and the pressure of H_2S is $P_{H_2S} = 2\epsilon = 1.75$ atm .

6.63 Titanium metal is to be used for a high-temperature process in which coking is possible. If elemental carbon is deposited, a carbide can form:

$$C(s) + Ti(s) = TiC(s)$$

Determine whether this reaction is spontaneous at 1500 K.

$$\Phi' = \Phi^0 + \frac{(H_m^\ominus(298.15) - H_0)}{T}$$. From Table 6.4, at T = 1500 K,

Φ^0(graphite) = 17.5 J K^{-1} and $H_m^\ominus(298.15) - H_0 = 1.05$ kJ so

that Φ'(graphite) = 18.2 J K^{-1} . $\Delta_{rxn}G^\ominus = \Delta H^\ominus(298.15) - T\Delta\Phi'$.

Using data for Ti (s) and TiC (s) from Table 6.5 ,

$\Delta_{rxn}H^\ominus = -185$ kJ and $\Delta\Phi' = -11.60$ J K^{-1} , so that with

T = 1500 K , $\Delta G^\ominus = -167.6$ kJ and the reaction is spontaneous,

since $K_a = 1$ and ΔG is then equal to $\Delta G^\ominus$.

6.64 (a) Use spectroscopic data from Chapter 5 for the reaction $Br_2(g) = 2\ Br(g)$ (using $\Delta H_0^\circ = 1.901 \times 10^5$ J) to derive the equation:

$$\ln K = 0.4057 + 1.5 \ln T + \ln(1 - e^{-470/T}) - \frac{22{,}864}{T} + 2 \ln(4 + 2e^{-5302/T})$$

(b) Calculate the degree of dissociation at 1 atm, 2200 K.

a) From Eq. 5.88:

$$\phi^0 = R\left\{2.5 \ln T + 1.5 \ln M - 3.6517 - \ln(\sigma\theta_r) - \sum \ln(1 - e^{-u}) + \ln z_{elec}\right\}$$

where 2.5 ln T is replaced by 3.5 ln T for diatomics. For Br_2 (g), $\theta_v = 470$ K, $\theta_r = 0.116$ K, $\sigma = 2$ and $g_0 = 1$. Then $\phi^0(Br_2) = R\{3.5 \ln T + 5.4204 - \ln(1 - e^{-470/T})\}$. For Br (g), the rotational and vibrational partition functions are 1. From Table 5.3, $z_{elec} = 4 + 2 \exp\left(-\frac{3685.24\ hc}{kT}\right)$. Then

$$\phi^0(Br) = R\left\{2.5 \ln T + 2.9196 + \ln\left[4 + 2 \exp\left(-\frac{5302}{T}\right)\right]\right\}.$$

From Eq. (6.25),

$$\ln K_a = \frac{\Delta\phi^0}{R} - \frac{\Delta H_0^\theta}{RT} = \frac{2\phi^0(Br) - \phi^0(Br_2)}{R} - \frac{\Delta H_0^\theta}{RT}$$

$$\ln K_a = 0.4057 + 1.5 \ln T + \ln\left(1 - e^{-470/T}\right) - \frac{22864}{T} + 2 \ln\left[4 + 2\ e^{-5302/T}\right].$$

b) At T = 2200 K, $K_a = 15.94$ atm. With the approximation

$K_a \cong K_p = \frac{P_{Br}^{\ 2}}{P_{Br_2}} = \frac{PX_{Br}^{\ 2}}{X_{Br_2}}$, α is given by Eq. (6.48),

$$\alpha = \left[\frac{K_p}{4P + K_p}\right]^{1/2} = \left[\frac{15.94}{4 + 15.94}\right]^{1/2} = 0.89 \text{ or } 89\% \text{ dissociation.}$$

6.65 (a) Calculate the equilibrium constant at 623 K for the ionization of cesium vapor:

$$Cs(g) = Cs^+(g) + e^-$$

from the ionization potential of Cs (3.89405 eV) and the mass of an electron (9.1094×10^{-28} g). (*Note:* 1 eV/molecule = 96,485 J/mol; Cs has an electronic degeneracy $g_0 = 2$ while Cs^+ has $g_0 = 1$; neither has any low-lying excited states; for the electron, use $g_0 = 2$.)
(b) At 623 K, the vapor pressure of Cs is 7.8×10^{-3} atm. Calculate the number of electrons per cubic centimeter in the vapor at this temperature.

a) From Table 5.4,

$\phi^0 = R\{2.5 \ln T + 1.5 \ln M - 3.6517 + \ln z_{elec}\}$. Since

Species	M(g)	z_{elec}
Cs (g)	132.905	2
$Cs^+(g)$	132.905	1
e^-	5.486×10^{-4}	2

then with T = 623 K , $\frac{\Delta\phi^0}{R} = 1.159$. The enthalpy of the reaction is

$$\Delta H_0^\theta = \text{I.P.} = (3.89405 \text{ eV})(96487 \text{ J eV}^{-1}) = 375.73 \text{ kJ} .$$

From Eq. (6.25), $\ln K_a = \frac{\Delta\phi^0}{RT} - \frac{\Delta H_0^\theta}{RT} = -71.38$,

or $K_a = 10 \times 10^{-32}$ atm .

b) From the ideal gas approximation, $K_p = K_a = \frac{P_{Cs^+} P_{e^-}}{P_{Cs}}$

or $P_{Cs^+} = P_{e^-} = \sqrt{K_p P_{Cs}}$ With $P_{Cs} = 7.8 \times 10^{-3}$ atm ,

$P_{e^-} = 2.79 \times 10^{-17}$ atm . From the ideal gas law,

$\frac{n}{V} = \frac{P}{RT} = 5.46 \times 10^{-22}$ moles/cm^3 or $n^*(e^-) = 329$ e-/cm^3 .

6.66 The table below lists the standard free energies of formation (P° = 1 atm) of several hydrates of $MgCl_2$ at 25°C. Which hydrate will be the stable form in air at 25° if the relative humidity is 80%? (The vapor pressure of water is 23.76 torr at 25°C.)

$MgCl_2$	$\Delta_f G^\circ =$	−592.33 kJ
$MgCl_2 \cdot H_2O$		−862.36
$MgCl_2 \cdot 2H_2O$		−1118.5
$MgCl_2 \cdot 4H_2O$		−1633.8
$MgCl_2 \cdot 6H_2O$		−1278.8

$$\Delta G = \Delta G^\theta - RT \ln P = \Delta G^\theta - (8.3143)(298.15) \ln\left[\frac{(0.8)(23.76)}{(760)}\right]$$

$$\Delta G = \Delta G^\theta + 9143.35 \text{ J} .$$

Using $\Delta_f G^\theta(H_2O\ (g)) = -228.593$ kJ ,

$MgCl_2 + H_2O = MgCl_2 \cdot H_2O$	$\Delta_{rxn}G(1) = -32.30$ kJ
$MgCl_2 + 2\ H_2O = MgCl_2 \cdot 2\ H_2O$	$\Delta_{rxn}G(2) = -59.84$ kJ
$MgCl_2 + 4\ H_2O = MgCl_2 \cdot 4\ H_2O$	$\Delta_{rxn}G(3) = -117.96$ kJ
$MgCl_2 + 6\ H_2O = MgCl_2 \cdot 6\ H_2O$	$\Delta_{rxn}G(4) = 694.23$ kJ

Formation of the tetrahydrate is the most favorable thermodynamically, so that $MgCl_2 \cdot 4\ H_2O$ will be the stable form.

6.67 What would be the minimum pressure of carbon dioxide required to change calcium oxide to calcium carbonate (calcite) at 25°C?

$$CO_2\ (g) + CaO\ (s) = CaCO_3\ (s)$$

Using data from Table 6.1, $\Delta_{rxn}G^\theta = -130.40$ kJ .

$\Delta G = \Delta G^\theta - RT \ln P_{CO}$. For the reaction to proceed to the right , $\Delta G \le 0$ or $P_{CO} \ge \exp\left(\frac{\Delta G^\theta}{RT}\right) = 1.4 \times 10^{-23}$ atm .

6.68 The formation of nitrogen oxides (collectively called NO_x) in internal combustion engines that use air is a significant factor in air pollution. Ignoring other reactions, determine the partial pressure of NO in a combustion chamber at 2000 K if there is 80 atm nitrogen and 10 atm oxygen present (before reaction).

$$N_2\ (g) + O_2\ (g) = 2\ NO\ (g)$$

Using data from Table 6.4 at $T = 2000$ K , $\Delta\Phi^0 = 24.7\ J\ K^{-1}$ and

$\Delta H_0^\ominus = 179.74$ kJ . $K_a = \exp\left(\frac{\Delta\Phi^0}{R} - \frac{\Delta H_0^\ominus}{RT}\right) = 3.94 \times 10^{-4}$.

Defining ϵ = extent of reaction , $P_{NO} = 2\epsilon$, $P_{N_2} = 80 - \epsilon$ and

$P_{O_2} = 10 - \epsilon$, so that $K_p = \frac{P_{NO}{}^2}{P_{N_2}P_{O_2}} = \frac{4\epsilon^2}{(10 - \epsilon)(80 - \epsilon)}$.

Assuming ideal behavior, $K_p = K_a$ and $\epsilon = 0.276$.

$$P_{NO} = 2\epsilon = 0.55 \text{ atm} .$$

6.69 In Problem 4.27 the pressure required to convert graphite to diamond at 298 K was estimated. For kinetic reasons this process is usually carried out at a higher temperature. Estimate the pressure required at 500 K. (You may assume enthalpies and densities to be independent of *T*.)

For C (gr) = C (d) , dG = V dP so that $d(\Delta_{rxn}G^\ominus) = \Delta_{rxn}V^\ominus\ dP$

and $\Delta_{rxn}G^\ominus(P) - \Delta_{rxn}G^\ominus(P_0) = \Delta_{rxn}V^\ominus(P - P_0)$. Using data from

Problem 4.27, $V(d) = \frac{M}{\rho} = \frac{12.011\ g}{3.513\ g\ cm^{-3}} = 3.419 \times 10^{-6}\ m^3$ and

$V(gr) = 5.315 \times 10^{-6}\ m^3$. Using data from Table 6.1,

$\Delta_{rxn}G^\ominus = 2.900$ kJ and $\Delta_{rxn}H^\ominus = 1.895$ kJ . From Eq. (6.30)

$\frac{\Delta G^\ominus(T_2)}{T_2} = \frac{\Delta G^\ominus(T_1)}{T_1} - \int_{T_1}^{T_2}\left(\frac{\Delta_{rxn}H^\ominus}{T^2}\right) dT$. Assuming $\Delta_{rxn}H^\ominus$ is

constant, $\frac{\Delta G^\ominus(T)}{T} = \frac{\Delta G^\ominus(298.15)}{298.15} + \Delta_{rxn}H^\ominus(298.15)\left(\frac{1}{T} - \frac{1}{298.15}\right)$.

We may thus calculate $\Delta G^{\theta}(500\text{ K, 1 atm}) = 3.52\text{ kJ}$. For a spontaneous reaction, $\Delta G^{\theta}(P) \leq 0$. Then, if we set $\Delta G^{\theta}(P) = 0$, $P = -\dfrac{\Delta_{rxn}G^{\theta}(P_0)}{\Delta_{rxn}V^{\theta}} + P_0 = 1.83 \times 10^4$ atm .

7
Solutions

7.1 Calculate the molality of a solution having $X_2 = 0.132$ in water.

From Eq. (7.4), $m = \dfrac{1000\ X_2}{M_1(1 - X_2)} = \dfrac{1000(0.132)}{18.01(1 - 0.132)} = 8.44\ \text{kg}^{-1}$.

7.2 0.15 mole of a solute is dissolved in 300 g of CCl_4 ($M = 153.823$). Calculate (a) the mole fraction of the solute, (b) the molality.

$X_s = \dfrac{n_s}{n_s + n_{CCl_4}} = \dfrac{0.15}{\left(0.15 + \dfrac{300}{153.823}\right)} = 0.0714$. The molality is

$$m = \frac{1000\ X_s}{(153.823)(1 - X_s)} = \frac{1000(0.0714)}{(153.823)(1 - 0.0714)} = 0.500\ \text{kg}^{-1}\ .$$

7.3 Use the data in Table 7.2 for 1-molal solutions of *n*-decane in *N*-methylacetamide (M_1 = 73.09 g/mol, $V^\bullet_{m1} = 77.03\ \text{cm}^3$/mole) to calculate $\overline{V}_1$ and $\Delta_{mix}V$ for one mole of this solution.

From Eq. (7.17),

$$V = n_2{}^{\Phi}V + n_1V^\bullet_{(1\ ml)} = (1)(199.75\ \text{cm}^3) + \left(\frac{1000\ g}{73.09\ g}\right)(77.03\ \text{cm}^3)$$

$$V = 1253.66\ \text{cm}^3\ .$$

From Eq. (7.15),

$$\overline{V}_1 = \frac{V - n_2\overline{V}_2}{n_1} = \frac{1253.66 - (1)(199.5)}{\left(\dfrac{1000\ g}{73.09\ g}\right)} = 77.06\ \text{cm}^3\ .$$

Thus

$$\Delta_{mix}V = n_1(\overline{V}_1 - V^{\bullet}_{m1}) + n_2(\overline{V}_2 - V^{\bullet}_{m2})$$
$$\Delta_{mix}V = 13.68(77.06 - 77.03) + (1)(199.5 - 196.9) = 3.0 \text{ cm}^3 .$$

7.4 The partial molar volumes of water and ethanol in a solution $X_{H_2O} = 0.6$ (25°C) are 17 and 57 cm^3 mol^{-1}, respectively. Calculate the volume change on mixing sufficient ethanol with two moles of water to give this composition. Use densities (H_2O) 0.997 g/cm^3 (EtOH) 0.7893 g/cm^3.

From Eq. (7.16), $\Delta_{mix}V = n_1(\overline{V}_1 - V^{\bullet}_{m1}) + n_2(\overline{V}_2 - V^{\bullet}_{m2})$.

Designating H_2O as 1 and C_2H_5OH as 2,

$V^{\bullet}_{m1} = \left(\frac{M_1}{\rho_1}\right) = \frac{18.01}{0.997} = 18.06 \text{ cm}^3$ and $V^{\bullet}_{m2} = 58.37 \text{ cm}^3$. With

$n_1 = 2$ and $n_2 = \frac{4}{3}$, we find $\Delta_{mix}V = -3.9 \text{ cm}^3$.

7.5 When n_2 moles of NaCl are added to 1 kg of water, the volume of the solution is (in cm^3):

$$V = 1001.38 + 16.6253n_2 + 1.7738n_2^{3/2} + 0.1194n_2^2$$

Calculate the partial molar volumes of NaCl and H_2O at $m = 1.5$ and 0 (that is, at infinite dilution).

From Eq. (7.8),

$$\overline{V}_2 = \left(\frac{\partial V}{\partial n_2}\right)_{T,P,n_1} = 16.6253 + \frac{3}{2}(1.7738\ n_2^{1/2}) + 2(0.1194\ n_2) .$$

For H_2O, $\overline{V}_1 = \frac{V - n_2\overline{V}_2}{n_1}$. Also, at $m = 1.5 \text{ mol kg}^{-1}$,

$n_1 = \frac{1000 \text{ g}}{18.01 \text{ g}} = 55.5$ and $n_2 = 1.5$. Then $\overline{V}_2 = 20.2422$,

$V = 1029.8453$ and $\overline{V}_1 = 18.0087$. With $m = 0$, $n_1 = 55.5$ and

$n_2 = 0$, thus $\overline{V}_2 = 16.6253$, $V = 1001.38$ and $\overline{V}_1 = 18.0429 \text{ cm}^3$.

7.6 A solution 0.1 molal $AgNO_3$ in water is saturated with AgCl and AgBr (that is, both solids are present). How many components are in this system? How many phases (name them)? How many degrees of freedom? If *P* is fixed, can *T* vary?

a) The minimum number of pure compounds required is four: $AgNO_3$ (s), AgCl (s), AgBr (s) and H_2O (l) . Thus, the number of components is 4 .

b) There are 4 phases: AgCl (s), AgBr (s), the aqueous phase and H_2O (vap) .

c) $F = c - p + 2 = 4 - 4 + 2 = 2$. Thus , if P is fixed, T may vary .

7.7 Solid I_2 is added to a mixture of water and CCl_4 (immiscible liquids) until saturated (solid present). How many components are there? Phases (including vapor)? Degrees of freedom?

There are 3 components: I_2 (s), CCl_4 (l) and H_2O (l) .

There are 4 phases:

1) vapor - I_2 (g), H_2O (g), CCl_4 (g)

2) liquid - H_2O (l), I_2 (aq)

3) liquid - CCl_4 (l), I_2

4) solid - I_2 (s). $F = c - p + 2 = 3 - 4 + 2 = 1$

7.8 How many components and phases are there in an equilibrium mixture of:
(a) $N_2O_4(g) = 2NO_2(g)$.
(b) $COCl_2(g) = CO(g) + Cl_2(g)$ (no excess CO or Cl_2 is added).
(c) $COCl_2$, CO, and Cl_2 with arbitrary amounts of CO and Cl_2.
(d) HCl, NH_3, NH_4Cl (solid) with arbitrary amounts of the gases.

Use the definition that c is the minimum number of pure compounds from which each phase could be created:

a) c = 1 , p = 1

b) c = 1 , p = 1

c) c = 2 , p = 1

d) c = 2 , p = 2

7.9 Assume that benzene and toluene form ideal solutions. Pure benzene boils at 80°C; at that temperature, toluene has a vapor pressure of 350 torr.
(a) Calculate the partial and total pressures of a solution at 80° with X(benzene) = 0.2.
(b) What composition of solution would boil at 80°C under a reduced pressure of 500 torr?

a) From Raoult's law, $P_i = X_i P_i^\bullet$. Then

$P_b = (0.2)(760) = 152$ torr and $P_t = (0.8)(350) = 281$ torr,

and $P = P_b + P_t = 433$ torr .

b) An ideal solution which boils at P has a vapor pressure

$P = X_b P_b^\bullet + X_t P_t^\bullet = X_b P_b^\bullet + (1 - X_b) P_t^\bullet$, thus

$$X_b = \left(\frac{P - P_t^\bullet}{P_b^\bullet - P_t^\bullet}\right) = \left(\frac{500 - 350}{760 - 350}\right) = 0.366 \text{ and } X_t = 0.634 .$$

7.10 Assuming ideal solution, calculate ΔG, ΔH, and ΔS of mixing 0.25 moles of benzene with 0.5 moles of toluene at 30°C.

From Eq. (7.35),

$$\Delta_{mix}G^{id} = RT\{n_1 \ln X_1 + n_2 \ln X_2\}$$

$$\Delta_{mix}G^{id} = (8.3143 \text{ J K}^{-1})(303.15 \text{ K})\{(0.25)\ln(0.33) + (0.50)\ln(67)\}$$

$$\Delta_{mix}G^{id} = -1.20 \text{ kJ} .$$

From Eq. (7.36), $\Delta_{mix}S^{id} = -R\{n_1 \ln X_1 + n_2 \ln X_2\} = 3.97 \text{ J K}^{-1}$.

From Eq. (7.38), $\Delta_{mix}H^{id} = 0$.

7.11 At 39.9°C a solution of ethanol (X_1 = 0.9006, $P_1^•$ = 130.4 torr) and isooctane ($P_2^•$ = 43.9 torr) forms a vapor phase with Y_1 = 0.6667, P = 185.9 torr.
(a) Calculate the activity and activity coefficient of each component.
(b) Calculate the vapor pressure of this solution using Raoult's law.

a) For ethanol, $P_1 = Y_1P = (0.6667)(185.9 \text{ torr}) = 123.9 \text{ torr}$.

For iso-octane, $P_2 = Y_2P = (0.3333)(185.9 \text{ torr}) = 61.97 \text{ torr}$.

Thus $a_1 = \frac{P_1}{P_1^•} = \frac{123.9}{130.4} = 0.9502$ and $a_2 = \frac{61.97}{43.9} = 1.412$. From

Eq. (7.42), $\gamma_1 = \frac{a_1}{X_1} = \frac{0.9502}{0.9006} = 1.055$. Similarly,

$\gamma_2 = \frac{a_2}{X_2} = \frac{1.412}{0.0994} = 14.20$.

b) $P = X_1P_1^• + X_2P_2^• = 122 \text{ torr}$.

7.12 At 90°C a solution of *n*-propanol (X_2 = 0.259, $P_2^•$ = 577.5 torr) and water ($P_1^•$ = 527.76 torr) has a vapor pressure of 820.3 torr; the vapor phase is 39.7% *n*-propanol.
(a) Calculate the vapor pressures, activities, and activity coefficients of each component.
(b) What should the vapor pressure of this solution be according to Raoult's law?

a) For H_2O, $P_1 = Y_1P = (0.603)(820.3 \text{ torr}) = 494.6 \text{ torr}$. For n-propanol, $P_2 = Y_2P = (0.397)(820.3 \text{ torr}) = 325.7 \text{ torr}$. The activities are given by Eq. (7.40), $a_1 = \frac{P_1}{P_1^•} = \frac{494.6}{527.76} = 0.9372$ and $a_2 = 0.5640$. Then $\gamma_1 = \frac{P_1}{X_1P_1^•} = \frac{494.6}{(0.741)(527.76)} = 1.26$ and $\gamma_2 = 2.18$.

b) $P = X_1P_1^• + X_2P_2^• = 541 \text{ torr}$.

7.13 Ratcliff and Chao [*Can. J. Chem. Eng.*, 47, 148 (1969)] measured vapor pressures of isopropanol ($P_1^\bullet$ = 1008 torr) and *n*-decane ($P_2^\bullet$ = 48.3 torr) at 90°C.
(a) Calculate the activity coefficients of *n*-decane and isopropanol at each concentration.
(b) Make a graph of $\Delta_{mix} G^{ex}$ vs. X_2.

	n-Decane	
P/torr	X_2	Y_2
942.6	0.1312	0.0243
909.6	0.2040	0.0300
883.3	0.2714	0.0342
868.4	0.3360	0.0362
830.2	0.4425	0.0411
786.8	0.5578	0.0451
758.7	0.6036	0.0489

a) From Eq. (7.42), $\gamma_i = \dfrac{P_i}{X_i P_i^\bullet}$. From Eq. (7.33), $\gamma_i = \dfrac{Y_i P}{X_i P_i^\bullet}$.

Also, $X_1 = 1 - X_2$, $Y_1 = 1 - Y_2$ and

$\Delta_{mix}G^{ex} = RT((1 - X_2) \ln \gamma_1 + X_2 \ln \gamma_2)$. We then draw up the following table :

P	γ_1	γ_2	$\Delta_{mix}G^{ex}$
942.6	1.050	3.615	637.0
909.6	1.100	2.769	856.4
883.3	1.162	2.305	1014.6
868.4	1.250	1.937	1118.1
830.2	1.417	1.593	1208.7
786.8	1.686	1.317	1161.1
758.7	1.806	1.273	1147.3

Note: 1 = isopropanol and 2 = n-decane .

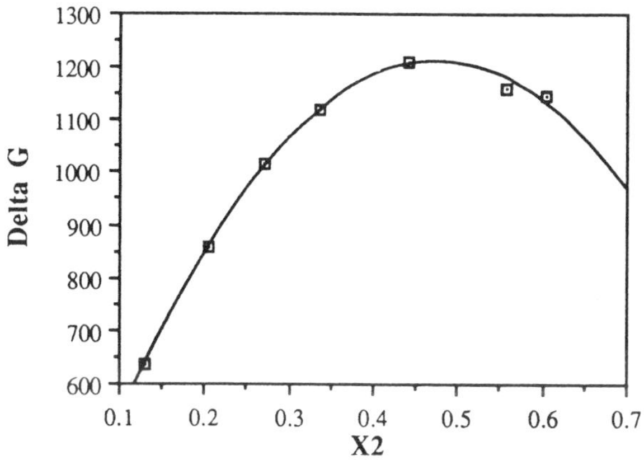

7.14 Below are given activity coefficients (25°C) for acetone (1)–chloroform (2) solutions. Do these data conform reasonably to Eq. (7.47)? If so, calculate *w*.

X_2	γ_1	γ_2
0.184	0.98	0.59
0.361	0.91	0.69
0.508	0.82	0.77
0.662	0.68	0.88

From Eq. (7.47), $w_1 = \frac{RT}{X_2^2} \ln \gamma_1$ and $w_2 = \frac{RT}{(1 - X_2)^2} \ln \gamma_2$.

Draw up the following table, with $\bar{w} = \frac{w_1 + w_2}{2} \cong w$:

X_2	w_1 (J)	w_2 (J)	$\bar{w}$ (J)
0.184	-1479	-1964	-1722
0.361	-1794	-2252	-2023
0.508	-1906	-2676	-2291
0.662	-2181	-2774	-2478

These data do not conform to Eq. (7.47) .

7.15 Use data from Table 7.3 to calculate *w* at 310 K for benzene + cyclohexane mixtures.

w(T) may be estimated as :

$$w(T) = w(T_0) + \left(\frac{\partial w}{\partial T}\right) \Delta T + \frac{1}{2}\left(\frac{\partial^2 w}{\partial T^2}\right) \Delta T^2 \text{ with } \Delta T = T - T_0 .$$

Then using the data in Table 7.3, w(310 K) = 1149 J .

7.16 Use the regular solution constants (Table 7.3) for CCl_4 + benzene to calculate ΔG, ΔS, and ΔH of mixing for a solution 4 moles CCl_4 with 6 moles of benzene at 25°C.

$$\Delta_{mix}G^{ex} = (n_c + n_b)X_cX_bw = (4 + 6)(0.4)(0.6)(324\text{ J}) = 777.6\text{ J} .$$

$$\Delta_{mix}S^{ex} = -(n_c + n_b)X_cX_b \frac{\partial w}{\partial T} = -(4 + 6)(0.4)(0.6)(-0.368\text{ J K}^{-1})$$

$$\Delta_{mix}S^{ex} = 0.883\text{ J K}^{-1} .$$

$\Delta_{mix}G^{id} = RT(n_b \ln X_b + n_c \ln X_c)$. At T = 298.15 K,

$\Delta_{mix}G^{id} = -16.68$ kJ , thus $\Delta_{mix}G = \Delta_{mix}G^{ex} + \Delta_{mix}G^{id} = -15.91$ kJ .

$\Delta_{mix}S^{id} = -R(n_b \ln X_b + n_c \ln X_c) = 55.95 \text{ J K}^{-1}$. Then

$\Delta_{mix}S = \Delta_{mix}S^{id} + \Delta_{mix}S^{ex} = 56.84 \text{ J K}^{-1}$.

$\Delta_{mix}H = \Delta_{mix}H^{ex} = \Delta_{mix}G^{ex} + T\Delta_{mix}S^{ex} = 1.036$ kJ at 298.15 K .

7.17 Derive Eqs. (7.47), (7.48), and (7.49) for a solution obeying Eq. (7.46).

Combining Eq. (7.46) for species 1 and 2,

$\mu_1 - \mu_1^{\bullet} = RT \ln X_1 + wX_2^2$ and $\mu_2 - \mu_2^{\bullet} = RT \ln X_2 + wX_1^2$, with

Eq. (6.13), $\mu_i - \mu_i^{\bullet} = RT \ln a_i = RT \ln (\gamma_i X_i)$, we have

$RT \ln (\gamma_1 X_1) = RT \ln X_1 + wX_2^2$ and $RT \ln (\gamma_2 X_2) = RT \ln X_2 + wX_1^2$.

These rearrange to Eq. (7.47), $\ln \gamma_1 = \frac{wX_2^2}{RT}$ and $\ln \gamma_2 = \frac{wX_1^2}{RT}$.

Since $\Delta_{mix}G^{ex} = RT(n_1 \ln \gamma_1 + n_2 \ln \gamma_2)$, then

$\Delta_{mix}G^{ex} = n_1 wX_2^2 + n_2 wX_1^2$. Dividing by $(n_1 + n_2)$,

$$\frac{\Delta_{mix}G^{ex}}{(n_1 + n_2)} = X_1 wX_2^2 + X_2 wX_1^2 = \frac{(n_1 + n_2)X_1X_2w}{(n_1 + n_2)} \quad \text{Thus}$$

$\Delta_{mix}G^{ex} = (n_1 + n_2)X_1X_2w$. Also,

$$\Delta_{mix}S^{ex} = -\left(\frac{\partial \Delta_{mix}G^{ex}}{\partial T}\right)_P = -(n_1 + n_2)X_1X_2\frac{\partial w}{\partial T} .$$

7.18 Use the data below for the solubility of 1-butene in benzyl alcohol at 0°C to calculate the Henry's law constant for this gas.

P_2/torr	X_2
200	0.040
400	0.087
600	0.151
700	0.193
760	0.226

The Henry's law constant is defined by $k_x = \lim_{X_2 \to 0} \left(\frac{P_2}{X_2} \right)$. Plot or regress $\frac{P_2}{X_2}$ vs. X_2 to find the intercept:

k = 5354.4 torr = 7.05 atm .

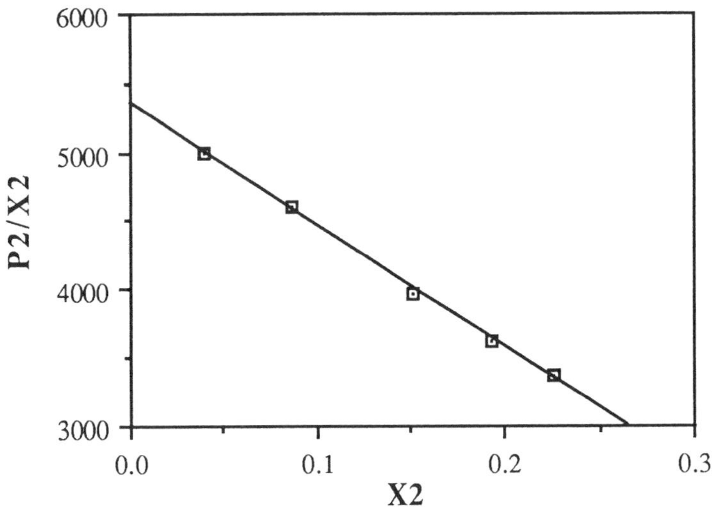

7.19 G. N. Lewis and H. Storch [*J. Am. Chem. Soc.*, 39, 2544 (1917)] measured the partial pressures of Br_2 above its solutions in CCl_4. Determine the Henry's law constant for Br_2 in CCl_4 from these data.

X_{Br_2}	P_{Br_2}/torr	X_{Br_2}	P_{Br_2}/torr
0.00394	1.52	0.0130	5.43
0.00420	1.60	0.0236	9.57
0.00599	2.39	0.0238	9.83
0.0102	4.27	0.025	10.27

From Eq. (7.51), $k_x = \lim_{X_2 \to 0} \left(\frac{P_2}{X_2} \right)$. Plot or regress

$\left(\frac{P}{X} \right)_{Br_2}$ vs. X_{Br_2} to find intercept = k = 390.9 torr = 0.514 atm .

7.20 Wood and Delaney [*J. Phys. Chem.*, 72, 4651 (1968)] measured the solubility of He in N-methylacetamide (NMA) at 1 atm and temperatures between 35° and 70°C. The results fit the equation:

$$\ln X_2 = -\frac{1152.5}{T} - 6.0579$$

Assuming ideal solution (HL), calculate ΔG° and ΔH° for one mole He(gas) → He(dilute solution in NMA) at 310 K.

μ_2 (gas) = μ_2 (soln) or

μ_2^θ (gas) + RT ln P_2 = μ_2^θ (soln) + RT ln a_2 . For an ideal solution, $a_i = X_i$, thus at P = 1 atm,

$$\Delta G^\theta (g \to s) = -RT \ln\left(\frac{X_2}{P_2}\right) = -RT \ln X_2 = -RT\left(\frac{1152.5}{T} + 6.0579\right) .$$

At T = 310 K, ΔG^θ (g → s) = 25.2 kJ .

$$\Delta H^\theta (g \to s) = \frac{\partial\left(\frac{\Delta G^\theta (g \to s)}{T}\right)}{\partial\left(\frac{1}{T}\right)} = 1152.5\ R = 9.58\ \text{kJ} .$$

7.21 The Henry's law constant (mole-fraction scale) for krypton in water is 2.00×10^4 atm at 20°C.
(a) How many grams of Kr would dissolve in 1000 g water at that temperature and P = 100 atm?
(b) How much would this solubility depress the vapor pressure of H_2O? Compare this effect to that of the applied pressure [Eq. (4.24)]. (Use $P^\bullet$ = 17.535 torr.)

a) The mole fraction of Kr is $X_2 = \frac{P_2}{k_x} = \frac{100}{2 \times 10^4} = 5 \times 10^{-3}$.

The number of moles of Kr is $n_2 = \frac{n_1 X_2}{(1 - X_2)}$. Since the number of moles of H_2O is $n_1 = \frac{1000\ \text{g}}{18.01\ \text{g mol}^{-1}} = 55.5$, then $n_2 = 0.279$. Thus n_2M_2 = 23.4 g is the amount soluble .

b) For H_2O, $P_1 = X_1P_1^\bullet$ = (0.994)(17.535) = 17.447 torr. Then

$\Delta P(\text{solubility}) = -0.09$ torr . From Eq. (4.24),

$$\ln\left(\frac{P_1}{P_1^0}\right) = \frac{V_m P_x}{RT} = \frac{(18.06\ \text{cm}^3)(100\ \text{atm})}{(82.06\ \text{cm}^3\ \text{atm}\ \text{K}^{-1})(293.15\ \text{K})}\ ,\ \text{thus}$$

$P_1 = 18.902$ torr and $\Delta P = 1.37$ torr .

7.22 If we assume an ideal dilute solution, the solvent activity $a_1(\text{RL}) = X_1$ and the solute activity (HL, mole fraction scale) $a_2(\text{HL}) = X_2$. Find the derivatives:

$$\frac{d(\ln X_1)}{dn_1} \quad \text{and} \quad \frac{d(\ln X_2)}{dn_1}$$

and prove that these conventions are consistent with the Gibbs-Duhem equation.

$X_1 = \dfrac{n_1}{n_1 + n_2}$. Since $\dfrac{d(\ln X_1)}{dn_1} = \dfrac{1}{X_1}\dfrac{dX_1}{dn_1}$ and

$$\frac{dX_1}{dn_1} = \frac{1}{n_1 + n_2} - \frac{n_1}{(n_1 + n_2)^2} = \frac{n_2}{n_1 + n_2} = X_1\ ,\ \text{then}$$

$$\frac{d(\ln X_1)}{dn_1} = \frac{X_2}{X_1}\frac{1}{(n_1 + n_2)} = \frac{n_2}{n_1(n_1 + n_2)}\ .\ \text{Similarly,}$$

$$\frac{d(\ln X_2)}{dn_1} = \frac{-1}{(n_1 + n_2)}\ .$$ The Gibbs - Duhem eq. states

$d(\ln X_2) = -\dfrac{n_1}{n_2}\, d(\ln X_1)$. We can see by inspection that the derivatives are consistent with this.

7.23 Vapor pressures of solvents containing nonvolatile solutes can be measured by bubbling dry nitrogen through the solution. If the exiting gas is saturated with solvent vapor, the vapor pressure can be calculated from the weight loss. 23.50 dm^3 of dry N_2 (P = 760.0 torr) is bubbled through an aqueous solution; the solution loses 0.5312 g. Calculate the vapor pressure of the water. (The outlet pressure also was 760.0 torr.)

From the ideal gas law, $P_{H_2O} = \dfrac{n_{H_2O}RT}{V} = \dfrac{n_{H_2O}RT}{V_{N_2} + V_{H_2O}}$. Using

$$n_{H_2O} = \frac{0.5312\ \text{g}}{18.01\ \text{g mol}^{-1}} = 2.95 \times 10^{-3}\ \text{mol},\ T = 298\ \text{K},$$

$$V_{N_2} = 23.50\ \text{dm}^3 \text{ and } V_{H_2O} = \frac{n_{H_2O}RT}{(1\ \text{atm})} = 0.72\ \text{dm}^3\ ,\ \text{then}$$

$$P_{H_2O} = 2.98 \times 10^{-2}\ \text{atm} = 22.6\ \text{torr}\ .$$

7.24 Q. Craft and R. H. Wood [*J. Solution Chem.*, 6, 525 (1977)] measured osmotic coefficients of N-methylacetamide in solution with *n*-nonane by freezing-point depression. The results were fitted by least squares to give:

$$\phi = 1 - 0.5035m + 0.2364m^2 - 0.1206m^3$$

Use this to calculate the activity coefficients of *n*-nonane at 0.01, 0.1, and 0.5 molal.

From Eq. (7.58), $\ln \gamma_{2m} = (\phi - 1) + \int_0^m \frac{\phi - 1}{m'}\,dm'$. Using ϕ of the problem statement and

$\frac{\phi - 1}{m} = -0.5035 + 0.2364\ m - 0.1206\ m^2$, we integrate to

find $\ln \gamma_{2m} = -2(0.5035)m + \frac{3}{2}(0.2364)m^2 - \frac{4}{3}(0.1206)m^3$. Then:

m	γ_{2m}
0.01	0.990
0.1	0.907
0.5	0.647

7.25 Calculate the freezing-point constant K_f for *n*-octane (C_8H_{18}) (use data from Table 4.2).

From Eq. (7.62),

$$K_f = \left[\frac{M_1R(T_f^{\bullet})^2}{1000\ \Delta_f H}\right] = \frac{(114.23\ \text{g})(8.3145\ \text{J K}^{-1})(216.36\ \text{K})^2}{1000\ \text{g/kg}(20.74 \times 10^3\ \text{J})}$$

$$K_f = 2.144\ \text{kg K}\ .$$

7.26 Use the data below for freezing point depression by *n*-decane in N-methylacetamide [Craft and Wood, *J. Solution Chem.*, 6, 525 (1977)] to determine the activity coefficient of *n*-decane when $m = 0.5$ mol/kg.

m	θ	m	θ
0.1753	0.9127	0.4069	1.8677
0.1742	0.9077	0.5699	2.3951
0.2708	1.3387	0.5633	2.3754
0.2697	1.3294		

Draw up the following table:

m	θ	$\Phi = \left(\frac{\theta}{K_f m}\right)$	$\frac{(\Phi - 1)}{m}$
0.1753	0.9127	0.902	-0.559
0.1742	0.9077	0.903	-0.557
0.2708	1.3387	0.857	-0.528
0.2697	1.3294	0.854	-0.541
0.4069	1.8677	0.796	-0.501
0.5699	2.3951	0.728	-0.477
0.5633	2.3754	0.731	-0.478

Regressing $\frac{(\Phi - 1)}{m}$ vs. m , we find

$\frac{(\Phi - 1)}{m} = a + bm = -0.591 + 0.205\ m$ so that, with

$\ln (\gamma_{2m}) = 2\ am + 1.5\ bm^2$ we have:

$\ln (\gamma_{2m}) = -1.183\ m + 0.3075\ m^2$. With m = 0.5 mol kg^{-1}:

$\ln (\gamma_{2m}) = -0.515$ and $\gamma_{2m} = 0.598$.

7.27 Show that the osmotic coefficient is related to the osmotic pressure as:

$$\phi = \frac{n_1 \overline{V}_1 \Pi}{n_2 RT}$$

From Eq. (7.65), $\ln a_1 = -\frac{\Pi \overline{V}_1}{RT}$, and from Eq. (7.57a),

$\Phi = -\frac{n_1}{n_2} \ln a_1$ or $\ln a_1 = -\frac{n_2}{n_1} \Phi$. Combining the two equations,

$$\Phi = \frac{n_1 \Pi \overline{V}_1}{n_2 RT} .$$

7.28 Use Eq. (7.66) to calculate the osmotic pressure of 0.20 moles/dm^3 solution of sucrose in water at 20°. The observed value is 5.06 atm.

From Eq. (7.66),

$$\Pi \cong cRT = (0.20 \text{ mol dm}^{-3})(293.15 \text{ K})R = 4.81 \text{ atm} .$$

7.29 Twenty milligrams of a protein is dissolved in 10 g water. The osmotic pressure at 25°C was 0.30 torr. Calculate the molecular weight, assuming ideal dilute solution.

Rearrange Eq. (7.66) to

$$n_2 = \frac{\Pi V}{RT} = \frac{(3.95 \times 10^{-4} \text{ atm})(0.01 \text{ dm}^3)}{(0.08206 \text{ dm}^3 \text{ atm K}^{-1})(298.15 \text{ K})} = 1.614 \times 10^{-7} \text{ mol} .$$

Then $M = \frac{m}{n_2} = \frac{20 \times 10^{-3} \text{ g}}{1.614 \times 10^{-7} \text{ mol}} = 1.24 \times 10^5 \text{ g mol}^{-1}$.

7.30 P. J. Flory [*J. Am. Chem. Soc.*, 65, 372 (1943)] reported the following osmotic pressure data for solutions of polyisobutylene at 25°C.

Concentration (g/dm^3)	Π (Pa, in C_6H_{12})	Π (Pa, in C_6H_6)
20.0	1187	210.3
15.0	667	150.4
10.0	306	100.5
7.5	176	
5.0	92	49.5
2.5	35	

Calculate the average molecular weight and second virial coefficients.

$\frac{\Pi}{cRT} = \frac{1}{\overline{M}} + Bc$. Plot or regress $\frac{\Pi}{cRT}$ vs. c for both C_6H_{12} and C_6H_6 to find:

$B(C_6H_{12}) = 1.06 \times 10^{-3}$ m^3/kg^2 $\quad\overline{M}(C_6H_{12}) = 463$ kg

$B(C_6H_6) = 1.47 \times 10^{-5}$ m^3/kg^2 $\quad\overline{M}(C_6H_6) = 256$ kg

The average molecular weight is $\overline{M}$(avg) = 360 kg .

7.31 If a pipe with a selective membrane on the end were inserted into the sea to a sufficient depth, the hydrostatic pressure of the water could cause reverse osmosis so that fresh water would flow into the pipe. Sea water has an osmotic pressure of 23 atm and a density of 1.03 g/cm^3. Estimate the depth below which the hydrostatic pressure of water would exceed the osmotic pressure; you may assume uniform density, temperature and salinity.

The hydrostatic pressure is simply the pressure exerted by a column of water of a specific height h: $P = \rho g h$.

$$\frac{23 \text{ atm}}{9.869 \times 10^{-6} \text{ N m}^{-2} \text{ atm}^{-1}} = (1030 \text{ kg m}^{-3})(9.8 \text{ m s}^{-2}) \text{ h}$$

Solving for h: h = 231 meters .

7.32 D'Orazio and Wood [*J. Phys. Chem.*, 67, 1435 (1963)] measured the solubility of hydrazoic acid (HN_3) in water as a function of $P(HN_3)$ and T. Use these results to calculate ΔG°, ΔS°, and ΔH° for $HN_3(g) \rightarrow HN_3(aq)$ at 24.42°C.

0°C		24.42°C		49.46°C	
$m(HN_3)$	$P(HN_3)$	m	P	m	P
1.807	33.3 torr	1.651	101.0	1.397	228.0
0.9473	16.8	0.9020	55.6	0.8187	134.8
0.3964	7.0	0.3922	24.5	0.3848	64.9
0.1023	1.8	0.1019	6.3	0.1008	17.7

According to Eq. (7.53), $K_m = \lim_{m \to 0} \left(\frac{P}{m}\right)$. Regressing $\frac{P}{m}$ vs. m, we find

$$\text{intercept} = K_m(0^\circ\text{C}) = 0.02413 \text{ atm kg}$$

$$K_m(24.42^\circ\text{C}) = 0.08190 \text{ atm kg}$$

$$K_m(49.46^\circ\text{C}) = 0.2290 \text{ atm kg}$$

Since $\Delta G^\theta = RT \ln K_m$, $\Delta G^\theta(0^\circ C) = -8.46$ kJ ,

$\Delta G^\theta(24.42^\circ C) = -6.19$ kJ and $\Delta G^\theta(49.46^\circ C) = -3.95$ kJ .

$\frac{\partial \Delta G}{\partial T} = -\Delta S$, thus at 24.42°C,

$$-\Delta S \cong \left(\frac{-3.95 + 8.46}{49.46}\right) 1000 = 91.2 \text{ J K}^{-1} . \quad \text{Also,} \quad \frac{\partial\left(\frac{\Delta G}{T}\right)}{\partial\left(\frac{1}{T}\right)} = \Delta H ,$$

so at 24.42°C , $\Delta H \cong \left(\dfrac{\dfrac{-3.95}{322.6} + \dfrac{8.46}{273.15}}{\dfrac{1}{322.6} - \dfrac{1}{273.15}} \right) = -33.4\ \text{kJ}$.

7.33 Bromine has a standard free energy of formation of 1.51 kJ/mol in CCl_4; in *n*-perfluoroheptane (npfh) it is −7.5 kJ/mol (both HL, mole fraction scale, 25°C). Assuming ideal solution, estimate the distribution constant: $X(Br_2 \text{ in npfh})/X(Br_2 \text{ in } CCl_4)$.

For the process $Br_2\ (CCl_4) \rightarrow Br_2\ (\text{npfh})$: $\Delta_{rxn}G = -9.01\ \text{kJ mol}^{-1}$.

$$K_a = \exp\left(-\frac{\Delta_{rxn}G}{RT}\right) .$$

$$K_a = \frac{a(Br_2 \text{ in npfh})}{a(Br_2 \text{ in } CCl_4)} \approx \frac{X(Br_2 \text{ in npfh})}{X(Br_2 \text{ in } CCl_4)}$$

$$K_a \approx \exp\left(\frac{9.01 \times 10^3\ \text{J mol}^{-1}}{(8.3143\ \text{J K}^{-1}\text{mol}^{-1})(298\ \text{K})}\right) = 37.9 .$$

7.34 Use data from Table 7.11 to estimate the solubility of H_2S in water at 25°C, 1 atm; assume ideal solution and neglect hydrolysis.

The process is: $H_2S\ (g) = H_2S\ (aq)$. For the solute in its standard state at 25°C, $\Delta_{rxn}G^{\ominus} = 5.60\ \text{kJ mol}^{-1}$.

The equilibrium constant is: $K_a = \dfrac{a(H_2S,\ aq)}{a(H_2S,\ g)} \approx \dfrac{m(H_2S,\ aq)}{\left(\dfrac{P(H_2S,\ g)}{P^{\ominus}}\right)}$.

Given $P(H_2S,\ g) = 1$ atm; from Table 7.11, $P^{\ominus} = 1$ atm .

$$K_a = \exp\left(-\frac{\Delta_{rxn}G}{RT}\right) = 0.104 \text{ and } K_a \sim m(H_2S,aq) = 0.104\ \text{mol kg}^{-1} .$$

7.35 For the equilibrium:

$$Br_2(\text{liquid}) = Br_2(\text{aq})$$

$\Delta H^\circ = -2.59$ kJ, $\Delta G^\circ = 3.93$ kJ at 25°C. Estimate the solubility of bromine in water at 25°C and 0°C. (Assume ideal solution; neglect hydrolysis.)

At 25°C, $\Delta G^\theta = 3.93$ kJ and $\Delta H^\theta = -2.59$ kJ:

$$K_a = \frac{a(Br_2,\ aq,\ 25°C)}{a(Br_2,\ liq,\ 25°C)} \approx m(Br_2,\ aq,\ 25°C)$$

$$m(Br_2,\ aq,\ 25°C) \approx K_a = \exp\left(-\frac{\Delta_{rxn}G^\theta}{RT}\right) = 0.205\ \text{mol kg}^{-1}\ .$$

At 0°C:

$$\ln K_a(0°C) = \ln K_a(25°C) + \frac{\Delta_{rxn}H^\theta}{R}\left(\frac{1}{298.15\ K} - \frac{1}{273.15\ K}\right) = -1.489$$

and $m(BR_2,\ aq,\ 0°C) \approx K_a = 0.226\ \text{mol kg}^{-1}$.

7.36 Calculate $\Delta_f G^\circ(aq)$ for H_2S in water at 25°C from the gas solubility data below:

$m(H_2S)$	P_{H_2S}/atm
0.050	0.486
0.101	0.992
0.150	1.474
0.204	2.049
0.254	2.514

From Eq. (7.71), $\Delta_f G^\theta(aq) = \Delta_f G^\theta(g) + RT \ln k_m$ where $k_m = \lim_{m \to 0}\left(\frac{P_{H_2S}}{m}\right)$. From Table 6.1 , for H_2S at 25°C, $\Delta_f G^\theta(g) = -33.56$ kJ . Regressing $\frac{P_{H_2S}}{m}$ vs. m , we find: intercept = $k_m = 9.689$ atm kg . At T = 298.15 K,

$$\Delta_f G^\theta(aq)\ -27.93\ \text{kJ}\ .$$

7.37 Use the data below (at 25°C) to calculate $\Delta_f G^\circ$ of Br_2 in CCl_4 (solute standard state, molal scale):

Molality	P_{Br_2}/torr
0.0257	1.52
0.0392	2.39
0.0670	4.27
0.0856	5.43

From Eq. (7.71), $\Delta_f G^\ominus(\text{soln}) = \Delta_f G^\ominus(g) + RT \ln k_m$. For Br_2 (g) at 298.15 K, from Table 6.1, $\Delta_f G^\ominus(g) = 3.11$ kJ. By definition, $k_m = \lim_{m \to 0} \left(\frac{P_{Br_2}}{m} \right)$. Regressing $\frac{P_{Br_2}}{m}$ vs. m, we find intercept = $k_m = 7.597 \times 10^{-2}$ atm kg. Thus

$$\Delta_f G^\ominus(\text{soln}) = -3.28 \text{ kJ} .$$

7.38 Glycine forms a saturated solution in water (25°C) at $m = 3.3$. At that concentration $\gamma_{2m} = 0.872$. Calculate the $\Delta_f G^\circ$ of glycine(aq) from that of the pure substance (Table 7.11). Compare your answer to that given in the table.

$$\Delta_f G^\ominus(aq) = \Delta_f G^\ominus(s) - RT \ln a_{sat} = \Delta_f G^\ominus(s) - RT \ln(m\gamma_{2m})$$

$$\Delta_f G^\ominus(aq) = -370.7 \text{ kJ} - (8.3143 \text{ J K}^{-1})(298.15 \text{ K}) \ln\{(3.3)(0.872)\}$$

$$\Delta_f G^\ominus(aq) = -373.3 \text{ kJ} .$$

7.39 The standard free energy of formation of L-serine (solid) is -508.8 kJ/mole at 25°C. This compound forms a saturated solution in water at 4.02 moles kg^{-1}, at which concentration $\gamma_m = 0.602$. Calculate $\Delta_f G^\circ$(aq).

$$\Delta_f G^\ominus(aq) = \Delta_f G^\ominus(s) - RT \ln a_{sat} = \Delta_f G^\ominus(s) - RT \ln(m\gamma_{2m})$$

$$\Delta_f G^\ominus(aq) = -508.8 \text{ kJ} - (8.3143 \text{ J K}^{-1})(298.15 \text{ K}) \ln\{(4.02)(0.602)\}$$

$$\Delta_f G^\ominus(aq) = -511.0 \text{ kJ} .$$

7.40 Use the data below for the distribution of H_3BO_3 between H_2O and amyl alcohol to calculate the thermodynamic K_a (water/alcohol) for the distribution equilibrium.

moles/dm^3 in H_2O	moles/dm^3 in alcohol
0.02602	0.00805
0.05140	0.01545

For H_3BO_3 distributed between H_2O and amyl alcohol,

$$K' = \frac{C(H_2O)}{C(\text{alcohol})} .$$

$C(H_2O)$	$C(\text{alcohol})$	k'
0.02602	0.00805	3.232
0.05140	0.01545	3.327

For both alcohol and water , extrapolate to C = 0 . Then

$$K_a = \lim_{C \to 0} (K') = 3.13 .$$

7.41 Amino acids can polymerize through the formation of peptide bonds:

$$RCOOH + R'NH_2 \longrightarrow R{-}\overset{\overset{\displaystyle O}{\|}}{C}{-}\overset{\overset{\displaystyle H}{|}}{N}{-}R' + H_2O$$

These form the primary structure of proteins. Calculate the concentration of the alanine-glycine dimer at equilibrium in water if alanine and glycine were initially at $0.1m$; assume ideal solution.

$$\text{ALA (aq)} + \text{GLY (aq)} = \text{DL (aq)} + H_2O\ (l)$$

Using data from Table 7.11, $\Delta_{rxn}G^{\ominus} = 27.75$ kJ . Then

$K_a = \exp\left(-\dfrac{\Delta_{rxn}G^{\ominus}}{RT}\right) = 1.37 \times 10^{-5}$. Assuming ideal solution behavior, $K_a = K_c = \dfrac{[DL]}{[ALA][GLY]}$. Defining an extent of reaction, x, in molality units, then $K_c = \dfrac{x}{(0.1 - x)^2}$ or

$$x^2 - \left(0.2 - \frac{1}{K_c}\right)x + 0.01 = 0 \ . \quad \text{With } K_c = 1.374 \times 10^{-5} \ ,$$

$$[DL] = x = 1.37 \times 10^{-7} \ m \ .$$

7.42 The freezing points (the temperature at which the first solid appears) of various Pb/Sn alloys are listed below. The eutectic temperature is 182°C. The Pb-rich solid in equilibrium with the eutectic liquid was analyzed and found to be a solid solution, 25% Sn in Pb. The Sn-rich solid was 5% Pb in Sn. Draw the phase diagram.

Wt % Pb	T_f	Wt % Pb	T_f
0	232°C	50	216°C
10	212°C	70	236°C
20	197°C	80	254°C
30	190°C	90	280°C
40	182°C	100	327°C

The phase diagram will be analogous to Fig. 7.19c:

α = solid solution = 25% Sn in Pb
β = solid solution = 5% Pb in Sn

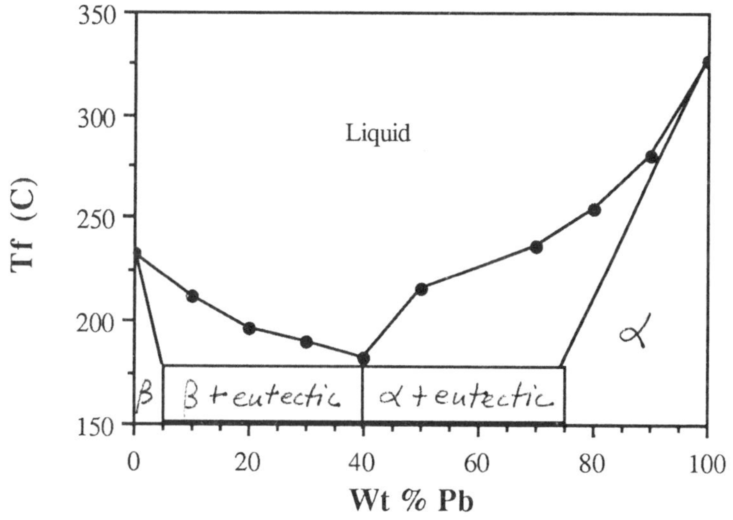

7.43 For the phase diagram below, label all areas. For the vertical dotted lines, describe the cooling history of a sample with that composition, naming the phases, their composition and the degrees of freedom for each area the line crosses.

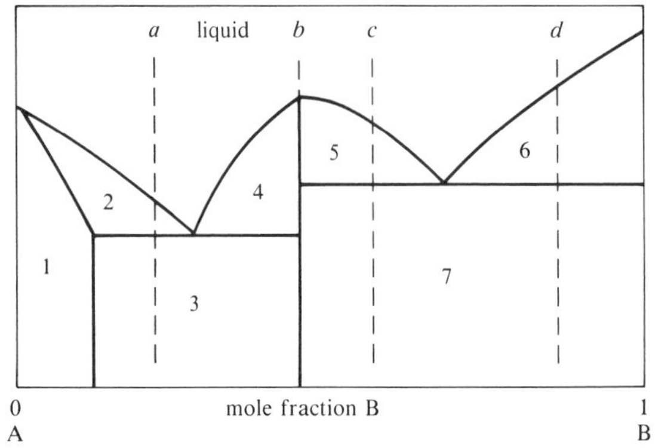

Areas are as follows:

1. Solid solution (α)

2. Liquid (L) + α

3. α + compound (C)

4. L + C

5. L + C

6. L + B

7. B + C

Cooling histories (degrees of freedom):

a. L (3) → L + α (2) → C + α (3)

b. L (3) → C (2)

c. L (3) → L + C (3) → C + B (2)

d. L (3) → L + B (2) → C + B (2)

7.44 For the phase diagram below, label all areas. For the vertical dotted lines, describe the cooling history of a sample with that composition, naming the phases, their composition and the degrees of freedom for each area the line crosses.

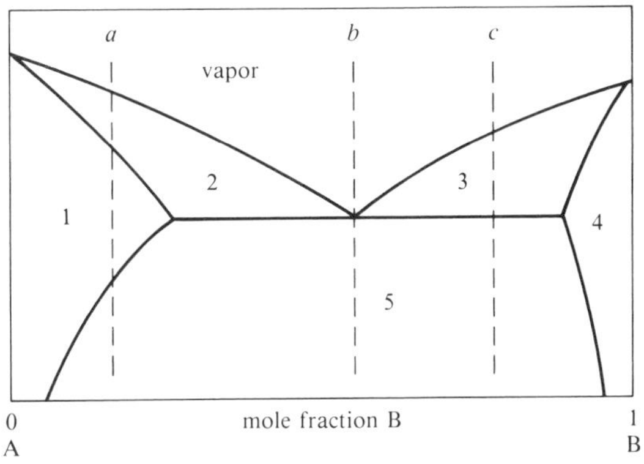

Areas are as follows:

1. A-rich solution (α)

2. α + vapor

3. B-rich solution (β) + vapor

4. β

5. Immisible solutions α + β

Cooling histories (degrees of freedom):

a. vapor (3) → α + vapor (2) → α + β (2)

b. vapor (3) → α + β (2)

c. vapor (3) → vapor + β (2) → α + β (2)

7.45 For the phase diagram below, label all areas. For the vertical dotted lines, describe the cooling history of a sample with that composition, naming the phases, their composition and the degrees of freedom for each area the line crosses.

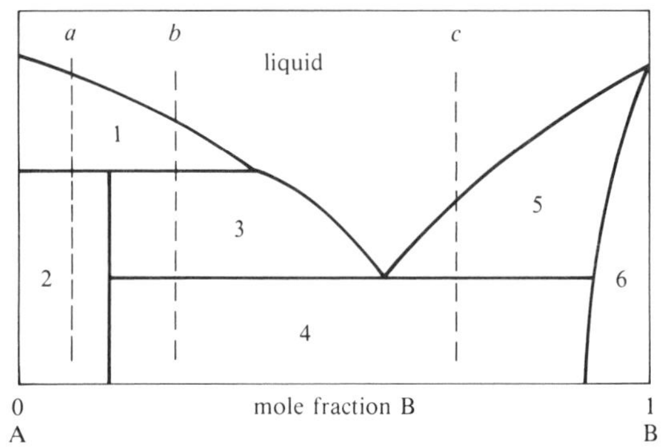

Areas are as follows:

1. L + A (s)

2. A (s) + Compound (C)

3. L + C

4. C + β

5. L + solid solution (β)

6. C + β

Cooling histories (degrees of freedom):

a. L (3) → A + L (2) → A + C (2)

b. L (3) → A + L (2) → C + L (3) → C + β (3)

c. L (3) → L + β (2) → C + β (3)

8
Ionic Solutions

8.1 A 0.01-molal solution of a weak acid in water depresses the freezing point of water by 0.0208 K. Calculate the percent ionization of this acid (assume ideal solution for all species present).

$$i = \frac{\theta}{K_f m} = \frac{0.0208}{(1.860)(0.1)} = 1.1183 \; .$$ The degree of dissociation is $$\alpha = \frac{(i - 1)}{(\nu - 1)} = \frac{(1.1183 - 1)}{(2 - 1)} = 0.1183 = 12\% \; .$$

8.2 Scatchard, Prentiss, and Jones [*J. Am. Chem. Soc.*, 56, 805 (1934)] measured freezing-point depressions of $KClO_4$ in H_2O. Use these data to calculate $\gamma_\pm$ at 0.001, 0.01, and 0.05 molal. (The concentrations given are low enough that it can be assumed that j/m vs. $1/\sqrt{m}$ is linear with reasonable accuracy.)

m	θ
0.003612	0.01316
0.006690	0.02421
0.009872	0.03509
0.016215	0.05712
0.030369	0.10541
0.048335	0.16359

From Eq. (8.8), $\phi \cong \frac{\theta}{\nu K_f m}$. Also, $j = 1 - \phi$ and $\frac{j}{m} \cong \frac{a}{\sqrt{m}} + b$. With $K_f = 1.860$, we have

ϕ	$\frac{j}{m}$	$\frac{1}{\sqrt{m}}$
0.97941	5.7004	16.639
0.97251	4.1079	12.224
0.95551	4.5067	10.065
0.94695	3.2717	7.8531
0.93306	2.2042	5.7383
0.90981	1.8659	4.5485

From least squares analysis a = 0.3124 and b = 0.6380 . From

Eq. (8.11), $\ln \gamma_\pm \cong -3a\sqrt{m} - 2\,bm$. Thus at $m = 0.001$, $\gamma_\pm = 0.970$. At $m = 0.01$, $\gamma_\pm = 0.899$ and at $m = 0.05$, $\gamma_\pm = 0.761$.

8.3 Use data in Table 8.1 to calculate the mean ionic activities ($a_\pm$) for 0.5-molal solutions of (a) KCl, (b) HCl, (c) $CuSO_4$, and (d) $Cr(NO_3)_3$.

From Eq. (8.6), $a_\pm^\nu = (m_+^{\nu_+}\, m_-^{\nu_-})\gamma_\pm^\nu$.

a) For KCl: $m_+ = m_- = m$, $\nu_+ = \nu_- = 1$, $\nu = 2$. Then

$a_\pm = m\gamma_\pm = (0.5)(0.649) = 0.325$.

b) For HCl: $m_+ = m_- = m$, $\nu_+ = \nu_- = 1$, $\nu = 2$. Then

$a_\pm = m\gamma_\pm = (0.5)(0.757) = 0.379$.

c) For $CuSO_4$: $m_+ = m_- = m$, $\nu_+ = \nu_- = 1$, $\nu = 2$. Then

$a_\pm = m\gamma_\pm = (0.5)(0.068) = 0.034$.

d) For $Cr(NO_3)_3$: $m_+ = m$, $m_- = 3m$, $\nu_+ = 1$, $\nu_- = 3$, $\nu = 4$.

Then $a_\pm = (27)^{1/4} m\gamma_\pm = (27)^{1/4}(0.5)(0.291) = 0.332$.

8.4 Calculate the ionic strength of a solution containing: 0.1m KNO_3, 0.15m K_2SO_4, and 0.023m $La_2(SO_4)_3$.

From Eq. (8.12), $I = \frac{1}{2} \sum_i (z_i)^2 m_i$. For KNO_3 ,

$I_1 = \frac{1}{2}(1)^2(0.1) + \frac{1}{2}(1)^2(0.1) = 0.1 \text{ mol kg}^{-1}$. For K_2SO_4 ,

$I_2 = \frac{1}{2}(1)^2[(2)(0.15)] + \frac{1}{2}(2)^2(0.15) = 0.45 \text{ mol kg}^{-1}$.

For $La_2(SO_4)_3$,

$I_3 = \frac{1}{2}(3)^2[(2)(0.023)] + \frac{1}{2}(2)^2[(3)(0.023)] = 0.345 \text{ mol kg}^{-1}$.

Then $I = I_1 + I_2 + I_3 = 0.895 \text{ mol kg}^{-1}$.

8.5 Use the Debye-Hückel theory to calculate the "distance of closest approach" from the experimental activity coefficients of KCl (Table 8.1). Note that the ionic radii from crystallography are 1.33 Å for K^+ and 1.81 Å for Cl^-.

Rearranging Eq. (8.13), $a_0 = -\frac{1}{B\sqrt{I}}\left[\frac{\alpha|z_+z_-|\sqrt{I}}{\ln \gamma_\pm} + 1\right]$. Using data for m(KCl) = 0.001, 0.005 and 0.01, and constants for H_2O at 25°C from Table 8.2, $a_0(\text{Å}) = -\frac{1}{0.329\sqrt{I}}\left[\frac{1.177\sqrt{I}}{\ln \gamma_\pm} + 1\right]$.

Then

m = I	$\gamma_\pm$	a_0 (Å)
0.001	0.9648	3.716
0.005	0.927	4.210
0.01	0.901	3.921

Then $\bar{a}_0 = 4$ Å .

8.6 Wood, Wicker, and Kreis [*J. Phys. Chem.*, **75**, 2313 (1971)] determined activity coefficients of $NaNO_3$ in N-methylacetamide. Plot these results vs. $\sqrt{I}$ to see if they fit the Debye-Hückel limiting law. For this solvent $\alpha = 0.32531$ [calculated with Eq. (8.14a)].

m	$\gamma_\pm$
0.01	0.970
0.05	0.937
0.10	0.915
0.20	0.886
0.30	0.864

The Debye - Hückel limiting law is $\ln \gamma_\pm = \alpha|z_+z_-|\sqrt{I}$. If we plot $\ln \gamma_\pm$ vs. $\sqrt{I} = \sqrt{m}$, the plot is linear , showing that the data fit the Debye - Hückel limiting law. The slope is

$$-\alpha = -0.2568 .$$

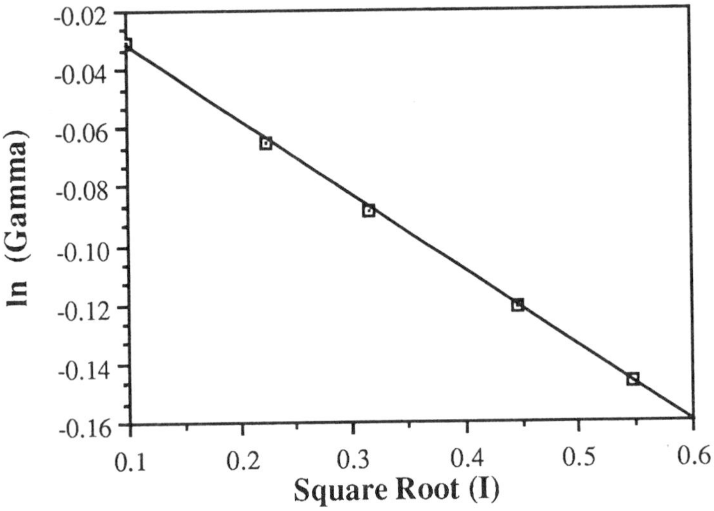

8.7 (a) Use data for $\gamma_\pm$ of HCl at 0.05 mol/kg (Table 8.1) to estimate the DHG β for this acid at 25°C.
(b) Use this β to calculate $\gamma_\pm$ from 0.01 to 0.5 mol/kg and compare the results to experimental.

a) For HCl, $z_+ = z_- = 1$ and $\nu_+ = \nu_- = 1$. Thus Eq. (8.15) reduces to $\ln \gamma_\pm = -\dfrac{\alpha \sqrt{m}}{1 + \sqrt{m}} + 2\,\beta m$. At 25°C, $\alpha = 1.177$ and at $m = 0.05$, $\gamma_\pm = 0.830$. Then

$$\ln(0.830) = -\frac{1.177\,\sqrt{0.05}}{1 + \sqrt{0.05}} + 2\,\beta(0.05) \quad \text{or } \beta = 0.288.$$

b) $\gamma_\pm = \exp\left[-\dfrac{1.177\,\sqrt{m}}{1 + \sqrt{m}} + 2(0.288)m\right]$. Thus for the m's given in Table 8.1:

m	$\gamma_\pm$ (calc.)	$\gamma_\pm$ (Table 8.1)
0.01	0.9037	0.904
0.02	0.8743	0.875
0.05	0.8300	0.830
0.1	0.7984	0.796
0.2	0.7800	0.767
0.5	0.8191	0.757

8.8 Use the DHG equation to calculate the mean ionic activity coefficient at 25°C of $CuSO_4$ at 0.001, 0.1, and 1 mol/kg. Compare your answers to the experimental values given as Table 8.1.

For $CuSO_4$, $z_+ = z_- = 2$, $\sqrt{I} = 2\sqrt{m}$, $\nu_+ = \nu_- = 1$ and $\alpha = 1.177$. We assume $\beta = 0$, thus Eq. (8.15) reduces to $\ln \gamma_\pm = -\dfrac{\alpha 4(2\sqrt{m})}{(1 + 2\sqrt{m})}$.

Then

m	$\gamma_\pm$ (calc.)	$\gamma_\pm$ (Table 8.1)
0.001	0.76	0.74
0.1	0.16	0.16
1.0	0.043	0.047

8.9 (a) The van't Hoff osmotic factor gives, for the freezing-point depression, $\theta = iK_f m$. Use the Debye-Hückel limiting law for a 1:1 electrolyte, $\ln \gamma_\pm = -\alpha\sqrt{m}$, to derive (to the same approximation):

$$i = \nu(1 - 0.378\sqrt{m})$$

(b) Calculate the freezing point of a 0.5-molal KCl solution; the observed value is 271.49.

a) From Eq. (8.10), to a first approximation, $j \cong c\sqrt{m}$ where c = constant . Using Eq. (8.9), with $\ln \gamma_\pm = -\alpha\sqrt{m}$,

$\alpha\sqrt{m} = c\sqrt{m} + \int \frac{c\sqrt{m}}{m}\, dm$ or $\alpha\sqrt{m} = c\sqrt{m} + 2\, c\sqrt{m} = 3\, c\sqrt{m}$. Thus

$c = \frac{\alpha}{3}$ and $j = \frac{\alpha\sqrt{m}}{3}$. From Eq. (8.8),

$\theta \cong \nu(1 - j)K_f m = \nu\left(1 - \frac{\alpha\sqrt{m}}{3}\right)$. Using $\theta = iK_f m$,

then $i = \nu\left(1 - \frac{\alpha\sqrt{m}}{3}\right) = \nu(1 - 0.378\sqrt{m})$.

b) Starting with $\theta = \nu(1 - 0.378\sqrt{m})K_f m$,

$\theta = 2(1 - 0.378\sqrt{0.5})(1.86)(0.5) = 1.363$. Since $\theta = T_f^0 - T_f$,

$1.363°C = 0°C - T_f$ or $T_f = -1.363°C = 271.79$ K .

8.10 TlCl has a solubility of 1.42×10^{-2} mol/kg in water at 25°C.
(a) Calculate K_a.
(b) Estimate the solubility of TlCl in 0.1-molal $NaNO_3$.
(c) Estimate the solubility of TlCl in 0.1-molal NaCl.

a) $K_a = (m_+^{\nu_+} m_-^{\nu_-})(\gamma_+^{\nu_+}\gamma_-^{\nu_-}) = s^2(\gamma_\pm)^\nu$. For a 1:1 electrolyte

$\ln \gamma_\pm = \frac{-\alpha\sqrt{m}}{1 + \sqrt{m}}$. Under equilibrium conditions (25°C, H_2O),

$m = S = 1.42 \times 10^{-2}$, thus

$$\gamma_\pm = \exp\left[-\frac{1.177\sqrt{1.42 \times 10^{-2}}}{1 + \sqrt{1.42 \times 10^{-2}}}\right] = 0.882 .$$

Then $K_a = 1.57 \times 10^{-4}$.

b) In this case, $I = S + I_{NaNO_3} = S + 0.1$. Using the ideal solubility, $I = 0.1142$. Then $\ln \gamma_{\pm} = -\frac{1.177\sqrt{0.1142}}{1 + \sqrt{0.1142}} = 0.743$. From part a), $K_a = 1.57 \times 10^{-4}$, thus $S = \frac{\sqrt{K_a}}{\gamma_{\pm}} = 1.69 \times 10^{-2}$.

c) For an ideal solution, $S = \frac{K_a}{0.1} = 0.00157$. Then $I = S + 0.1 = 0.10157$, $\gamma_{\pm} = \exp\left[-\frac{\alpha\sqrt{I}}{1 + \sqrt{I}}\right] = 0.752$ and $K_{sp} = \frac{K_a}{(\gamma_{\pm})^2} = 2.77 \times 10^{-4}$. S is then

$$S = \frac{K_{sp}}{(0.1 + S)} = 2.70 \times 10^{-3} .$$

8.11 The thermodynamic solubility product (K_a) of Ag_2CrO_4 is 2.0×10^{-7} at 25°C. Calculate the solubility of this salt in a solution with 0.1 moles $AgNO_3$/kg (a) assuming ideal solutions and (b) more accurately.

a) $K_{sp} \cong (0.1)^2 s$. For an ideal solution, $K_{sp} = K_a$. Then

$$S = \frac{K_a}{0.01} = \frac{2.0 \times 10^{-7}}{0.01} = 2.0 \times 10^{-5} .$$

b) $I = \frac{1}{2}(1)^2 2S + \frac{1}{2}(2)^2 S = 3S$. If $AgNO_3$ completely dissociates, $I = 0.1 + 3S$. If $3S >> 1$, $I \cong 0.1$. From Eq. (8.15), $\gamma_{\pm} = 0.568$. Since $K_{sp} = \frac{K_a}{(\gamma_{\pm})^3}$, then $K_{sp} = 1.09 \times 10^{-6}$. We then have $S = \frac{K_{sp}}{0.01} = 1.1 \times 10^{-4}$.

8.12 MgF_2 has $K_{sp} = 6.4 \times 10^{-9}$ (in water at 25°C).
(a) Calculate the solubility.
(b) Estimate the thermodynamic solubility product (K_a) from K_{sp}.
(c) Use this K_a to estimate the standard free energy of formation of MgF_2(s).

a) $K_{sp} = (S)(2S)^2 = 4S^3$ or $S = \left(\frac{K_{sp}}{4}\right)^{1/3} = 1.2 \times 10^{-3}$ mol kg^{-1} .

b) $K_a = K_{sp}\gamma_\pm^\nu$ where for MgF_2 , $\nu = 3$, and

$\ln \gamma_\pm = -\dfrac{1.177(2)\sqrt{I}}{1 + \sqrt{I}}$. Since

$I = \frac{1}{2}(1)^2 2S + \frac{1}{2}(2)^2 S = 3S = 3.51 \times 10^{-3}$, $\gamma_\pm = 0.877$ and

$$K_a = (6.4 \times 10^{-9})(0.877)^3 = 4.3 \times 10^{-9} .$$

c) For the reaction MgF_2 (s) = Mg^{2+} (aq) + 2 F^- (aq):

$$\Delta_{rxn}G^\theta = \Delta_f G^\theta(Mg^{2+}(aq)) + 2\Delta_f G^\theta(F^-(aq)) - \Delta_f G^\theta(MgF_2(s))$$

Using $\Delta_{rxn}G^\theta = -RT \ln K_a = 47.76$ kJ , $\Delta_f G^\theta(F^-(aq)) = -278.79$ kJ

and $\Delta_f G^\theta(Mg^{2+}(aq)) = -454.8$ kJ , we find

$$\Delta_f G^\theta(MgF_2(s)) = -1060.14 \text{ kJ} .$$

8.13 (a) Use data from Tables 6.1 and 8.4 to calculate K_a for the solubility of CaF_2 in water at 25°C. (b) Estimate the solubility of this salt in water at this temperature.

a) For the reaction $CaF_2\,(s) = Ca^{2+}\,(aq) + 2\,F^-\,(aq)$:

$\Delta_{rxn}G^{\Theta} = 56.14$ kJ so that $\ln K_a(298.15) = -22.65$ and

$$K_a\,(298.15) = 1.46 \times 10^{-10}\ .$$

b) If the solubility is S, then: $K_a = \gamma_\pm^3(S)(2S)^2 = 4S^3\gamma_\pm^3$.

Assume $\gamma_\pm \sim 1$, so that: $S \sim 3.3175 \times 10^{-4}$ mol kg^{-1} and

$I = 3S = 9.953 \times 10^{-4}$ kg . Then:

$$\ln \gamma_\pm = -\frac{1.177(2)\sqrt{I}}{1 + \sqrt{I}} = -0.07169 \text{ and } \gamma_\pm = 0.931\ .$$

$$\frac{K_a}{\gamma_\pm^{\ 3}} = 1.811 \times 10^{-10}\ . \quad S = 3.56 \times 10^{-4} \text{ mol kg}^{-1}\ .$$

8.14 Estimate the molality of HCl in water for a solution for which pH = 2.00.

As a first approximation we take $a_{H^+} = m = 10^{-2}$. Then using Eq. (8.15) for HCl in H_2O,

$$\ln \gamma_\pm = \left[-\frac{1.177\sqrt{0.01}}{1 + \sqrt{0.01}}\right] + \left[2\left\{\frac{2}{2}\right\} 0.27(0.1)\right] \text{ or } \gamma_\pm = 0.903\ .$$

Since $a_{H^+} = [H^+]\gamma_\pm$, $m = [H^+] = \dfrac{a_{H^+}}{\gamma_\pm} = \dfrac{0.01}{0.903} = 1.11 \times 10^{-2}$.

Substituting back into Eq. (8.15) to get a new $\gamma_\pm$, $\gamma_\pm = 0.899$

which gives $m = 1.11 \times 10^{-2}$ mol/kg .

8.15 Dichloroacetic acid has an acid dissociation constant $K_a = 3.32 \times 10^{-2}$. Calculate the degree of dissociation and pH of a 0.01-mol/kg solution (a) for an ideal solution, (b) using the DHG formula for $\gamma_\pm$ ($\beta = 0$).

a) For the equilibrium $HA = H^+ + A^-$, $[H^+] = [A^-] = \alpha m_0$ and $[HA] = m_0(1 - \alpha)$. Assuming an ideal solution,

$$K_a' = \frac{[H^+][A^-]}{[HA]} = \frac{\alpha^2 m_0^2}{m_0(1 - \alpha)} = \frac{\alpha^2 m_0}{1 - \alpha}$$. Substituting in,

$$3.32 \times 10^{-2} = \frac{\alpha^2(0.01)}{1 - \alpha}$$. The solution is $\alpha = 0.805$. Thus for an ideal solution, $pH = -\log_{10}[H^+] = 2.09$.

b) Using the DHG eq. with $B = 0$ and $I = m \cong 0.01$,

$$\ln \gamma_\pm = -\frac{1.177\sqrt{0.01}}{1 + \sqrt{0.01}}$$ or $\gamma_\pm = 0.899$. Then

$$K_a' = \frac{K_a}{(\gamma_\pm)^2} = \frac{3.32 \times 10^{-2}}{(0.899)^2} = 4.11 \times 10^{-2}$$. Since $K_a' = \frac{\alpha^2 m_0}{1 - \alpha}$,

$$4.11 \times 10^{-2} = \frac{\alpha^2(0.01)}{1 - \alpha}$$. The solution is $\alpha = 0.832$

and $pH = -\log_{10}(\alpha m_0 \gamma_\pm) = 2.13$.

8.16 Calculate the degree of dissociation of chloroacetic acid ($K_a = 1.38 \times 10^{-3}$ at 25°C) when it is in solution at 0.1 mol/kg with 0.05 mol/kg HCl (a) using ideal solution and (b) using DHG ($\beta = 0$).

a) $$K_a' = K_a = 1.38 \times 10^{-3} = \frac{[H^+][A^-]}{[HA]} = \frac{[0.1\alpha + 0.05][0.1\alpha]}{0.1(1 - \alpha)}$$.

This has the solution $\alpha = 0.0256$ or 2.6% .

b) Using $I \cong 0.05$ in the DHG eq., $\ln \gamma_{\pm} = -\dfrac{1.177\sqrt{0.05}}{1 + \sqrt{0.05}}$ or

$\gamma_{\pm} = 0.807$. $K_a' = \dfrac{K_a}{(\gamma_{\pm})^2} = \dfrac{1.38 \times 10^{-3}}{(0.807)^2} = 2.12 \times 10^{-2}$. From

part a) , $K_a = 1.38 \times 10^{-3} = \dfrac{[0.1\alpha + 0.05][0.1\alpha]}{0.1(1 - \alpha)}$,

thus $\alpha = 0.0378$ or 3.8% .

8.17 Use data in Table 8.4 to estimate the solubility of PbI_2 in water at 25°C (use DHG, $\beta = 0$).

For the reaction $PbI_2\,(s) = Pb^{2+}\,(aq) + 2\,I^-\,(aq)$:

$\Delta_{rxn}G^{\theta}(298.15) = 46.07$ kJ . Thus

$$K_a = \exp\left(-\frac{\Delta_{rxn}G^{\theta}}{RT}\right) = 8.49 \times 10^{-9} = 4\gamma_{\pm}^3 s^3 \text{ and}$$

$\ln \gamma_{\pm} = -\dfrac{1.177(2)\sqrt{I}}{1 + \sqrt{I}}$. Assuming that $K_a = K_{sp}$:

$I = 3\left(\dfrac{K_a}{4}\right)^{1/3} = 3.86 \times 10^{-3}$ mol kg^{-1} , $\ln \gamma_{\pm} = -0.1377$ and

$\gamma_{\pm} = 0.8714$. Using this value:

$S = \dfrac{1}{\gamma_{\pm}}\left(\dfrac{K_a}{4}\right)^{1/3} = 1.47 \times 10^{-3}$ mol kg^{-1} . A second iteration

gives $S = 1.48 \times 10^{-3}$ mol kg^{-1} .

8.18 Repeat the calculation of the previous problem for 100°C.

For the reaction PbI_2 (s) = Pb^{2+} (aq) + 2 I^- (aq):

$\Delta_{rxn}G(298.15) = 46.07$ kJ and $\Delta_{rxn}H(298.15) = 63.40$ kJ .

$$\ln K_a(373.15\ K) = \ln K_a(298.15\ K) - \frac{\Delta_{rxn}H}{R}\left(\frac{1}{373.15} - \frac{1}{298.15}\right)$$

$$\ln K_a(373.15\ K) = -13.44$$

$K_a = 1.45 \times 10^{-6}$. Using the procedure of the previous problem with the new value for K_a we find:

$I = 2.14 \times 10^{-2}$ mol kg^{-1} , $\gamma_\pm = 0.7405$ and

$S = 0.9629 \times 10^{-2}$ mol kg^{-1} . A second iteration gives:

$I = 0.02888$, $\gamma_\pm = 0.7104$ and $S = 1.00 \times 10^{-2}$ mol kg^{-1} .

8.19 Calculate the ratio of I_3^-/I^- ions in a saturated solution of iodine in water at 25°C. Assume ideal solution for neutral species and DHG ($\beta = 0$) for ions.

For the reaction I_2 (s) = I_2 (aq):

$\Delta_{rxn}G^\ominus(298.15) = 16.4$ kJ , so that $K_a(298.15) = 1.34 \times 10^{-3}$.

For the reaction I_2 (aq) + I^- (aq) = I_3^- (aq):

$\Delta_{rxn}G^\ominus(298.15) = -16.23$ kJ so that $K_a(298.15) = 6.97 \times 10^2$.

For the first reaction:

$$K_a = \frac{a(I_2,\ aq)}{a(I_2,\ s)} \approx m(I_2,\ aq) = [I_2] .$$

For the second reaction:

$$K_a = \frac{a(I_3^-, aq)}{a(I^-, aq)a(I_2, aq)} \approx \frac{m(I_3^-, aq)}{m(I^-, aq)m(I_2, aq)} = \frac{[I_3^-]}{[I_2][I^-]} .$$

Therefore : $\dfrac{[I_3^-]}{[I^-]} = 697(1.34 \times 10^{-3}) = 0.934$.

8.20 (a) Calculate the equilibrium constant at 25°C for the reaction:

$$I_2(aq) + I^-(aq) = I_3^-(aq)$$

(b) Solid iodine is added to a solution 0.01 mol/kg I^- until it is saturated (solid present). Calculate the molality of all species present.
(c) How many moles of iodine (per kg water) will dissolve? (Assume ideal solution for neutral species and DHG, $\beta = 0$, for ions.)

a) For the reaction I_2 (aq) + I^- (aq) = I_3^- (aq):

$\Delta_{rxn}G^{\theta}(298.15) = -16.23$ kJ , so that $K_a(298.15) = 697$.

b) The overall reaction is: I_2 (s) + I^- (aq) = I_3^- (aq)

with $\Delta_{rxn}G^{\theta}(298.15) = 0.17$ kJ and $K_a(298.15) = 0.934$. With an extent of reaction ϵ: $K_a = \dfrac{\epsilon}{(0.01 - \epsilon)} = \dfrac{[I_3^-]}{[I^-]}$ Thus

$\epsilon = [I_3^-] = 4.83 \times 10^{-3}$ mol kg^{-1} and

$$(0.01 - \epsilon) = [I^-] = 5.17 \times 10^{-3} \text{ mol kg}^{-1} .$$

For the reaction I_2 (s) = I_2 (aq):

$$K_a(298.15) = [I_2] = 1.34 \times 10^{-3} \text{ mol kg}^{-1} .$$

c) The total I_2 (s) dissolved is

$$1.34 \times 10^{-3} + 4.83 \times 10^{-3} = 6.16 \times 10^{-3} \text{ mol kg}^{-1} .$$

8.21 Calculate the equilibrium constant for the ionization of methanol in water:

$$CH_3OH(aq) = CH_3O^- + H^+$$

(a) at 25°C; (b) at 0°C.

For the reaction $CH_3OH\ (aq) = CH_3O^-\ (aq) + H^+\ (aq)$:

$\Delta_{rxn}G^\theta(298.15) = 104.41$ kJ and $\Delta_{rxn}H^\theta(298.15) = 52.46$ kJ ,

so that $K_a(298.15) = 5.10 \times 10^{-19}$.

$$\ln K_a(273.15) = \ln K_a(298.15) - \frac{\Delta_{rxn}H}{R}\left(\frac{1}{273.15} - \frac{1}{298.15}\right) .$$

Thus : $\ln K_a(273.15) = -44.06$ and $K_a(273.15) = 7.35 \times 10^{-20}$.

8.22 (a) Calculate the ionization constant at 25°C for

$$H_2S(aq) = H^+(aq) + HS^-(aq)$$

(b) Estimate the pH of a solution 0.01 mol/kg of H_2S in water at 25°C (use DHG, $\beta = 0$, for ions, ideal for neutrals).

a) For the reaction $H_2S\ (aq) = H^+\ (aq) + HS^-\ (aq)$:

$\Delta_{rxn}G^\theta(298.15) = 39.91$ kJ , so that $K_a(298.15) = 1.02 \times 10^{-7}$.

b) Assuming an ideal solution, with degree of dissociation α:

$$K_a = \frac{[H^+][HS^-]}{[H_2S]} = \frac{\alpha^2 m_0}{1 - \alpha}$$ with $m_0 = 0.01$ and $\alpha = 3.19 \times 10^{-3}$.

Thus, $[H^+] \sim \alpha m_0 = 3.19 \times 10^{-5}$ and

$pH = -\log[a_{H^+}] \sim -\log[H^+] = 4.50$.

8.23 (a) Calculate the equilibrium constant for the solubility of AgSCN in water at 25°C.
(b) Calculate the solubility of AgSCN at this temperature.
(c) Estimate the solubility of AgSCN at 25°C in water that contains 0.004 mol/kg $NaNO_3$.

a) For the reaction AgSCN (s) = Ag^+ (aq) + SCN^- (aq):

$\Delta_{rxn}G^\theta(298.15) = 68.43$ kJ , so that $K_a(298.15) = 1.03 \times 10^{-12}$.

b) $K_a = \gamma_\pm^2 S^2$. Assuming an ionic strength $I = \sqrt{K_a}$ or

$I = 1.014 \times 10^{-6}$ we calculate: $\ln \gamma_\pm = \dfrac{-1.177\sqrt{I}}{1 + \sqrt{I}} = -1.184 \times 10^{-3}$

and $\gamma_\pm = 0.999$, so that $S = \dfrac{\sqrt{K_a}}{\gamma_\pm} = 1.015 \times 10^{-6}$ mol kg^{-1} .

c) The ionic strength changes to $I \cong 0.004$ so that $\gamma_\pm = 0.932$

and $S = 1.088 \times 10^{-6}$ mol kg^{-1} .

8.24 Estimate the solubility of AgCN in water at (a) 25°C and (b) 50°C.

a) For the reaction AgCN (s) = Ag^+ (aq) + CN^- (aq):

$\Delta_{rxn}G^\theta(298.15) = 92.61$ kJ and $\Delta_{rxn}H^\theta(298.15) = 110.179$ kJ ,

so that $K_a(298.15) = 5.96 \times 10^{-17}$. Assuming $\gamma_\pm \sim 1$:

$S = \sqrt{K_a} = 7.72 \times 10^{-9}$ mol kg^{-1} .

b) $\ln K_a(323.15) = \ln K_a(298.15) - \dfrac{\Delta_{rxn}H}{R}\left(\dfrac{1}{323.15} - \dfrac{1}{298.15}\right)$

so that $K_a(323.15) = 1.86 \times 10^{-15}$

and $S = \sqrt{K_a} = 4.31 \times 10^{-8}$ mol kg^{-1} .

8.25 (a) Calculate the equilibrium constant for the hydrolysis of methyl amine in water at 25°C:

$$CH_3NH_2(aq) + H_2O(liq) = CH_3NH_3^+ + OH^-$$

(b) Estimate the concentration of OH^- ion in a 0.05 mol/kg solution of methyl amine in water at 25°C. Neglect ionization of water and assume ideal solution for all neutral species.

a) For the hydrolysis of methylamine:

$\Delta_{rxn}G^\theta(298.15) = 19.255$ kJ , so that $K_a(298.15) = 4.23 \times 10^{-4}$.

b) With degree of dissociation α :

$$K_a = \frac{\gamma_\pm^2[CH_3NH_3^+][OH^-]}{[CH_3NH_2]} \sim \frac{\alpha^2 m_0}{1-\alpha} .$$ With $m_0 = 0.05$:

$\alpha = 8.785 \times 10^{-2}$, $I \sim m_0\alpha = 4.39 \times 10^{-3}$ mol kg^{-1} and

$\ln \gamma_\pm = \frac{-1.177\sqrt{I}}{1 + \sqrt{I}} = -0.07314$, so that $\gamma_\pm = 0.9295$. Using

$\frac{K_a}{\gamma_\pm^2} = \frac{\alpha^2 m_0}{1-\alpha}$, we find $\alpha = 0.0942$ and

$$m_0\alpha = [OH^-] = 4.71 \times 10^{-3} \text{ mol kg}^{-1} .$$

8.26 Calculate the degree of ionization of formic acid (HCOOH) at (a) 25°C and (b) 100°C.

a) For the reaction HCOOH (l) = $HCOO^-$ (aq) + H^+ (aq):

$\Delta_{rxn}G^\theta(298.15) = 21.3$ kJ and $\Delta_{rxn}H^\theta(298.15) = -0.12$ kJ , so that $K_a(298.15) = 1.855 \times 10^{-4}$. With degree of dissociation α:

$K_a \sim \frac{\alpha^2 m_0}{1-\alpha}$. With $m_0 = 0.025$, we find $\alpha = 0.0825$ and

$I \sim m_0\alpha = 2.06 \times 10^{-3}$ mol kg^{-1} . $\ln \gamma_\pm = \frac{-1.177\sqrt{I}}{1 + \sqrt{I}} = -0.05113$

and $\gamma_\pm = 0.9502$. Now with $\frac{K_a}{\gamma_+^2} = \frac{\alpha^2 m_0}{1-\alpha}$, we find $\alpha = 0.0867$.

b) At 100°C:

$$\ln K_a(373.15) = \ln K_a(298.15) - \frac{\Delta_{rxn}H}{R}\left(\frac{1}{373.15} - \frac{1}{298.15}\right) .$$

Thus: $\ln K_a(373.15) = -8.602$ and $K_a(373.15) = 1.837 \times 10^{-4}$.

Using the procedure of part a) with DH constant = 1.372, we find: $I \sim 2.05 \times 10^{-3}$, $\gamma_{\pm} = 0.942$ and $\alpha = 0.0869$.

8.27 (a) Calculate the equilibrium constants at 25°C for the solubility of carbon dioxide in water:

$$CO_2(g) = CO_2(aq)$$

(b) for the hydrolysis of carbon dioxide:

$$CO_2(aq) + H_2O(liq) = H^+(aq) + HCO_3^-(aq)$$

(c) Calculate the pH of a solution saturated in CO_2 at a constant $P(CO_2) = 0.1$ MPa. Assume ideal gas and ideal solution for neutrals.

a) For the reaction $CO_2\ (g) = CO_2\ (aq)$:

$\Delta_{rxn}G^{\theta}(298.15) = 8.379$ kJ , so that

$$K_a(298.15) = \frac{a(CO_2,\ aq)}{a(CO_2,\ g)} \approx \frac{m(CO_2)}{\left(\frac{P_{CO_2}}{P^{\theta}}\right)} .\quad \text{Since } P = P^{\theta} ,$$

$$K_a = a(CO_2) \approx m(CO_2) = 0.034 .$$

b) For the reaction $CO_2\ (aq) + H_2O\ (l) = H^+\ (aq) + HCO_3^-\ (aq)$:

$\Delta_{rxn}G^{\theta}(298.15) = 36.34$ kJ , so that

$$K_a(298.15) = 4.30 \times 10^{-7} = \frac{a_+a_-}{a_{CO_2}} .$$

c) Assume $a_+ = a_-$ so $a_+ = \sqrt{(4.3 \times 10^{-7})(0.034)} = 1.21 \times 10^{-4}$.

$$pH = -\log a_+ = 3.917 .$$

8.28 (a) Use data in Table 8.4 to calculate the equilibrium constant at 25°C for:

$$Fe^{2+}(aq) + Cu^{2+} = Fe^{3+}(aq) + Cu^{+}(aq)$$

(b) Estimate the molality of Cu^{+} in a solution with (initially) 0.001 mol/kg Fe^{2+} and 0.001 mol/kg Cu^{2+}(assume ideal solution and neglect other possible reactions).

a) For the reaction:

$$Fe^{2+}\ (aq) + Cu^{2+}\ (aq) = Fe^{3+}\ (aq) + Cu^{+}\ (aq)$$

$\Delta_{rxn}G^{\theta}(298.15) = 58.69$ kJ , so that $K_a(298.15) = 5.22 \times 10^{-11}$.

b) Assuming ideal solutions with an extent of reaction ϵ:

$K_a = \dfrac{\epsilon^2}{(0.001 - \epsilon)^2}$. As $\epsilon \to 0$, $K_a = 10^6\epsilon^2$. The solution is

$$\epsilon = 7.2 \times 10^{-9} \text{ mol kg}^{-1} .$$

8.29 In their famous book, Lewis and Randall (1923) tell of a "distinguished chemist" who attempted to measure the hydrolysis of nitrogen in water:

$$N_2(g) + 2\ H_2O(liq) = NH_4^+(aq) + NO^{2-}(aq)$$

With a simple calculation, they calculated that, to achieve a "minimum detectable" concentration of 0.001 mol/kg for the ions, the pressure of nitrogen would need to be impossibly high. Repeat this calculation using $\Delta_f G^{\circ}(NO_2^-, aq) = 51.31$ kJ/mol, and other data as needed.

For the hydrolysis of N_2: $\Delta_{rxn}G^{\theta}(298.15) = 446.26$ kJ, so that

$K_a = 6.57 \times 10^{-79}$. $K_a = \dfrac{a_{NO_2^-}a_{NH_4^+}}{a_{N_2}} \sim \dfrac{(0.001)^2}{\left(\dfrac{P_{N_2}}{P^{\theta}}\right)}$. The

solution is $P_{N_2} = 1.5 \times 10^{72}$ atm .

8.30 Show that Henry's law for a gas such as HCl that ionizes in solution should be written:

$$k_m = \lim_{m \to 0} \left(\frac{P}{m^2 P^{\ominus}} \right)$$

Henry's law states $k = \lim_{m \to 0} \left(\frac{P}{mP^{\theta}} \right)$. With $m = \frac{a}{\gamma}$, $k = \lim_{m \to 0} \left(\frac{\gamma P}{aP^{\theta}} \right)$.

For HCl , $a = m^2 \gamma_{\pm}^2$. Also $\lim_{m \to 0} \gamma_{\pm} = \lim_{m \to 0} \gamma = 1$,

so that $k = \lim_{m \to 0} \left(\frac{P}{m^2 P^{\theta}} \right)$.

8.31 Calculate the resistance (25°) of a conductivity cell with plates 1.2 cm apart and plate area 7.2 cm^2, if it is filled with a 0.1-mol/dm^3 solution of NaCl.

From Eq. (8.32), $\kappa = \frac{1}{AR}$ where κ is given by Eq. (8.36),

$\Lambda = \frac{1000\ \kappa}{\tilde{c}}$. In our case , $\tilde{c} = \nu_i |z_i| c = 0.1$ M . Then

$\kappa = \frac{\Lambda(0.1)}{1000} = \frac{(106.4)(0.1)}{1000} = 1.067 \times 10^{-2}\ \Omega^{-1}\ cm^{-1}$ and

$$R = \frac{1.2}{(7.2)(1.607 \times 10^{-2})} = 15.6\ \Omega\ .$$

8.32 The cell of Problem 8.31 was used to measure the concentration of a $Ca(NO_3)_2$ solution. The measured resistance was 13 Ω. Assuming $\Lambda = \Lambda°$, calculate the concentration of this salt.

$\kappa = \frac{1}{AR} = \frac{1.2}{(7.2)(13)} = 1.282 \times 10^{-2}\ \Omega^{-1}\ cm^{-1}$. The equivalent conductivity of $Ca(NO_3)_2$ is:

$$\Lambda^{\circ}_{Ca(NO_3)_2} = \lambda^{\circ}_{\frac{1}{2}Ca^{2+}} + \lambda^{\circ}_{NO_3^-} = 59.50 + 71.44 = 130.94\ cm^2\ S\ .$$

$\tilde{c} = \frac{1000\ \kappa}{\Lambda^{\circ}} = 9.79 \times 10^{-2}\ mol\ dm^3$. For $Ca(NO_3)_2$,

$\tilde{c} = \nu_i |z_i| c = 2c$ so that: $c = \frac{1}{2}\tilde{c} = 4.90 \times 10^{-2}\ mol\ dm^{-3}$.

8.33 Calculate the equivalent conductivity and cation transference number of the following at infinite dilution: (a) rubidium acetate, (b) ammonium sulphate, (c) $K_3Fe(CN)_6$.

a) Using data from Table 8.7 at 25°C,

$\Lambda^\circ_{RbAc} = \lambda^\circ_{Rb^+} + \lambda^\circ_{Ac^-} = 118.7\ cm^2\ S$. The cation transferance number is $\lambda_+ = t_+\Lambda$. At infinite dilution $\Lambda = \Lambda^\circ$, thus

$$t_+ = \frac{\lambda^\circ_+}{\Lambda^\circ} = \frac{77.8}{118.7} = 0.66\ .$$

b) For $(NH_4)_2SO_4$, $\Lambda^\circ = \lambda^\circ_{NH_4^+} + \lambda^\circ_{\frac{1}{2}SO_4^{2-}} = 153.4\ cm^2\ S$ and

$$t_+ = \frac{73.4}{153.4} = 0.48\ .$$

c) For $K_3Fe(CN)_6$, $\Lambda^\circ = \lambda^\circ_{K^+} + \lambda^\circ_{\frac{1}{3}Fe(CN)_6^{3-}} = 172.6\ cm^2\ S$ and

$$t_+ = \frac{73.5}{172.6} = 0.43\ .$$

8.34 Use data in this chapter to calculate the mobility of K^+ for (a) infinite dilution, (b) 0.1 mol/kg KCl, (c) 0.1 mol/kg KNO_3.

a) From Eq. (8.39), $u_i = \frac{\lambda_i}{\mathcal{F}}$ At infinite dilution, we take $\lambda^\circ_{K^+}$ from Table 8.7 and $u^\circ_{K^+} = \frac{73.50\ cm^2\ S}{96487\ C} = 7.618 \times 10^{-4}\ cm^2\ V^{-1}\ s^{-1}$.

b) Using the value of Λ from Table 8.6, $\Lambda = 128.96\ cm^2\ S$. From Eq. (8.39) and Table 8.5,

$\lambda_{K^+} = t_{K^+}\Lambda = (0.4898)(128.96) = 63.165\ cm^2\ S$ and

$$u_{K^+} = \frac{\lambda_{K^+}}{\mathcal{F}} = \frac{63.165}{96487} = 6.547 \times 10^{-4}\ cm^2\ V^{-1}\ s^{-1}\ .$$

c) For 0.1 m KNO_3 , $\Lambda = \lambda_{K^+} + \lambda_{NO_3^-} = 120.40\ cm^2\ S$.

$\lambda_{K^+} = (0.5103)(120.40) = 61.440 \text{ cm}^2 \text{ S}$ and

$$u_{K^+} = \frac{\lambda_{K^+}}{\mathcal{F}} = \frac{61.440}{96487} = 6.368 \times 10^{-4} \text{ cm}^2 \text{ V}^{-1} \text{ s}^{-1} .$$

8.35 The equivalent conductances in ethanol (25°) are:

$$\Lambda°(LiCl) = 39.2$$

$$\Lambda°(NaCl) = 42.5$$

$$\Lambda°(LiI) = 43.4$$

Calculate $\Lambda°$ for NaI in this solvent.

Since $\Lambda^\circ_{NaCl} - \Lambda^\circ_{LiCl} + \Lambda^\circ_{LiI} = \lambda^\circ_{Na^+} + \lambda^\circ_{I^-} = \Lambda^\circ_{NaI}$, then

$$\Lambda^\circ_{NaI} = 42.5 - 39.2 + 43.4 = 46.7 \text{ cm}^2 \text{ S}.$$

8.36 The data below give values for the equivalent conductivity of NaBr in methanol at 25°C. Determine $\Lambda°$ for this salt in methanol.

$10^4 c$	Λ
1	99.19
2	98.11
5	96.04
10	93.80
20	90.86

(Plot data; do not use linear regression.)

From Eq. (8.42), $\Lambda \cong \Lambda° + k\sqrt{\tilde{c}}$. For NaBr, $c = \tilde{c}$, thus a plot of Λ vs. $\sqrt{\tilde{c}}$ should have y-intercept = $\Lambda°$. From the graph, $\Lambda° = 101.50 \text{ cm}^2 \text{ S}$.

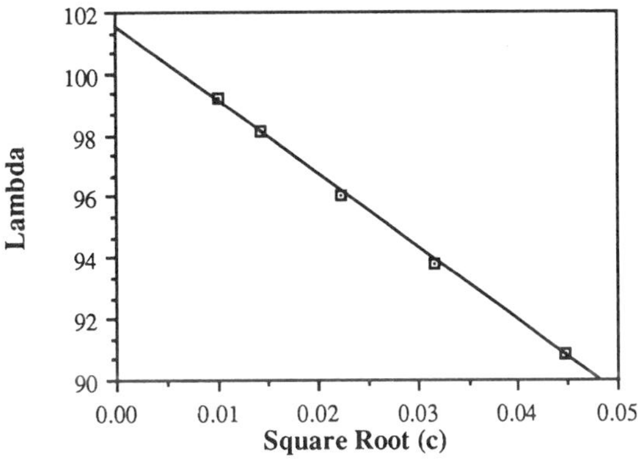

8.37 Use the data below for the equivalent conductivity of NaI in water (25°C) to calculate $\Lambda°$ (use the Onsager equation).

c	Λ
0.005	121.25
0.01	119.24
0.02	116.70
0.05	112.79

From Eq. (8.44), $\Lambda° \cong \dfrac{\Lambda + \sigma\sqrt{c}}{1 - \theta\sqrt{c}} \equiv \Lambda'$ and Eq. (8.45), $\Lambda' = \Lambda° + Bc$, a plot of c vs. Λ' has a slope of $\Lambda°$. Using

Λ'	c
127.57	0.005
128.20	0.01
129.40	0.02
133.06	0.05

From a least squares analysis,

slope = 126.97 cm^2 S with σ = 0.01 cm^2 S and r = 1.000 .

8.38 The following are degrees of dissociation measured (by conductance) for picric acid in methanol (25°). Calculate the thermodynamic dissociation constant. (The DH constant $\alpha = 4.58$ for methanol at 25°C.)

c	α
0.001563	0.3131
0.003125	0.2408
0.00625	0.1820
0.0125	0.1379

$K_a'' = \dfrac{c\alpha^2}{1 - \alpha}$ and $K_a = K_a''\gamma_{\pm}^2$ where $\gamma_{\pm} = \exp\left[\dfrac{-\alpha\sqrt{\alpha c}}{1 + \sqrt{\alpha c}}\right]$. Then:

K_a''	K_a
2.23×10^{-4}	1.83×10^{-4}
2.39×10^{-4}	1.87×10^{-4}
2.53×10^{-4}	1.88×10^{-4}
2.76×10^{-4}	1.91×10^{-4}

As $c \to 0$, $K_a \cong 1.83 \times 10^{-4}$.

8.39 Calculate the thermodynamic ionization constant of chloroacetic acid (in water) from the data:

$10^3 c$	Λ (Ω^{-1} cm^2)
0.11010	362.10
0.30271	328.92
0.58987	295.58
1.3231	246.15

For chloroacetic acid, $\Lambda^\circ = \lambda^\circ_{H^+} + \lambda^\circ_{chloroacetate} = 389.6\ cm^2\ S$.

Since $\alpha' = \frac{\Lambda}{\Lambda^\circ}$ and $K_a'' = \frac{c(\alpha')^2}{1 - \alpha}$:

α'	K_a''	$\sqrt{c}$
0.9306	1.374×10^{-3}	0.0105
0.8443	1.386×10^{-3}	0.0174
0.7587	1.407×10^{-3}	0.0243
0.6318	1.434×10^{-3}	0.0364

A plot of K_a'' vs. $\sqrt{c}$ extrapolated to zero concentration has intercept K_a .

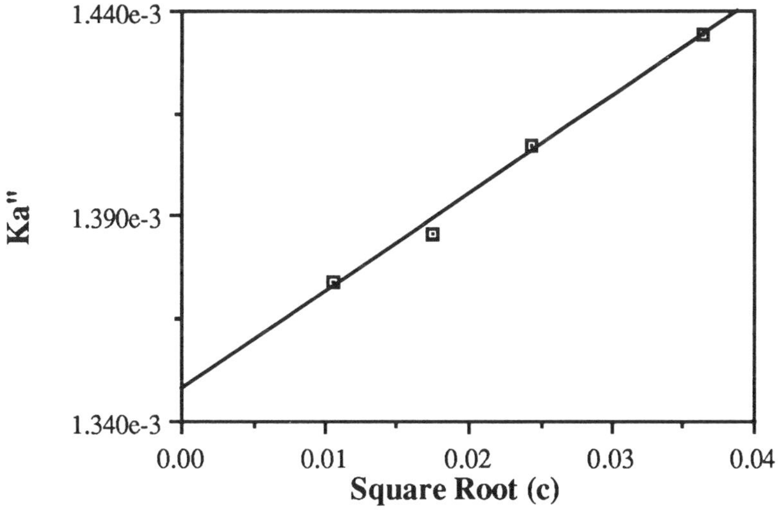

Thus $K_a = 1.346 \times 10^{-3}$.

8.40 The cell:

$$\text{Pt, H}_2\text{(1 atm)}\,|\,\text{HCl(aq}, m = 1.5346)\,|\,\text{AgCl(s)}\,|\,\text{Ag}$$

has $\mathscr{E} = 0.20534$ volts.
(a) Use $\mathscr{E}^{\circ}$ from Table 8.10 to calculate $\gamma_\pm$ for HCl.
(b) What is the pH of this solution?

a) The cell as written has the reaction:

$$\frac{1}{2}\,H_2 = H^+ + e^-$$
$$AgCl + e^- = Ag + Cl^-$$

$$AgCl + \frac{1}{2}\,H_2 = H^+ + Cl^- + Ag$$

$\mathscr{E}_{cell}$ is given by $\mathscr{E}_{cell} = \mathscr{E}_R - \mathscr{E}_L$. From Table 8.10,

$\mathscr{E}^{\ominus} = 0.2225 - 0 = 0.2225$. From Eq. (8.56c),

$$m^2\gamma_\pm^{\,2} = \exp\left[-\frac{(\mathscr{E} - \mathscr{E}^{\ominus})\mathscr{F}}{RT}\right] = \exp\left[-\frac{(0.20534 - 0.2225)96485}{(8.3145)(298.15)}\right]$$

Using m = 1.5346, we obtain $\gamma_\pm = 0.910$.

b) The pH is

$$pH = -\log_{10}a_{H^+} = -\log_{10}[H^+]\gamma_\pm = -\log_{10}(1.5346)(0.910) = -0.145 \ .$$

8.41 The emf of the cell:

$$Hg(liq) \mid Hg_2Cl_2(s) \mid HCl(aq, 0.1m) \mid Cl_2(g, P), (Pt\text{-}Ir)$$

was measured with the chlorine pressure reduced in nitrogen to prevent hydrolysis of Cl_2 in the water. When $P_{Cl_2} = 0.0124$ atm, $\mathscr{E} = 1.0330$ volts. Calculate the standard emf of this cell from this datum.

From Eq. (8.53), $\mathscr{E}^{\ominus} = \mathscr{E} + \frac{RT}{n\mathscr{F}} \ln Q$. For the reaction:

$$2\ Cl^- + 2\ Hg = 2\ e^- + Hg_2Cl_2$$
$$Cl_2 + 2\ e^- = 2\ Cl^-$$

$$Cl_2 + 2\ Hg = Hg_2Cl_2$$

n = 2 and $Q = \frac{P^{\ominus}}{P_{Cl_2}} = \frac{1\ \text{atm}}{0.0124\ \text{atm}}$. Thus

$$\mathscr{E}^{\ominus} = 1.0330\ \ V + \frac{(8.3145)(298.15)}{2(96485)} \ln \frac{1}{0.0124} = 1.0894\ V\ .$$

8.42 Use data in this chapter to calculate the emf of the cell:

$$Zn(s) \mid ZnCl_2(aq, m = 0.05) \mid Cl_2(g, P = 0.5\ \text{atm}), (Pt\text{-}Ir)$$

$$Zn = Zn^{2+} + 2\ e^-$$
$$e^- + Cl_2 = 2\ Cl^-$$

$$Zn + Cl_2 = Zn^{2+} + 2\ Cl^-$$

$\mathscr{E}^{\ominus} = \mathscr{E}_R - \mathscr{E}_L = 1.3595 + 0.7628 = 2.1223$ V . From Eq. (8.53), $\mathscr{E} = \mathscr{E}^{\ominus} + \frac{RT}{n\mathscr{F}} \ln Q$. Since n = 2 and

$$Q = \frac{P^{\ominus}}{P_{Cl_2}}(a_{Zn^{2+}})(a_{Cl^-})^2 = \frac{P^{\ominus}}{P_{Cl_2}}(m_+)(m_-)^2\gamma_{\pm}^3$$

$$Q = \frac{1}{0.5}\ (0.05)(0.10)^2(0.556)^3 = 1.719 \times 10^{-4}\ ,$$

then

$$\mathscr{E} = 2.1223 - \frac{(8.3145)(298.15)}{2(96485)} \ln[1.719 \times 10^{-4}] = 2.2337\ V\ .$$

8.43 Use data in this chapter to calculate the emf (25°C) of the cell:

$$Cu(s)\,|\,CuSO_4(aq, m = 0.2)\,|\,PbSO_4(s)\,|\,Pb(s)$$

$$Cu = Cu^{2+} + 2\ e^-$$

$$PbSO_4 + 2\ e^- = Pb + SO_4^{2-}$$

$$PbSO_4 + Cu = Pb + Cu^{+2} + SO_4^{-2}$$

$$\mathcal{E}^\ominus = \mathcal{E}_R - \mathcal{E}_L = -0.3546 - 0.337 = -0.6916\ V\ .$$

$$Q = (a_{Cu^{2+}})(a_{SO_4^{2-}}) = a_{CuSO_4} = (m_+m_-)\gamma_\pm^2$$

$$Q = (0.2)^2(0.11)^2 = 4.84 \times 10^{-4}\ .$$

Using Eq. (8.53),

$$\mathcal{E} = -0.6916 - \frac{(8.3145)(298.15)}{2(96485)}\ \ln[4.84 \times 10^{-4}] = -0.594\ V\ .$$

8.44 The cell:

$$Pb(Hg)\,|\,PbSO_4(s)\,|\,H_2SO_4(aq, 0.001m)\,|\,H_2(1\ atm), Pt$$

has $\mathcal{E}^\circ = 0.3505$ and $\mathcal{E} = 0.09589$. Calculate $\gamma_\pm$ for the electrolyte.

$$Pb + SO_4^{2-} = PbSO_4 + 2\ e^-$$

$$2\ H^+ + 2\ e^- = H_2$$

$$Pb + 2\ H^+ + SO_4^{2-} = PbSO_4 + H_2$$

$$Q = \frac{P_{H_2}}{P^\ominus}\left(\frac{1}{(a_{H^+})^2(a_{SO_4^{2-}})}\right) = \frac{P_{H_2}}{P^\ominus}\left(\frac{1}{4m^3\gamma_\pm^3}\right) = \frac{1}{1}\left(\frac{1}{4(0.001)^3(\gamma_\pm)^3}\right)\ .$$

Since $\mathcal{E}^\ominus - \mathcal{E} = 0.2546 = \frac{RT}{n\mathcal{F}}\ \ln Q$, we may solve for $\gamma_\pm$ and obtain $\gamma_\pm = 0.851$.

8.45 Use the selected data (25°C) below [Harned and Ehlers, *J. Am. Chem. Soc.*, **54**, 1350 (1932)] to calculate $\mathscr{E}^\ominus$ for the cell:

$$\mathrm{Pt, H_2(g, 1\ atm) | HCl(aq,} m\mathrm{) | AgCl(s) | Ag(s)}$$

m	$\mathscr{E}$/volts
0.003215	0.52053
0.005619	0.49257
0.009138	0.46860
0.013407	0.44974
0.02563	0.41824

From Eq. (8.58), $\mathscr{E}'' \equiv \mathscr{E} + \frac{2RT}{\mathscr{F}}\left(\ln m - \frac{1.177\sqrt{m}}{1 + \sqrt{m}}\right) = \mathscr{E}^\ominus + Bm$.

We draw up the following table:

$\mathscr{E}''$	m
0.22268	0.003215
0.22247	0.005619
0.22243	0.009138
0.22223	0.013407
0.22175	0.02563

Regressing $\mathscr{E}''$ vs. m , we obtain $\mathscr{E}^\ominus$ = 0.2228 V with

$\sigma = 3.98 \times 10^{-5}$ V and r = -0.99223 .

8.46 Use the emf data below [E. W. Canning and M. G. Bowman, *J. Am. Chem. Soc.*, **68**, 2042 (1946)] for the cell (25°C):

$$\mathrm{Pt, H_2(g, 1\ atm) | H_2SO_4(}m\mathrm{, CH_3OH) | Hg_2SO_4(s) | Hg(liq)}$$

to calculate the standard emf of this cell. Note that sulfuric acid in a dilute solution in methanol acts as a 1 : 1 electrolyte—that is, it ionizes to H^+ and HSO_4^-. Also, the Debye-Hückel constant for methanol at 25°C is $\alpha = 4.065$.

10^3m	$\mathscr{E}$/volts	10^3m	$\mathscr{E}$/volts
0.700	0.7289	8.111	0.6711
1.1184	0.7174	22.385	0.6509
2.412	0.6996	43.217	0.6388
5.475	0.6805	96.88	0.6249
6.778	0.6756		

As in problem 8.45, use Eq. (8.58) with n = 2 and α = 4.065 ,

$\mathscr{E}'' \equiv \mathscr{E} + \frac{RT}{\mathscr{F}}\left(\ln m - \frac{4.065\sqrt{m}}{1 + \sqrt{m}}\right) = \mathscr{E}^\ominus + Bm$. Regress $\mathscr{E}''$ vs. m to

find $\mathscr{E}^\ominus$ = 0.5394 V , σ = 0.0001 V and r = 0.6341 .

8.47 Calculate the standard emf of the cell:

$$Zn \mid ZnSO_4(aq, m) \mid PbSO_4(s) \mid Pb(Hg)$$

from these data:

m	$\mathscr{E}$/volts
0.0005	0.61144
0.001	0.59714
0.002	0.58319
0.005	0.56598
0.01	0.55353

n = 2, so Eq. (8.58) is $\mathscr{E}'' \equiv \mathscr{E} + \frac{RT}{\mathscr{F}}\left(\ln m - \frac{9.416\sqrt{m}}{1 + \sqrt{m}}\right) = \mathscr{E}^{\theta} + Bm$.

Then

$\mathscr{E}''$	m
0.41559	0.0005
0.41886	0.001
0.42238	0.002
0.43164	0.005
0.43265	0.01

Linear regression gives $\mathscr{E}^{\theta}$ = 0.412 V , σ = 0.0007 V and r = 0.8294 .

8.48 The standard potentials listed below are for:

$$Pt, H_2(g) \mid HBr(aq) \mid AgBr(s) \mid Ag(s)$$

(a) What is the cell reaction?
(b) Calculate ΔG°, ΔS°, and ΔH° for this reaction at 25°C.

t/°C	$\mathscr{E}^\circ$/volts
5	0.07991
15	0.07595
25	0.07131
35	0.06597
45	0.05995

a)

$$\frac{1}{2} H_2 = H^+ + e^-$$

$$AgBr + e^- = Ag + Br^-$$

$$AgBr + \frac{1}{2} H_2 = Ag + H^+ + Br^-$$

b) From Eq. (8.59),

$\Delta_{rxn}G^{\theta} = -n\mathcal{F}\mathcal{E}^{\theta} = -(1)(96485)(0.07131) = -6.88\ kJ$. From Eq. (8.60), $\Delta_{rxn}S^{\theta} = n\mathcal{F}\left(\frac{d\mathcal{E}^{\theta}}{dT}\right)$. Using the 5-point formula (AI.21c) at 25°C, $\frac{d\mathcal{E}^{\theta}}{dT} = -4.99 \times 10^{-4}$. Thus

$$\Delta_{rxn}S^{\theta} = (96485)(-4.99 \times 10^{-4}) = -48.15\ J\ K^{-1} .$$

$$\Delta_{rxn}H^{\theta} = n\mathcal{F}\left[T\ \frac{d\mathcal{E}^{\theta}}{dT} - \mathcal{E}^{\theta}\right]$$

$$\Delta_{rxn}H^{\theta} = 96485[(298)(-4.99 \times 10^{-4}) - 0.07131] = -21.24\ kJ .$$

8.49 The standard potentials of the cell:

Pt, $H_2(g)$ | HCl(solution) | AgCl(s) | Ag(s)

in 20% dioxane/water are $\mathcal{E}^{\circ}$ = 0.20674 volts at 20°C, 0.20303 at 25°C, 0.19914 at 30°C. Calculate the standard entropy and free energy of $H^{+}Cl^{-}$ in this solvent at 25°C.

$$\Delta_{rxn}G^{\theta} = -n\mathcal{F}\mathcal{E}^{\theta} = -(1)(96485)(0.20303) = -19.59\ kJ .$$

$$\Delta_{rxn}S^{\theta} = n\mathcal{F}\left(\frac{d\mathcal{E}^{\theta}}{dT}\right) .$$

With $\frac{d\mathcal{E}^{\theta}}{dT} = \frac{0.19914 - 0.20674}{10} = -7.60 \times 10^{-4}\ J\ K^{-1}$

$$\Delta_{rxn}S^{\theta} = -73.33\ J\ K^{-1} .$$

$$S^{\theta}(Cl^{-}) = \Delta_{rxn}S^{\theta} - S^{\theta}(H^{+}) - S^{\theta}(Ag) + \frac{1}{2}\ S^{\theta}(H_2) + S^{\theta}(AgCl)$$

$$S^{\theta}(Cl^{-}) = (-73.33) - (0) - (42.55) + \frac{1}{2}\ (130.684) + (96.2)$$

$S^{\ominus}(Cl^-) = 45.66 \text{ J K}^{-1}$.

$$\Delta_f G^{\ominus}(Cl^-) = \Delta_{rxn} G^{\ominus} - \Delta_f G^{\ominus}(H^+) - \Delta_f G^{\ominus}(Ag) + \frac{1}{2}\Delta_f G^{\ominus}(H_2) + \Delta_f G^{\ominus}(AgCl)$$

$$\Delta_f G^{\ominus}(Cl^-) = (-19.59) - (0) - (0) + \frac{1}{2}(0) + (-109.789)$$

$$\Delta_f G^{\ominus}(Cl^-) = -129.38 \text{ kJ} .$$

8.50 (a) What is the cell reaction for:

$$Pb(s)\,|\,PbCl_2(s)\,|\,HCl(aq, m = 0.1)\,|\,Hg_2Cl_2(s)\,|\,Hg(liq)\ ?$$

(b) Calculate the emf (25°C) of this cell from thermodynamic data in this text.
(c) Estimate the emf of this cell at 18°C.
(d) How much heat would be released if the cell were charged reversibly (at 25°C) with 2 faradays of electricity?
(e) How much heat would be released if the cell were discharged irreversibly (2 faradays, at 25°C) through a short circuit?

a)

$$Pb + 2\,Cl^- = PbCl_2 + 2\,e^-$$
$$Hg_2Cl_2 + 2\,e^- = 2\,Hg + 2\,Cl^-$$
$$\overline{\quad Hg_2Cl_2 + Pb = PbCl_2 + 2\,Hg \quad}$$

b) $$\Delta_{rxn} G^{\ominus} = -n\mathcal{F}\mathcal{E}^{\ominus} = \Delta_f G^{\ominus}(PbCl_2) + 2\Delta_f G^{\ominus}(Hg) - \Delta_f G^{\ominus}(Hg_2Cl_2) - \Delta_f G^{\ominus}(Pb)$$

$$\Delta_{rxn} G^{\ominus} = (-314.10) + 2(0) - (-210.745) - (0) = -103.355 \text{ kJ}$$

so that: $$\mathcal{E}^{\ominus} = \frac{103.355 \times 10^3}{2(96485)} = 0.5356 \text{ V} .$$

c) $$\frac{d\mathscr{E}}{dT} = \frac{\Delta S^{\theta}}{n\mathscr{F}}$$

$$\Delta_{rxn}S^{\theta} = -S^{\theta}(Hg_2Cl_2) - S^{\theta}(Pb) + S^{\theta}(PbCl_2) + 2S^{\theta}(Hg)$$

$$\Delta_{rxn}S^{\theta} = -196 - 64.81 + 136.0 + 2(76.02) = 27.23 \text{ J K}^{-1} \text{ mol}^{-1}$$

and $$\Delta\mathscr{E}^{\theta} = \frac{\Delta S^{\theta}\Delta T}{n\mathscr{F}} = \frac{(27.23)(298.15 - 291.15)}{2(96485)} = 0.0010$$

$$\mathscr{E}^{\theta} = 0.5366 \text{ V} .$$

d) For a reversible process: $Q = -T\Delta S = -8.12$ kJ .

e) $w = 0$, so that $\Delta U = Q = \Delta H$. From Table 6.1,

$$\Delta_{rxn}H^{\theta} = -359.41 - (-265.22) = -94.19 \text{ kJ} = Q .$$

8.51 The cell:

$$Pb(s)\,|\,PbBr_2(s)\,|\,CuBr_2(aq, m = 0.01)\,|\,Cu(s)$$

has $\mathscr{E} = 0.442$ volts at 25°.
(a) Calculate $\mathscr{E}^\circ$. (Use the DHG formula to calculate the activity coefficient.)
(b) Calculate the thermodynamic solubility product of $PbBr_2$.

a)

$$Pb + 2\,Br^- = PbBr_2 + 2\,e^-$$
$$Cu^{2+} + 2\,e^- = Cu$$

$$Pb + 2\,Br^- + Cu^{2+} = PbBr_2 + Cu$$

$Q = \dfrac{1}{a_{CuBr_2}} = \dfrac{1}{4m^3\gamma_\pm^3}$. From Eq. (8.15),

$\ln \gamma_\pm = \dfrac{-\alpha|z_+z_-|\sqrt{I}}{1 + \sqrt{I}} = -\dfrac{1.177(2)\sqrt{3m}}{1 + \sqrt{3m}}$. For m = 0.01, $\gamma_\pm = 0.706$.

Substituting into the Nernst eq.,

$$\mathscr{E}^\ominus = 0.442 - \frac{(8.3145)(298.15)}{2(96485)} \ln\left[\frac{1}{4(0.01)^3(0.706)^3}\right] = 0.615\ \text{V}\ .$$

b) $\mathscr{E}^\ominus_{cell} = \mathscr{E}^\ominus_R - \mathscr{E}^\ominus_L$ or $\mathscr{E}^\ominus_L = 0.337 - 0.615 = -0.278$ V . We combine the following reactions to get the solubility reaction:

$PbBr_2 + 2\,e^- = Pb + 2\,Br^-$	$\mathscr{E}^\ominus = -0.278$ V
$Pb = 2\,e^- + Pb^{2+}$	$-\ (\mathscr{E}^\ominus = -0.126$ V)
$PbBr_2 = Pb^{2+} + 2\,Br^-$	$\mathscr{E}^\ominus = -0.152$ V

When $\mathscr{E} = 0$, $Q = K_{sp}$, thus $\mathscr{E}^\ominus = \dfrac{RT}{n\mathscr{F}} \ln K_{sp}$ or

$$K_{sp} = \exp\left(\frac{-0.152(2)(96485)}{(8.3145)(298.15)}\right) = 7.26 \times 10^{-6}\ .$$

8.52 Use the standard emf (Table 8.10) to calculate the solubility product of AgBr.

$$AgBr + e^- = Ag + Br^- \qquad \mathcal{E}^\ominus = 0.0711\ \text{V}$$
$$Ag = Ag^+ + e^- \qquad -(\mathcal{E}^\ominus = 0.7991\ \text{V})$$
$$AgBr = Ag^+ + Br^- \qquad \mathcal{E}^\ominus = -0.7280\ \text{V}$$

At equilibrium, $K_{sp} = Q$ and $\mathcal{E} = 0$, thus $\mathcal{E}^\ominus = \frac{RT}{n\mathcal{F}} \ln K_{sp}$

or $K_{sp} = \exp\left(\frac{-0.7280(1)(96485)}{(8.3145)(298.15)}\right) = 4.94 \times 10^{-13}$.

8.53 The solubility product of AgSCN is $K_{sp} = 1.16 \times 10^{-12}$ (25°C). Calculate the standard emf of the electrode:

$$SCN^- | AgSCN(s) | Ag(s)$$

(The actual value is 0.0859 V.)

The electrode reaction is $AgSCN + e^- = Ag + SCN^-$. The K_{sp} reaction is

$$AgSCN + e^- = Ag + SCN^- \qquad \mathcal{E}^\ominus = x$$
$$Ag = Ag^+ + e^- \qquad -(\mathcal{E}^\ominus = 0.7991\ \text{V})$$
$$AgSCN = Ag^+ + SCN^- \qquad \mathcal{E}^\ominus = x - 0.7991$$

V

For the K_{sp} reaction, $\mathcal{E}^\ominus = \frac{RT}{n\mathcal{F}} \ln K_{sp}$ or

$$x - 0.7991 = \frac{(8.3145)(298.15)}{1(96485)} \ln(1.16 \times 10^{-12}) \text{ or}$$

$$x = \mathcal{E}^\ominus_{electrode} = 0.0931\ \text{V} .$$

8.54 The solubility product of $BaSO_4$ is 1.08×10^{-10} at 25°C. Calculate the standard emf of the cell:

$$\text{Pt, } H_2(\text{g, 1 atm}) \,|\, H_2SO_4(\text{aq}) \,|\, BaSO_4(\text{s}) \,|\, \text{Ba(s)}$$

Is this a practical cell?

The cell reaction is

$$H_2 = 2\,H^+ + 2\,e^- \qquad \mathcal{E}^\ominus = 0$$

$$BaSO_4 + 2\,e^- = Ba + SO_4^{2-} \qquad -\,(\mathcal{E}^\ominus = -x)$$

$$H_2 + BaSO_4 = Ba + 2\,H^+ + SO_4^{2-} \qquad \mathcal{E}^\ominus_c = x$$

The solubility reaction is

$$BaSO_4 + 2\,e^- = Ba + SO_4^{2-} \qquad \mathcal{E}^\ominus = x$$

$$Ba = Ba^{2+} + 2\,e^- \qquad -\,(\mathcal{E}^\ominus = -2.906\ \text{V})$$

$$BaSO_4 = Ba^{2+} + SO_4^{2-} \qquad \mathcal{E}^\ominus_c = x + 2.096$$

For this reaction, when $Q = K_{sp}$ and $\mathcal{E} = 0$,

$$\mathcal{E}^\ominus_s = \frac{RT}{n\mathcal{F}} \ln K_{sp} = \frac{(8.3145)(298.15)}{1(96485)} \ln(1.08 \times 10^{-10})$$

$$\mathcal{E}^\ominus_s = -0.2949 = \mathcal{E}^\ominus_c + 2.906 \,.$$

or $\mathcal{E}^\ominus_c = -3.201$ V . This is not a practical cell since Ba reacts with acid .

8.55 Calculate the ion product of water from the standard emf of $OH^- | H_2 | Pt$ (Table 8.10). (Devise a hypothetical cell and give the cell reaction.)

$$2\ H_2O + 2\ e^- = H_2 + 2\ OH^- \qquad \mathcal{E}^\ominus = -0.82806$$

$$H_2 = 2\ e^- + 2\ H^+ \qquad -\ (\mathcal{E}^\ominus = 0)$$

$$2\ H_2O = 2\ H^+ + 2\ OH^- \qquad \mathcal{E}^\ominus = -0.82806$$

At equilibrium $K = \exp\left(\frac{\mathcal{E}^\ominus n\mathcal{F}}{RT}\right) = 1.006 \times 10^{-14}$.

8.56 Calculate the fugacity coefficient (γ) for H_2(gas) at the pressures given, from the emf of the cell (at 25°C):

$$\text{Pt, } H_2(g, P)\,|\,HCl(aq, m = 0.1)\,|\,Hg_2Cl_2(s)\,|\,Hg(liq)$$

$P(H_2)$/atm	$\mathcal{E}$/volts
1.0	0.3990
110.2	0.4596
556.8	0.4844
1035.2	0.4975

$$H_2 = 2\ H^+ + 2\ e^- \qquad \mathcal{E}^\ominus = 0$$

$$Hg_2Cl_2 + 2\ e^- = 2\ Hg + 2\ Cl^- \qquad -\ (\mathcal{E}^\ominus = -0.2680)$$

$$H_2 + Hg_2Cl_2 = 2\ Hg + 2\ H^+ + 2\ Cl^- \qquad \mathcal{E}^\ominus = 0.2680$$

From the Nernst equation, $\exp\left(\frac{-(\mathcal{E} - \mathcal{E}^\ominus)n\mathcal{F}}{RT}\right) = \frac{(a_{HCl})^2}{a_{H_2}} = \frac{(a_{HCl})^2}{P_{H_2}\gamma}$.

From Table 8.1, $(a_{HCl})^2 = (m_+m_-)\gamma_\pm^2 = 3.99 \times 10^{-5}$, thus

$$\gamma = \frac{3.99 \times 10^{-5}}{P_{H_2} \exp\left(-\frac{(\mathcal{E} - 0.268)(2)(96485)}{(8.3145)(298.15)}\right)}$$ and $\gamma(P = 1\text{ atm}) = 1.07$,

$\gamma(P = 110.2\text{ atm}) = 1.09$, $\gamma(P = 556.8\text{ atm}) = 1.49$,

$\gamma(P = 1035.2\text{ atm}) = 2.21$.

8.57 Calculate the emf of the cell (using the ideal gas approximation):

(Pt-Ir), Cl_2(g, 1 atm) | HCl(aq, m = 0.1) | Cl_2(g, 0.3 atm), (Pt-Ir)

From the Nernst eq. with $\mathcal{E}^{\ominus} = 0$,

$$\mathcal{E} = -\frac{RT}{n\mathcal{F}} \ln \frac{a_{Cl_2(1\ atm)}}{a_{Cl_2(0.3\ atm)}} \cong -\frac{(8.3145)(298.15)}{2(96485)} \ln \frac{1}{0.3}$$

$\mathcal{E} = -0.0155$ V .

8.58 (a) Devise a cell that could be used to measure activity coefficients of $ZnCl_2$.
(b) What is the Nernst equation for your cell?

a)

$$Zn = Zn^{2+} + 2\ e^- \qquad \mathcal{E}^{\ominus} = 0.7628$$

$$Hg_2Cl_2 + 2\ e^- = 2\ Hg + 2\ Cl^- \qquad -\ (\mathcal{E}^{\ominus} = -0.2680)$$

$$Hg_2Cl_2 + Zn = Zn^{2+} + 2\ Cl^- + 2\ Hg \qquad \mathcal{E}^{\ominus} = 1.0308$$

or Zn | $ZnCl_2$ (m, aq) | Hg_2Cl_2 (s) | Hg .

b) $Q = a_{ZnCl_2} = (m)(2m)^2\gamma_{\pm}^3 = 4m^3\gamma_{\pm}^3$. From the Nernst equation , $\mathcal{E} = 1.0380 - \frac{RT}{2\mathcal{F}} \ln 4m^3\gamma_{\pm}^3$.

8.59 The Ruben cell, which is frequently used in applications such as hearing aids, has a cell reaction:

$$Zn(s) + HgO(s) + H_2O + 2\,KOH = Hg(liq) + K_2Zn(OH)_4$$

(a) Diagram this cell and calculate its standard emf.
(b) Assuming $\mathscr{E} = \mathscr{E}^{\circ}$, calculate the minimum weight of a cell that would last two weeks with a load of 5 mW.

a) $Zn\ (s)\ |\ K_2Zn(OH)_4\ (m,\ aq)\ |\ HgO\ (s)\ |\ Hg\ (liq)$

$$Zn + 4\ OH^- = Zn(OH)_4^{2-} + 2\ e^-$$
$$HgO + H_2O + 2\ e^- = Hg + 2\ OH^-$$

$$Zn + HgO + H_2O + 2OH^- = Zn(OH)_4^{2-} + Hg$$

$$\mathscr{E}^{\ominus} = 1.215 - -(0.097) = 1.312\ V\ .$$

b) $\Delta G^{\ominus}$ is the electrical work done, thus $Pt = -\Delta G^{\ominus} = n\mathscr{F}\mathscr{E}^{\ominus}$ or $(5 \times 10^{-3}\ W)(1.2096 \times 10^{6}\ s) = n(96487)(1.312\ V)$. This gives n = 0.0478 moles, which is the number of moles of e- required for the cell to last two weeks. The weight of the cell components per mole of e- transferred is

$$M = \frac{MW\ of\ (K_2Zn(OH)_4 + Hg)}{2\ moles\ e^-} = \frac{412.21\ g}{2\ mol}\ .$$

Then the weight of the cell required is $\frac{412.21\ g}{2}(0.0478) = 9.85\ g$.

8.60 Show that a concentration cell with a salt that has ν ions per "molecule" and transfers n equivalents of electricity per mole has an emf:

$$\mathscr{E} = \pm \frac{\nu t_i RT}{n\mathscr{F}} \ln \frac{a_{\pm 1}}{a_{\pm 2}}$$

where $t_i = t_+$ (+ sign) if the cell is anion reversible and $t_i = t_-$ (− sign) if the cell is cation reversible.

Let us take for an example a cation reversible cell with the salt MA_2:

$$\begin{array}{lrcl} \text{Left (ox.):} & M & = & M^{2+}(m_1) + 2\,e^- \\ \text{L. J.:} & t_+M^{2+}(m_1) & = & t_+M^{2+}(m_2) \\ & 2t_-A^-(m_2) & = & 2t_-A^-(m_1) \\ \text{Right (red.):} & M^{2+}(m_2) + 2\,e^- & = & M \end{array}$$

$$M^{2+}(m_2) + 2t_-A^-(m_2) + t_+M^{2+}(m_1) = M^{2+}(m_1) + t_+M^{2+}(m_2) + 2t_-A^-(m_1)$$

Thus $t_-MA_2(m_2) = t_-MA_2(m_1)$. $\mathscr{E}$ is then

$\mathscr{E} = -\frac{RT}{2\mathscr{F}} \ln\left(\frac{a_1}{a_2}\right)^{t_-} = -\frac{RTt_-}{2\mathscr{F}} \ln\left(\frac{a_1}{a_2}\right)$. Since $a_{MA_2} = m^3\gamma_\pm^{\,3} = (a_\pm)^3$,

then $\mathscr{E} = -\frac{RT3t_-}{2\mathscr{F}} \ln\left(\frac{m_1\gamma_{\pm 1}}{m_2\gamma_{\pm 2}}\right)$. Generalizing this formula,

$\mathscr{E} = -\frac{RT\nu t_-}{2\mathscr{F}} \ln\left(\frac{a_{\pm 1}}{a_{\pm 2}}\right)$. For t_+ we have $\mathscr{E} = \frac{RT\nu t_+}{2\mathscr{F}} \ln\left(\frac{a_{\pm 1}}{a_{\pm 2}}\right)$.

Note that the minus sign disappears in the t_+ expression since a_1 and a_2 are inverted in the expression for Q .

8.61 The emf of the cell:

$$Zn(Hg)|ZnI_2(m = 0.3, \gamma_\pm = 0.564)|ZnI_2(m = 0.1, \gamma_\pm = 0.581)|Zn(Hg)$$

is -0.02689 V (at 25°C). Calculate the cation transference number. (The electrodes are identical.)

For a cation reversible cell, $\mathcal{E} = -\frac{t_- RT\nu}{n\mathcal{F}} \ln\left(\frac{a_{m1}}{a_{m2}}\right)$. For ZnI_2 , $\nu = 3$, $n = 2$ and $a_{ZnI_2} = m(2m)^2\gamma_\pm^3 = 4m^3\gamma_\pm^3$. Then

$$0.02689 = -\frac{3t_-(8.3145)(298.15)}{2(96485)} \ln\left(\frac{0.3(0.564)}{0.1(0.581)}\right) \text{ or } t_- = 0.653 .$$

Thus $t_+ = 1 - t_- = 0.347$.

8.62 Calculate the emf of the cell:

$$(Pt\text{-}Ir), Cl_2(g, 1\ atm)|NaCl(m = 0.1)|NaCl(m = 0.02)|Cl_2(g, 1\ atm), (Pt\text{-}Ir)$$

From Eq. (8.71b), $\mathcal{E} = \frac{2t_+RT}{\mathcal{F}} \ln\left(\frac{m_1\gamma_{\pm1}}{m_2\gamma_{\pm2}}\right)$. Taking an average value for t_+ from Table 8.5,

$$\mathcal{E} = \frac{2(0.3878)(8.3145)(298.15)}{96485} \ln\left(\frac{0.1(0.778)}{0.02(0.875)}\right) = 0.0297 \text{ V} .$$

8.63 Estimate the liquid-junction potential for:

$$KOH(c = 0.1)|KCl(c = 0.2)$$

(Use conductivities at infinite dilution, $\Lambda°$.)

From Eq. (8.74b),

$$\mathcal{E}_J = \frac{RT}{\mathcal{F}}\left\{\frac{c_1(\lambda_+ - \lambda_-) - c_2(\lambda_+' - \lambda_-')}{c_1\Lambda - c_2\Lambda'}\right\} \ln\left\{\frac{c_1\Lambda}{c_2\Lambda'}\right\} .$$

For c_1 , $\Lambda = \lambda^\circ_{K^+} + \lambda^\circ_{OH^-} = 73.5 + 197.6 = 271.10$ and for c_2, $\Lambda' = \lambda^\circ_{K^+} + \lambda^\circ_{Cl^-} = 73.5 + 76.34 = 149.84$. Then

$$\mathscr{E}_J = \frac{(8.3145)(298.15)}{96485}\left\{\frac{0.1(-124.1) - 0.2(-2.84)}{0.1(271.1) - 0.2(149.84)}\right\}\ln\left\{\frac{0.1(271.1)}{0.2(149.84)}\right\}$$

$$\mathscr{E}_J = 0.0107 \text{ V} .$$

8.64 Calculate the junction potential for:

$$NH_4Cl(c = 0.1)|LiCl(c = 0.1)$$

Using Eq. (8.75) and data from Table 8.6 ,

$$\mathscr{E}_J = \frac{RT}{\mathscr{F}} \ln \frac{\Lambda}{\Lambda'} = \frac{(8.3145)(298.15)}{96485} \ln \left(\frac{128.75}{95.86}\right) = 7.6 \text{ mV} .$$

8.65 Devise a cell that could be used to measure the Nernst potential of:

$$Zn|ZnSO_4(aq)||CuSO_4(aq)|Cu$$

(that is, a cell without a liquid junction).

One such cell, sensitive to SO_4^{-2} , is:

$$Zn \mid ZnSO_4 \text{ (aq)} \mid PbSO_4 \text{ (s)} \mid Pb \text{ (s)} \mid PbSO_4 \text{ (s)} \mid CuSO_4 \text{ (aq)} \mid Cu.$$

8.66 A solution 0.02 mol/kg KCl in water is divided by a membrane permeable to both ions. On one side of the membrane (the "left"), 0.0001 mol/kg of a polyelectrolyte is dissolved. The polymer has a net charge number $z = +63$, and cannot pass through the membrane. Calculate the ratio $[K^+(\text{right})]/[K^+(\text{left})]$ at equilibrium.

If $[K^+]$ refers to the "left" and $[K^+]'$ to the "right," then:

$$\frac{[K^+]'}{[K^+]} = \left[1 + \frac{zc_p}{[K^+]}\right]^{1/2} , \quad [K^+]' = 0.02 + x , \quad [K^+] = 0.02 - x ,$$

$z = 63$ and $c_p = 0.0001$. The solution is $x = 1.46 \times 10^{-3}$, so

that $\frac{[K^+]'}{[K^+]} = \left(\frac{0.02 + x}{0.02 - x}\right) = 1.1575$.

9

Transport Properties

9.1 Calculate the collision frequency for a molecule of neon ($\sigma = 0.2749 \times 10^{-9}$ m) in a gas at 1 atm and $T = 473$ and 673 K.

From Eqs. (9.8), (9.2) and (9.3), $z = \sqrt{2}\bar{v}\pi\sigma^2 n^*$, $\bar{v} = \sqrt{\frac{8RT}{\pi M}}$ and $n^* = \frac{PL}{RT}$. For neon at 473 K,

$$\bar{v} = \left(\frac{8(8.3145 \text{ J K}^{-1})(473 \text{ K})}{\pi(0.02018 \text{ kg})}\right)^{1/2} = 704.5 \text{ ms}^{-1} .$$

Also,

$$n^* = \frac{(101325 \text{ Pa})(6.02214 \times 10^{23})}{(8.3145 \text{ J K}^{-1})(473 \text{ K})} = 1.552 \times 10^{25} \text{ m}^{-3} .$$

Then

$$z = \sqrt{2}(704.5 \text{ ms}^{-1})\pi(0.2749 \times 10^{-9} \text{ m})^2(1.552 \times 10^{25} \text{ m}^{-3})$$

$$z = 3.67 \times 10^9 \text{ s}^{-1} .$$

Similarly, at 673 K, $\bar{v} = 840.3 \text{ ms}^{-1}$, $n^* = 1.091 \times 10^{25} \text{ m}^{-3}$ and

$$z = 3.08 \times 10^9 \text{ s}^{-1} .$$

9.2 Calculate the mean free path of N_2 ($\sigma = 0.37$ nm) at 273 K, for $P = 1$ atm and $P = 1$ torr.

The mean free path λ is $\lambda = \frac{RT}{\sqrt{2}PL\pi\sigma^2}$ With P = 101325 Pa, $\sigma = 3.7 \times 10^{-10}$ m and T = 273 K: $\lambda(1 \text{ atm}) = 6.12 \times 10^{-8}$ m .

λ is inversely proportional to pressure, so that at 1 torr:

$$\lambda(1 \text{ torr}) = 760\ \lambda(1 \text{ atm}) = 4.65 \times 10^{-5} \text{ m} .$$

9.3 Calculate the mean free path and the frequency of collisions of one molecule for He at 1 atm and T = 300 and 1000 K.

$$\lambda = \frac{RT}{\sqrt{2}PL\pi\sigma^2} = \frac{(8.3145\ \text{J K}^{-1})(300\ \text{K})}{\sqrt{2}(101325\text{Pa})L\pi(0.263 \times 10^{-9}\ \text{m})^2} = 1.33 \times 10^{-5}\ \text{cm} .$$

Similarly, at T = 1000 K , $\lambda = 4.43 \times 10^{-5}$ cm .

$$\bar{v} = \left(\frac{8RT}{\pi M}\right)^{1/2} = \left(\frac{8(8.3145)(300\ \text{K})}{\pi(4.002 \times 10^{-3})}\right)^{1/2} = 1259.8\ \text{ms}^{-1} .$$

At T = 1000 K , $\bar{v} = 2300.1\ \text{ms}^{-1}$. $n^* = \frac{PL}{RT}$. Substituting,

$n^*(300\ \text{K}) = 2.446 \times 10^{25}\ \text{m}^{-3}$ and $n^*(1000\ \text{K}) = 7.339 \times 10^{24}\ \text{m}^{-3}$.

From Eq. (9.8) , we find $z(300\ \text{K}) = 9.47 \times 10^{9}\ \text{s}^{-1}$

and $z(1000\ \text{K}) = 5.188 \times 10^{9}\ \text{s}^{-1}$.

9.4 Treating air as a uniform gas with molecular weight $\overline{M}$ = 28.8 g and $\sigma = 3.67 \times 10^{-8}$ cm, calculate the mean free path at 25°C for P = 1 atm, 1 torr, 10^{-3} torr.

From Eq. (9.9c),

$$\lambda = \frac{RT}{\sqrt{2}PL\pi\sigma^2} = \frac{(8.3145\ \text{J K}^{-1})(298.15\ \text{K})}{\sqrt{2}(101325\ \text{Pa})L\pi(3.67 \times 10^{-10}\ \text{m})^2} = 6.79 \times 10^{-6}\ \text{cm} .$$

Since $\lambda \propto \frac{1}{P}$, $\lambda(1\ \text{torr}) = 760\ \lambda(1\ \text{atm})$ and

$\lambda(1\ \text{torr}) = 5.16 \times 10^{-3}$ cm, $\lambda(10^{-3}\ \text{torr}) = 5.16$ cm .

9.5 Calculate the average velocities and average relative velocities (A-A, B-B, and A-B) for a mixture of CO and H_2 at STP.

From Eqs. (9.2) and (9.11), $\bar{v} = \left(\frac{8RT}{\pi M}\right)^{1/2}$ and

$\langle v_{ab} \rangle = \left(\frac{8RT}{\pi(L\mu)}\right)^{1/2}$ where $L\mu = \frac{M_A M_B}{M_A + M_B}$. At STP,

$$\bar{v}_{(CO)} = \left(\frac{8(8.3145 \text{ J K}^{-1})(273.15 \text{ K})}{\pi(0.02801 \text{ kg})} \right)^{1/2} = 4.54 \times 10^4 \text{ cm s}^{-1} .$$

Also, $\bar{v}_{(H_2)} = 1.69 \times 10^5 \text{ cm s}^{-1}$. The molar reduced masses are

$L\mu(H_2, CO) = 1.881$ g , $L\mu(H_2, H_2) = 1.008$ g , and

$L\mu(CO, CO) = 14.005$ g . Thus

$$\langle v_{H_2, CO} \rangle = \left(\frac{8(8.3145)(273.15)}{\pi(0.001881)} \right)^{1/2} = 1.753 \times 10^5 \text{ cm s}^{-1} .$$ Also

$\langle v_{H_2, H_2} \rangle = 2.395 \times 10^5 \text{ cm s}^{-1}$ and $\langle v_{CO, CO} \rangle = 6.426 \times 10^4 \text{ cm s}^{-1}$.

9.6 For an equimolar mixture of H_2 and CO at STP, calculate the total H_2-H_2 CO-CO, and H_2-CO collisions per unit volume per second. (You may use the results of Problem 9.5.) Why is the last number so much larger than the first two?

From Eqs. (9.14) and (9.15), $Z_{AA} = \dfrac{\pi \bar{v}_A \sigma_A^2 (n_A^*)^2}{\sqrt{2}}$ and

$Z_{AB} = \pi \langle v_{AB} \rangle \sigma_{AB}^2 \, n_A^* \, n_B^*$, where $\sigma_{AB} = \frac{1}{2}(\sigma_A + \sigma_B)$. n^* is

given by the ideal gas law,

$$n_A^* = n_B^* = \frac{P_A L}{RT} = \frac{1}{2} \frac{(101325 \text{ Pa}) \, L}{(8.3145 \text{ J K}^{-1})(273.15 \text{ K})} = 1.344 \times 10^{25} \text{ m}^{-3} .$$

Using data from Table 1.7 for σ_{H_2} and σ_{CO} , and average and

relative velocities from problem 9.5,

$Z_{H_2,H_2} = 5.593 \times 10^{34} \text{ m}^{-3} \text{ s}^{-1}$ and $Z_{CO,CO} = 2.580 \times 10^{34} \text{ m}^{-3} \text{ s}^{-1}$.

From Eq. (9.12), $\sigma_{H_2,CO} = 0.3317 \times 10^{-9}$ m , thus

$$Z_{H_2,CO} = 1.094 \times 10^{35} \text{ m}^{-3} \text{ s}^{-1} .$$

9.7 Into a 1-m^3 container at 300 K are placed 20 moles of CH_4 and 5 moles of H_2. Calculate the number of H_2-CH_4 collisions in the container which occur in one second.

From Eq. (9.15), $Z_{AB} = \pi \langle v_{AB} \rangle \sigma_{AB}^2 n_A^* n_B^*$.

$\sigma_{H_2, CH_4} = \frac{1}{2}(\sigma_{H_2} + \sigma_{CH_4}) = 0.3344 \times 10^{-9}$ m . $\langle v_{ab} \rangle$ is given by

$\langle v_{ab} \rangle = \left(\frac{8RT}{\pi(L\mu)}\right)^{1/2}$ where

$$(L\mu)_{H_2, CH_4} = \frac{(2.016)(16.04)}{(2.016 + 16.04)} = 0.001791 \text{ kg} .$$

Thus at T = 300 K, $\langle v_{H_2,CH_4} \rangle = 1883.2 \text{ m s}^{-1}$.

$n_{H_2}^* = \frac{N_{H_2}}{V} = \frac{5(6.02214 \times 10^{23})}{1 \text{ m}^3} = 3.011 \times 10^{24} \text{ m}^{-3}$. Similarly,

$n_{CO}^* = 1.204 \times 10^{25} \text{ m}^{-3}$. Plugging into Eq. (9.15),

$$Z_{H_2,CH_4} = 2.3984 \times 10^{34} \text{ m}^{-3} \text{ s}^{-1} .$$

9.8 For N_2 gas at 298 K and 1 atm, $\bar{v} = 454.2 \text{ ms}^{-1}$, $\lambda = 6 \times 10^{-8}$ m, $z = 7.57 \times 10^9 \text{ s}^{-1}$. Calculate the rms mean distance (x) traveled by an N_2 molecule in one minute under these conditions.

From Eq. (9.24),

$$(\Delta x)_{rms} = \sqrt{zt}\ \lambda = ((7.57 \times 10^9 \text{ s}^{-1})(60 \text{ s}))^{1/2}(6 \times 10^{-6} \text{ cm})$$

$$(\Delta x)_{rms} = 4.04 \text{ cm} .$$

9.9 An indecisive professor sets out toward the dean's office (500 paces away) to ask for a raise. After each step he stops and flips a coin to decide whether to continue or return (this takes about 4 seconds). What is the probability that he will reach the dean's office in 8 hours?

Use Eq. (9.25) to find the probability that the professor will be at the dean's office in exactly 8 hours:

$W(m, N) = \frac{2}{\sqrt{2\pi N}} \exp\left(-\frac{m^2}{2N}\right)$. Here,

$N = \#$ of steps $= \frac{(8 \text{ hrs})(3600 \text{ s/hr})}{(4 \text{ s/step})} = 7200$ steps and $m = 500$.

Then $W(500, 7200) = 2.71 \times 10^{-10}$.

9.10 Compare the predictions of Eqs. (9.18) and (9.25), the latter being an approximation of the former, that a random walk of 50 steps will end on the 10th step. What is the probability that it will end on the 9th step?

From Eq. (9.18), $W(m, N) = \left(\frac{1}{2}\right)^N C_p^N$ where $C_p^N = \frac{N!}{p!\ (N - p)!}$

and $p = \frac{N + m}{2}$. In the present case we have $m = 10$, $N = 50$, and $p = 30$ so that $W(10, 50) = 4.1859 \times 10^{-2}$. The Gaussian approximation is: $W(m, N) \sim \frac{2}{\sqrt{2\pi N}} \exp\left(-\frac{m^2}{2N}\right)$ so that

$W(10, 50) \sim 4.1511 \times 10^{-2}$. $W(9, 50) = 0$ because the walk couldn't end on an odd step after an even number of steps .

9.11 For a random walk of 1000 steps, with a step length of 0.125, calculate the probability that the walk will end between $x = 5$ and $x = 10$.

The probability that the walk will end between x = 5 and 10 is approximated by the integral:

$$\int_5^{10} P(x)dx = \frac{1}{(2\pi\sigma^2)^{1/2}} \int_5^{10} \exp\left(-\frac{x^2}{2\sigma^2}\right)dx \quad \text{where } \sigma = (N\lambda^2)^{1/2} .$$

Here we have N = 1000 and λ = 0.125 so that σ = 3.9528 .

Numerical integration using Simpson's rule with a step size of 0.5 gives: $\int_5^{10} \exp\left(-\frac{x^2}{31.25}\right)dx = 0.96353$

and $\int_5^{10} P(x)dx = 9.725 \times 10^{-2} = 9.72\%$.

9.12 A drunken sailor, leaning on a lamp post, begins a random walk and takes 100 steps before falling down. 20 paces down the street is an alcoholic rehabilitation center. What is the probability that he is in the center when he falls down? Assume that all distances $x = +20$ or greater are within the rehab center.

The probability that the drunken sailor will end up in the center is:

$$\int_{20}^{100} P(x)dx = \frac{1}{(2\pi\sigma^2)^{1/2}} \int_{20}^{100} \exp\left(-\frac{x^2}{2\sigma^2}\right)dx \quad \text{where} \quad \sigma = (N\lambda^2)^{1/2} .$$

Here we have N = 100 and λ = 1 so that σ = 10 and:

$\int_{20}^{100} P(x)dx = \frac{1}{\sqrt{200\pi}} \int_{20}^{100} \exp\left(-\frac{x^2}{200}\right)dx$. Numerical integration using Simpson's rule with a step size of 5 gives:

$\int_{20}^{100} \exp\left(-\frac{x^2}{200}\right)dx = 0.5715$ and $\int_{20}^{100} P(x)dx = 0.0228 = 2.28\%$.

9.13 The random-walk arguments, which imply that the rms length of a polymer chain is $\sqrt{2N\lambda^2}$, presume that the links are universal. For N links with a fixed angle ϕ, the result is:

$$\langle r^2 \rangle \cong N\lambda^2 \frac{1 - \cos\phi}{1 + \cos\phi}$$

Estimate the rms average length of a polyethylene chain with molecular weight 10,000 assuming a C-C bond length of 1.54 Å, and the tetrahedral angle.

With $N = \dfrac{10000 \text{ g}}{14 \text{ g/seg.}} = 714$, $\langle r^2 \rangle \cong 714(1.54 \text{ Å})^2 \dfrac{(1 - \cos 109.5)}{(1 + \cos 109.5)}$

or $\langle r^2 \rangle = 3386.6 \text{ Å}^2$. Then $\sqrt{\langle r^2 \rangle} = 58 \text{ Å}$.

9.14 Show that, for a random walk on a surface, the probability that in time t the distance is between r and $r + dr$ is:

$$W(r, t)\, dr = (1/2Dt)e^{-r^2/4Dt} r\, dr$$

where $D = z\lambda^2/2$, and z is the number of steps per unit time.

For a random walk in two dimensions:

$$W(x, y, t) = W(x, t)\; W(y, t) .$$

With $r^2 = x^2 + y^2$: $W(x, y, t)dx\, dy = \dfrac{1}{4\pi Dt} \exp\left(-\dfrac{r^2}{4Dt}\right)dx\, dy$.

Now $dx\, dy = r\, dr\, d\Phi$. Integrating over $\Phi(0 \text{ to } 2\pi)$:

$$W(r, t) = \frac{1}{2Dt} \exp\left(-\frac{r^2}{4Dt}\right)r\, dr .$$

9.15 Using the result of the previous problem for a random walk on a surface, calculate the average distance traveled in time t.

$\langle r \rangle = \displaystyle\int_0^{\infty} \frac{r^2}{2Dt} \exp\left(-\frac{r^2}{4Dt}\right)dr$. From the Table of Integrals:

$$\langle r \rangle = \frac{1}{2Dt}(Dt)\sqrt{4\pi Dt} = \sqrt{\pi Dt} .$$

9.16 Using the result of problem 9.14 for a random walk on a surface, calculate the rms distance traveled in time *t*.

$$r_{rms} = \langle r^2\rangle^{1/2} = \left[\int_0^\infty \frac{r^3}{2Dt}\exp\left(-\frac{r^2}{4Dt}\right)dr\right]^{1/2}$$

. From the Table of Integrals: $\langle r^2\rangle = \frac{1}{2Dt}\left(\frac{1}{2}\right)(4Dt)^2 = 4Dt$ and $r_{rms} = \sqrt{4Dt}$.

9.17 Using the result of problem 9.14 for a random walk on a surface, derive a formula for the probability that the walk will end between r_1 and r_2 after time *t*. Use this result, for the case $D = 6 \times 10^{-5}$ cm^2/sec, to calculate the probability that the walk will go farther than 0.5, 1.0, 1.5, and 2 cm in one hour.

$$P(r_1 \text{ to } r_2) = \int_{r_1}^{r_2} W(r, t)dr = \int_{r_1}^{r_2}\frac{r}{2Dt}\exp\left(-\frac{r^2}{4Dt}\right)dr$$

. This may be integrated directly: $P(r_1 \text{ to } r_2) = -\exp\left(-\frac{r^2}{4Dt}\right)\Big|_{r_1}^{r_2}$ and

$$P(r_1 \text{ to } r_2) = \exp\left(-\frac{r_1^2}{4Dt}\right) - \exp\left(-\frac{r_2^2}{4Dt}\right)$$

. If $r_2 = \infty$, then:

$$P(r > r_1) = \exp\left(-\frac{r_1^2}{4Dt}\right)$$

. With $D = 6 \times 10^{-5}$ cm^2 s^{-1} and $t = 3600$ s , we find: $P(r > r_1) = (75\%, 31\%, 7\%, 1\%)$ for

$$r_1 = (0.5, 1.0, 1.5, 2.0) \text{ cm} .$$

9.18 For a 3-dimensional random walk, derive a formula for the average distance traveled: $\langle r\rangle$. What is the ratio of the rms average to the average distances? Compare this to the result of Chapter 1 for the ratio of the rms average and average speeds of a molecule in a gas.

In three dimensions: $\langle r\rangle = \int_0^\infty \frac{4\pi r^3}{(4\pi Dt)^{3/2}}\exp\left(-\frac{r^2}{4Dt}\right)dr$. From the Table of Integrals: $\langle r\rangle = \left(\frac{4\pi}{(4\pi Dt)^{3/2}}\right)\frac{(4Dt)^2}{2} = 4\sqrt{\frac{Dt}{\pi}}$.

$r_{rms} = \sqrt{6Dt}$ so that the ratio is: $\frac{\langle r^2\rangle^{1/2}}{\langle r\rangle} = \sqrt{\frac{3\pi}{8}} = 1.0854$.

9.19 The diffusion constant of water (liquid) at 25°C is 2.26×10^{-5} cm^2 s^{-1}. How long would it take a molecule of water to travel across a container 1 cm wide? This can be estimated as the time required to have an rms displacement (Δx) of 1 cm.

Rearranging Eq. (9.28),

$$t = \frac{(x_{rms})^2}{2D} = \frac{(1\ cm)^2}{2(2.26 \times 10^{-5}\ cm^2\ s^{-1})} = 22{,}123.9\ s = 6.15\ hr\ .$$

9.20 Tobacco mosaic virus has a diffusion coefficient (water, 20°C) of 5.3×10^{-8} cm^2 s^{-1}. What times would be required for this material to have rms displacements of 1 mm and 2 mm?

$t = \frac{(x_{rms})^2}{2D}$. For $x_{rms} = 0.1$ cm:

$$t(1\ mm) = \frac{(0.1\ cm)^2}{2(5.3 \times 10^{-8}\ cm^2\ s^{-1})} = 94{,}340\ s = 26.2\ hr\ .$$

t is proportional to x_{rms}^2 , so that:

$$t(2\ mm) = 4t(1\ mm) = 104.8\ hr\ .$$

9.21 Calculate the diffusion coefficient for the molecules in air (assume $\overline{M} = 28.8$ g, $\sigma = 3.67 \times 10^{-8}$ cm) when $P = 1$ atm and $P = 1$ torr for $T = 300$ K and 1000 K.

From Eq. (9.37), $D = 0.599\ \lambda\overline{v}$ where $\overline{v} = \sqrt{\frac{8RT}{\pi M}}$. Substituting, $\overline{v}(300\ K) = 469.6\ m\ s^{-1}$ and $\overline{v}(1000\ K) = 857.4\ m\ s^{-1}$. Using Eq. (9.9c) for λ,

$$\lambda(1\ atm,\ 300\ K) = \frac{RT}{\sqrt{2}PL\pi\sigma^2} = \frac{(8.3145\ J\ K^{-1})(300\ K)}{\sqrt{2}(101325\ Pa)L\pi(3.67 \times 10^{-10})^2}$$

$$\lambda(1\ atm,\ 300\ K) = 6.831 \times 10^{-8}\ m\ .$$

Similarly, $\lambda(1\ torr,\ 300\ K) = 5.192 \times 10^{-5}\ m$,

$\lambda(1\ atm,\ 1000\ K) = 2.277 \times 10^{-7}\ m$,

$$\lambda(1 \text{ torr}, 1000 \text{ K}) = 1.731 \times 10^{-4} \text{ m} .$$

Thus $$D(1 \text{ atm}, 300 \text{ K}) = 0.192 \text{ cm}^2 \text{ s}^{-1} ,$$

$$D(1 \text{ torr}, 300 \text{ K}) = 146 \text{ cm}^2 \text{ s}^{-1} ,$$

$$D(1 \text{ atm}, 1000 \text{ K}) = 1.17 \text{ cm}^2 \text{ s}^{-1} ,$$

$$D(1 \text{ torr}, 1000 \text{ K}) = 889 \text{ cm}^2 \text{ s}^{-1} .$$

9.22 The diffusion curves of Fig. 9.7 can be used to answer this question. If a solution of sucrose in water ($C_0 = 1$) is in contact with pure water, how long would it take for the concentration at a point 0.18 cm into the water to reach 0.1?

From Figure 9.7 , $\frac{C}{C_0} = 0.1$ at $x = 0.18$ when $Dt = 0.01$. If $D = 0.4586 \times 10^{-5} \text{ cm}^2 \text{ s}^{-1}$ (Table 9.1), then $t = 2181 \text{ s} = 0.6 \text{ hr}$.

9.23 A solvent is layered over a solution ($C_0 = 1$). The diffusion coefficient of the solute is $2 \times 10^{-5} \text{ cm}^2 \text{ s}^{-1}$. After 24 hours, what will be the concentration 1.7 cm into the solution or solvent?

From Eq. (9.38), $C(x, t) = C_0\left\{\frac{1}{2}\left[1 - \frac{2}{\sqrt{\pi}}\int_0^{\xi} e^{-y^2} dy\right]\right\}$ where $\xi = \frac{x}{\sqrt{4Dt}}$. Using the error function to solve the integral, $\xi_{solution} = -0.65$. Similarly, $\xi_{solvent} = 0.65$. Using Simpson's rule, Eq. (AI.12), with $n = \frac{0.65}{2} = 0.325$:

$$\int_0^{0.65} e^{-y^2} dy = \frac{0.325}{3} [1 + 3.599 + 0.655] = 0.569 .$$

Thus, for the solution: $C(-1.7 \text{ cm}, 24 \text{ hr}) = 0.82$. For the solvent: $C(1.7 \text{ cm}, 24 \text{ hr}) = 0.18$.

9.24 Hydrogen is in an iron container at 500°C. The diffusion coefficient for H_2 in iron is 1.5×10^{-5} cm^2 s^{-1}. If the container is a cylinder with radius 100 cm, height 1000 cm, and wall thickness 1 cm, how long would it take for half of the hydrogen to escape?

Fick's first law states: $\frac{1}{A}\frac{dn}{dt} = -D\frac{dC}{dx}$. Assume the concentration inside the pipe to be uniform and outside the pipe to be zero. Then the concentration gradient at steady state is $\frac{dC}{dx} = \frac{C}{\Delta x}$. Since $n = V_C$, where V is the internal volume of the pipe, then $\frac{V}{A}\frac{dC}{dt} = -\frac{DC}{\Delta x}$ or $\frac{dC}{C} = -\frac{DA}{V\Delta x}dt$. Integrating from C_0 to C and from 0 to t gives $\ln\frac{C}{C_0} = -\frac{DA}{V\Delta x}t$ or $C = C_0\exp\left(-\frac{DAt}{V\Delta x}\right)$. When $C = \frac{C_0}{2}$, $t = -\frac{V\Delta x}{DA}\ln\left(\frac{1}{2}\right)$ or

$$t = \frac{\pi r^2 h\Delta x \ln(2)}{D(2\pi rh + 2\pi r^2)} = 2.1 \times 10^6 \text{ s} = 583.5 \text{ hrs} = 24.3 \text{ days}.$$

9.25 In constructing a flow viscometer, the tube diameter must be chosen to give reasonable flow rates, neither too fast nor too slow, for the range of viscosities to be measured. What would be the flow rate (cm^3/min) through a tube (length 5 cm, diameter 2 mm) for a liquid with a viscosity of 0.01 poise if the pressure head were 3 torr? (3 torr is a water head of approximately 4 cm.)

$\frac{\Delta V}{\Delta t} = \frac{\pi r^4 \Delta P}{8\eta l}$. With $\Delta P = 3$ torr $= 3999.6$ dyne cm^{-2}, $r = 0.1$ cm, $l = 5$ cm and $\eta = 0.01$ poise, we find

$$\frac{\Delta V}{\Delta t} = \frac{\pi(0.1 \text{ cm})^4(3999.6 \text{ dyne cm}^{-2})}{8(0.01 \text{ poise})(5 \text{ cm})}$$

$$\frac{\Delta V}{\Delta t} = 3.14 \text{ cm}^3 \text{ s}^{-1} = 188.5 \text{ cm}^3 \text{ min}^{-1}.$$

9.26 A 1.50-cm radius spherical aluminum ball (density 2.70 g/cm^3) is dropped through a fluid of density 1.26 g/cm^3. Its terminal velocity was measured as 15.1 cm/s. What is the viscosity of the fluid?

From Eq. (9.44),

$$\eta = \frac{2r^2(\rho - \rho_0)g}{9\ v_S} = \frac{2(1.50\ \text{cm})(2.7 - 1.96)\ \text{g cm}^{-3})(980\ \text{cm s}^{-2})}{9(15.1\ \text{cm s}^{-1})}$$

$$\eta = 46.7\ \text{poise}\ .$$

9.27 The biological macromolecule lactalbumin has a diffusion coefficient in water (20°C) of 1.06 × 10^{-6}cm^2/s. Assuming the molecule to be spherical, calculate its radius using the Stokes-Einstein law.

Rearrange the Stokes - Einstein law to

$$r = \frac{kT}{6\pi\eta D} = \frac{(1.38 \times 10^{-23}\ \text{J K}^{-1})(293.15\ \text{K})}{6\pi(1.005 \times 10^{-3}\ \text{kg m}^{-1}\ \text{s}^{-1})(1.06 \times 10^{-10}\ \text{m}^2\ \text{s}^{-1})}$$

$$r = 2.015 \times 10^{-9}\ \text{m} = 20 \times 10^{-8}\ \text{cm}\ .$$

9.28 Estimate the diffusion coefficient of sucrose in water at 50°C from its diffusion constant at 20°C. (Data: Tables 9.1 and 9.2.)

Using Eq. (9.47) at 20°C for sucrose in H_2O,

$$\left(\frac{D\eta}{T}\right)_{20°C} = \frac{(0.4568 \times 10^{-5}\ \text{cm}^2\ \text{s}^{-1})(10.05 \times 10^{-3}\ \text{poise})}{(293.15\ \text{K})}$$

$$\left(\frac{D\eta}{T}\right)_{20°C} = 1.566 \times 10^{-10}\ \text{g cm s}^{-2}\ \text{K}^{-1}\ .$$

This quantity is a constant so at 50°C,

$$D(50°C) = \frac{323.15\ \text{K}}{5.494 \times 10^{-3}\ \text{poise}}\ (1.566 \times 10^{-10}\ \text{g cm s}^{-2}\ \text{K}^{-1})$$

$$D(50°C) = 9.211 \times 10^{-6}\ \text{cm}^2\ \text{s}^{-1}\ .$$

9.29 Chlorine and ethylene (C_2H_4) have similar diameters (to judge from their van der Waals b, Table 1.1) but greatly different masses. Which will have the higher viscosity, and by how much?

From Eq. (9.51), $\eta = \dfrac{M\bar{v}}{2\sqrt{2}\pi\sigma^2 L}$. Assuming $\sigma^2(Cl_2) = \sigma^2(C_2H_4)$,

then $\dfrac{\eta(Cl_2)}{\eta(C_2H_4)} = \dfrac{(M\bar{v})_{Cl_2}}{(M\bar{v})_{C_2H_4}}$. From Eq. (9.2), $\bar{v} = \sqrt{\dfrac{8RT}{\pi M}}$,

$$\frac{\eta(Cl_2)}{\eta(C_2H_4)} = \left(\frac{M_{Cl_2}}{M_{C_2H_4}}\right)^{1/2} = \left(\frac{70.91}{28.05}\right)^{1/2} = 1.59 \ .$$

9.30 The viscosity of CO_2 at 1500 K is:

$$\eta = 505.2 \times 10^{-6} \text{ poise}$$

Estimate the molecular diameter (σ) and compare it to the value given in Table 1.7 [from $B(T)$ data]. (Use the simple formula, which neglects intermolecular forces.)

From Eq. (9.51), $\sigma = \left[\dfrac{M\bar{v}}{2\sqrt{2}\pi\eta L}\right]^{1/2}$.

$$\bar{v} \text{ is } \bar{v}_{CO_2}\text{, 1500 K} = \sqrt{\frac{8RT}{\pi M}} = \left(\frac{8(8.3145)(1500)}{\pi(44.01 \times 10^{-3})}\right)^{1/2} = 849.5 \text{ m s}^{-1} \ .$$

$$\text{Then } \sigma = \left[\frac{0.04401 \text{ kg}(849.5 \text{ m s}^{-1})}{2\sqrt{2}\pi(505.2 \times 10^{-7} \text{ kg m}^{-1}\text{s}^{-1})L}\right]^{1/2} = 3.72 \times 10^{-8} \text{ cm} \ .$$

9.31 Estimate the molecular diameter (σ) of CH_4 from each of the following:

van der Waals: $b = 42.8\ \text{cm}^3$

viscosity: $\eta = 1.116 \times 10^{-4}\ \text{g cm}^{-1}\ \text{s}^{-1}$ (at 300 K)

diffusion: $D = 0.189\ \text{cm}^2\ \text{s}^{-1}$ (at 273 K, 1 atm)

From Eq. (1.4),

$$\sigma_b = \left(\frac{3b}{2\pi L}\right)^{1/3} = \left(\frac{3(42.8\ \text{cm}^3)}{2\pi L}\right)^{1/3} = 3.24 \times 10^{-8}\ \text{cm}\ .$$

From Eq. (9.51), $\sigma_\eta = \left(\dfrac{M\bar{v}}{2\sqrt{2}\pi\eta L}\right)^{1/2}$. Since $\bar{v} = \sqrt{\dfrac{8RT}{\pi M}}$, then

$$\bar{v} = \left(\frac{8(8.3145)(300)}{\pi(0.01643)}\right)^{1/2} = 692.2\ \text{m s}^{-1}\ \text{and}\ \sigma_\eta = 4.11 \times 10^{-8}\ \text{cm}\ .$$

For the diffusion data, we use Eqs. (9.37) and (9.9c) rearranged to give

$$\sigma_d = \left(\frac{0.599\ RT\bar{v}}{\sqrt{2}\pi PLD}\right)^{1/2} = \left(\frac{0.599(8.3145)(273)(600.2)}{\sqrt{2}\pi(101325)(0.189 \times 10^{-4})}\right)^{1/2}$$

$$\sigma_d = 3.99 \times 10^{-10}\ \text{m} = 3.99 \times 10^{-8}\ \text{cm}\ .$$

9.32 An experimental study of viscosities of ammonia (gas) in the range 300–400 K gave a Sutherland constant $k_s = 202.7 \times 10^{-7}\ \text{p K}^{-1/2}$. Estimate the collision diameter of ammonia from this datum.

From Eq. (9.55), $\sigma = \left(\dfrac{(RM)^{1/2}}{\pi^{3/2}k_s L}\right)^{1/2}$. Substituting,

$$\sigma = \left(\frac{(8.3145 \times 0.01703)^{1/2}}{\pi^{3/2}L(20.27 \times 10^{-7})}\right)^{1/2} = 2.353 \times 10^{-10}\ \text{m}$$

$$\sigma = 2.353 \times 10^{-8}\ \text{cm}\ .$$

9.33 Use the data below for viscosity of Ar to calculate the Sutherland constants. Then estimate the parameters for the Sutherland potential.

T	η/μp
100	83.9
200	153.4
300	227.0
800	462.1

Rearrange Eq. (9.53) to $\frac{\sqrt{T}}{\eta} = \frac{1}{k_S} + \frac{S}{k_S}\left(\frac{1}{T}\right)$. We now regress $\frac{\sqrt{T}}{\eta}$ vs. $\frac{1}{T}$ to find intercept $= \frac{1}{k_S} = 5.494 \times 10^4\ K^{1/2}\ p^{-1}$ and slope $= \frac{S}{k_S} = 6.595 \times 10^6\ K^{3/2}\ p^{-1}$. Thus $k_S = 1.82 \times 10^{-5}\ p\ K^{-1/2}$ and $S = 120.0\ K$. From Eq. (9.54), $\frac{\xi}{k} = \frac{S}{c} \cong \frac{S}{0.2} = 600\ K$. From Eq. (9.55),

$$\sigma = \left(\frac{(RM)^{1/2}}{\pi^{3/2}k_S L}\right)^{1/2} = \left(\frac{(8.3145\ J\ K^{-1})^{1/2}(0.03995\ kg)^{1/2}}{\pi^{3/2}L(1.82 \times 10^{-6}\ kg\ m^{-1}\ s^{-1}\ K^{-1/2})}\right)^{1/2}$$

$$\sigma = 3.07 \times 10^{-10}\ m\ .$$

9.34 Estimate the viscosity of a solution of polystyrene ($\overline{M} = 1 \times 10^6$) in cyclohexane at 35°C, if the concentration is 20 mg/cm^3.

Using data from Table 9.3,

$$[\eta] = KM^{\alpha} = (8.1 \times 10^{-2}\ cm^3\ g^{-1})(10^6)^{0.5} = 81\ cm^3\ g^{-1}\ .$$

$$\eta_{sp} = C_m[\eta] = (0.02\ g\ cm^{-3})(81\ cm^3\ g^{-1}) = 1.62\ .$$

Since $\eta = \eta_0(1 + \eta_{sp})$ and from Table 9.2, $\eta_0 = 7.5 \times 10^{-3}$ p,

thus $\eta = 20$ mp .

9.35 The molecular weight of polystyrene was determined by measuring the viscosity of its solutions in benzene and using the Mark-Houwink equation ($\alpha = 0.74$) and found to be 12,500. Calculate the number-average molecular weight (M_n).

The Mark - Hoowink equation is: $[\eta] = KM_V^{\alpha}$ where M_V is the viscosity - average molecular weight . The number average molecular weight is:

$$M_n = \frac{M_V}{[(1+\alpha)\Gamma(1+\alpha)]^{1/\alpha}} = \frac{12500}{[(1.74)\Gamma(1.74)]^{1/0.74}}$$

$$M_n = 6.6 \times 10^3 \text{ g mol}^{-1} .$$

9.36 Use the viscosity data below for a polystyrene sample in benzene (25°C, $\alpha = 0.74$) to calculate the viscosity-average and number-average molecular weights of the sample.

$c/(\text{mg/cm}^3)$	η/mp
0	6.04
2	6.41
5	6.98
10	8.02
20	10.38
50	19.69

With $\eta_{sp} = \dfrac{\eta - \eta_0}{\eta_0}$ and $[\eta] = \lim\limits_{c_m \to 0}\left(\dfrac{\eta_{sp}}{c_m}\right)$, we have

$$[\eta] = \lim_{c_m \to 0}\left\{\frac{\frac{\eta}{\eta_0} - 1}{c_m}\right\} .$$ Also , $[\eta] = KM_V^{\alpha}$, so that:

$$M_v = \left[\frac{1}{K}\lim_{c_m \to 0}\left\{\frac{\frac{\eta}{\eta_0} - 1}{c_m}\right\}\right]^{1/\alpha} .$$ Regress $\left\{\dfrac{\frac{\eta}{\eta_0} - 1}{c_m}\right\}$ vs. c_m to

find the intercept = $[\eta] = 0.298 \text{ cm}^3 \text{ mg}^{-1}$. Using

$K = 0.95 \times 10^{-2} \text{ cm}^3 \text{ g}^{-1}$ and $\alpha = 0.74$,

we find $M_V = 5.3 \times 10^4 \text{ g mol}^{-1}$.

$$M_n = \frac{M_V}{[(1.74)\Gamma(1.74)]^{1/0.74}} = \frac{5.3 \times 10^4 \text{ g mol}^{-1}}{[(1.74)(0.91682)]^{1/0.74}}$$

$$M_n = 2.8 \times 10^4 \text{ g mol}^{-1} .$$

9.37 Estimate the gravity sedimentation rate for rabbit papilloma virus in water (Table 9.1) assuming a buoyancy correction of 0.25.

Using data from Table 9.1 and Eq. (9.63),

$$\frac{dx}{dt} = \frac{MDg}{RT} \quad (b)$$

$$\frac{dx}{dt} = \frac{(4.7 \times 10^{7}\ g)(5.9 \times 10^{-8}\ cm^{2}\ s^{-1})(980\ cm\ s^{-2})(0.25)}{(8.3143 \times 10^{7}\ erg\ K^{-1})(293.15\ K)}$$

$$\frac{dx}{dt} = 2.8 \times 10^{-8}\ cm\ s^{-1} = 0.002\ cm/day\ .$$

9.38 In an ultracentrifuge with a speed of 60,000 rpm, the boundary of a solution (6 cm average distance from the axis) moved 5.1 mm in 3 hours. Calculate the sedimentation coefficient of the solute.

From Eq. (9.68), $s \equiv \frac{dx/dt}{\omega^{2}x}$. Approximating $\frac{dx}{dt} \cong \frac{\Delta x}{\Delta t}$,

$$\frac{dx}{dt} \cong \frac{0.51\ cm}{(3\ hr)(3600\ s\ hr^{-1})} = 4.72 \times 10^{-5}\ cm\ s^{-1}\ .$$

Since $\omega = 2\pi(60{,}000\ min^{-1})(1\ min/60\ s) = 2\pi(10^{3}\ s^{-1})$, then

$$s = \frac{4.72 \times 10^{-5}\ cm\ s^{-1}}{(2\pi \times 10^{3}\ s^{-1})^{2}(6\ cm)} = 1.99 \times 10^{-13}\ s\ .$$

9.39 Serum globulin has a sedimentation coefficient in water ($\rho_0 = 0.9982$ g/cm^3 at 20°C), $s = 7.1 \times 10^{-13}$ sec. Its diffusion constant (20°C) is 4.0×10^{-7} cm^2 s^{-1} and its partial specific volume is 0.75 cm^3/g. Calculate the molecular weight.

From Eq. (9.69),

$$M = \frac{RTs}{D(1 - \rho_0 \bar{v}_s)}$$

$$M = \frac{(8.3143 \times 10^{7}\ erg\ K^{-1})(293.15\ K)(7.1 \times 10^{-13}\ s^{-1})}{(4.0 \times 10^{-7}\ cm^{2}\ s^{-1})(1 - (0.9982)(0.75))}$$

$$M = 1.72 \times 10^{5}\ g\ .$$

9.40 (a) Calculate the sedimentation coefficient for sucrose ($C_{12}H_{22}O_{11}$) (partial specific volume 0.630 cm^3/g) in water at 20°C (ρ_0 = 0.9982 g/cm^3). (Data: Table 9.1.)
(b) What angular velocity (rpm) would be required to obtain a sedimentation rate of 1 mm/hour if the radius is 5 cm?

a) $b = (1 - \bar{v}_s\rho_0) = (1 - (0.630)(0.9982)) = 0.37$.

$$s = \frac{MDb}{RT} = \frac{(342.3 \text{ g})(0.4586 \times 10^{-5} \text{ cm}^2 \text{ s}^{-1})(0.37)}{(8.3145 \times 10^7 \text{ erg K}^{-1})(293.15 \text{ K})}$$

$s = 2.38 \times 10^{-14}$ s .

b) From Eq. (9.68),

$$\omega = \sqrt{\frac{dx/dt}{sx}} = \left(\frac{(2.78 \times 10^{-5} \text{ cm s}^{-1})}{(2.38 \times 10^{-14} \text{ s})(5 \text{ cm})}\right)^{1/2}$$

$\omega = 1.53 \times 10^4 \text{ s}^{-1} = 1.46 \times 10^5$ rpm .

9.41 For a sedimentation experiment to be useful, the sedimentation must be fast compared to diffusional mixing. For a macromolecule with $D = 10^{-7}$ cm^2 s^{-1}, $M = 10^5$ g, and a buoyancy correction $b = 0.25$, calculate the width of the $\partial c/\partial x$ curve after 10 hours. If the boundary started 5 cm from the axis, how far would it move in 10 hours if ω = 4000 radians/sec?

From Eq. (9.67),

$$\delta x_{1/2} = [4Dt \ln 2]^{1/2} = [4(10^{-7} \text{ cm}^2 \text{ s}^{-1})(3.6 \times 10^4 \text{ s})\ln 2]^{1/2}$$

$\delta x_{1/2} = 1.0 \times 10^{-1}$ cm = 1 mm .

For the second part , $\frac{dx}{dt} \cong \frac{\Delta x}{\Delta t}$, and

$$\Delta x \cong \frac{MD\omega^2 xb\Delta t}{RT}$$

$$\Delta x \cong \frac{(10^5 \text{ g})(10^{-7} \text{ cm}^2 \text{ s}^{-1})(4000 \text{ s}^{-1})^2(5 \text{ cm})(0.25)(3.6 \times 10^4 \text{ s})}{(8.3145 \times 10^7 \text{ erg K}^{-1})(293.15 \text{ K})}$$

$\Delta x \cong 0.3$ cm = 3 mm .

9.42 An equilibrium sedimentation was carried out in an ultracentrifuge (80,000 rpm) in a 3-mm tube mounted with its bottom 1 cm from the rotation axis. The temperature was 23°C. The solute had a specific volume of 0.750 cm^3/g and the solvent was water (ρ_0 = 0.9951 g/cm^3 at 23°C). The solute concentration at the bottom of the tube was 4.2 times that at the top. Calculate the molecular weight.

Rearranging Eq. (9.70),

$$M = \frac{2RT\ \ln\left(\frac{c_2}{c_1}\right)}{(x_2^2 - x_1^2)(1 - \rho_0\overline{v}_s)\omega^2} =$$

$$\frac{2(8.3145 \times 10^7\ \text{erg K}^{-1})(296.15\ \text{K})\ \ln(4.2)}{((0.70)^2 - (1.00)^2)\text{cm}^2(1 - (0.9951)(0.75))(2\pi[1.33 \times 10^3\ \text{s}^{-1}])^2}$$

M = 7783 g .

9.43 (a) Show that, in a gravitational equilibrium sedimentation, the concentration ratio (c_1 at x_1, c_2 at x_2) is given by:

$$\frac{\ln(c_2/c_1)}{x_2 - x_1} = \frac{Mg(1 - \rho_0\overline{v}_s)}{RT}$$

(b) Calculate the concentration ratio between the top and bottom of a 10-cm tube containing urease in water ($M = 4.9 \times 10^5$ g/mol, $\overline{v}_s$ = 0.73 cm^3/g, ρ_0 = 0.9982 g/cm^3, t = 20°C).

a) At equilibrium the fluxes due to diffusion and sedimentation will cancel: $J_{sed} + J_{diff} = 0$. With $J_{diff} = - D\,\frac{dc}{dx}$ and $J_{sed} = c\,\frac{dx}{dt}$, we may use Eq. (9.63) for $\frac{dx}{dt}$ so that

$D\,\frac{dc}{dt} = \frac{cMDg}{RT}\,(1 - \overline{v}_s\rho_0)$. Then $\int_{c_1}^{c_2} \frac{dc}{c} = \int_{x_1}^{x_2} \frac{Mg}{RT}(1 - \overline{v}_s\rho_0)dx$

or $$\frac{\ln\left(\frac{c_2}{c_1}\right)}{(x_2 - x_1)} = \frac{Mg(1 - \overline{v}_s\rho_0)}{RT} .$$

b) Using the data of the problem statement,

$\ln\left(\frac{c_2}{c_1}\right) = 5.345 \times 10^{-2}$ and $\frac{c_2}{c_1} = 1.055$. Then $\frac{c_{top}}{c_{bottom}} = \frac{c_1}{c_2} = 0.95$.

10

Chemical Kinetics

10.1 What would be the units for the rate constant of a $\frac{3}{2}$-order reaction? Use concentrations in mol/dm^3, time in seconds.

Since $v = k[C]^{3/2}$, then $\frac{\text{mole}}{\text{dm}^3\ \text{s}}$ [=] $k\left[\frac{\text{mole}}{\text{dm}^3}\right]^{3/2}$, or

$$k\ [=]\ \text{mole}^{-1/2}\ \text{dm}^{3/2}\ \text{s}^{-1} .$$

10.2 The decomposition of dimethyl ether:

$$CH_3OCH_3 = CH_4 + CO + H_2$$

was studied by C. N. Hinshelwood and P. J. Askey [*Proc. Roy. Soc.* (London), **A115**, 215 (1927)] by measuring the time required for the total pressure to double. Use the data below to determine the order of this reaction.

Initial P/torr	t/s	Initial P/torr	t/s
28	1980	321	625
58	1500	394	590
150	900	422	508
171	824	509	465
261	670	586	484

Define an extent of reaction x such that $P_{CH_3OCH_3} = P_0 - x$,

$P_{CH_4} = P_{CO} = P_{H_2} = x$. Then $P = P_0 + 2x$ and when $P = 2\ P_0$,

$x = \frac{P_0}{2}$. Using Eq. (10.28) with $C_0 = \frac{P_0}{RT}$,

$t_{1/2} = \frac{(2^{n-1} - 1)(RT)^{n-1}}{(n - 1)P_0^{n-1}k}$. Taking ln on both sides and

rearranging, $\ln t_{1/2} = \ln\left\{\frac{(2^{n-1} - 1)(RT)^{n-1}}{(n - 1)k}\right\} - (n - 1) \ln P_0$.

Regressing $\ln t_{1/2}$ vs. $\ln P_0$, slope = $-(n - 1) = -0.5$ with

$r = -0.9960$. Then $n = 1.5$.

10.3 Use the data below for the decomposition of diacetylene at 1173 K [K. C. Hou and H. B. Palmer, *J. Phys. Chem.*, **69**, 858 (1965)] to determine the reaction order.

$10^7 C/(mol/cm^3)$	t/s	$10^7 C/(mol/cm^3)$	t/s
0.532	0	0.298	0.150
0.454	0.030	0.267	0.200
0.420	0.050	0.237	0.250
0.364	0.100		

Assuming $\frac{dC}{dt} = \frac{\Delta C}{\Delta t}$, then

$\bar{v} = -\frac{\Delta C}{\Delta t}$	$10^7 \bar{C}$
2.60×10^{-7}	0.493
1.70×10^{-7}	0.437
1.12×10^{-7}	0.392
1.32×10^{-7}	0.331
6.20×10^{-8}	0.283
6.00×10^{-8}	0.252

Since $\ln \bar{v} = \ln k + n \ln \bar{C}$, a plot of $\ln \bar{v}$ vs. $\ln \bar{C}$ should have slope = n. From linear regression n = 2.09 ≅ 2 with r = 0.944.

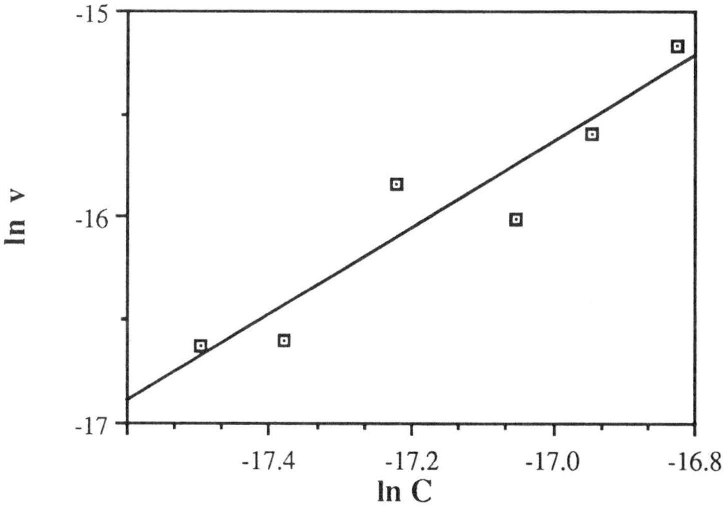

10.4 T. Y. Chin and R. E. Connich [*J. Phys. Chem.*, **63**, 1518 (1959)] measured the data below for the OH^--catalyzed reaction:

$$OCl^- + I^- = OI^- + Cl^-$$

Determine the rate law and rate constant.

$[OCl^-]$ (mol dm^{-3})	$[I^-]$ (mol dm^{-3})	$[OH^-]$ (mol dm^{-3})	Initial velocity (mol dm^{-3} s^{-1})
0.0017	0.0017	1.00	1.75×10^{-4}
0.0034	0.0017	1.00	3.50×10^{-4}
0.0017	0.0034	1.00	3.50×10^{-4}
0.0017	0.0017	0.50	3.50×10^{-4}

We assume the rate law has the form $v = k[OCl^-]^x[I^-]^y[OH^-]^z$ and the initial velocity is $v_0 = k[OCl^-]_0^x[I^-]_0^y[OH^-]_0^z$. From the first two sets of data we see that doubling $[OCl^-]_0$ doubles v_0 . Thus x = 1 . Combination of the first and third sets similarly tells us y = 1 . Finally, from the first and fourth sets, we see that halving $[OH^-]_0$ doubles v_0 , thus z = -1 .

Then $v = \frac{k[OCl^-][I^-]}{[OH^-]}$. We may determine k by plugging in any of the 4 sets of data: $k = 60.5\ s^{-1}$.

10.5 Use the data below for the partial pressure of N_2O_5 during a thermal decomposition at 45°C to determine the rate constant, assuming a first-order reaction.

t/min	P (N_2O_5)/torr
0	348.4
20	185.2
40	105.4
60	58.6
80	33.1
100	18.6
160	2.8

For a first-order decomposition, $\ln\left(\frac{P_0}{P}\right) = kt$ so that a plot of $\ln\left(\frac{P_0}{P}\right)$ vs. t should have slope k. Draw up the following table:

$\frac{P_0}{P}$	$\ln\left(\frac{P_0}{P}\right)$	t (min)
1	0	0
1.881	0.632	20
3.306	1.196	40
5.945	1.783	60
10.526	2.354	80
18.73	2.930	100
124.43	4.824	160

From linear regression we find $k = 2.99 \times 10^{-2}$ min^{-1} with $\sigma = 3.0 \times 10^{-4}$ min^{-1} and $r^2 = 0.9995$.

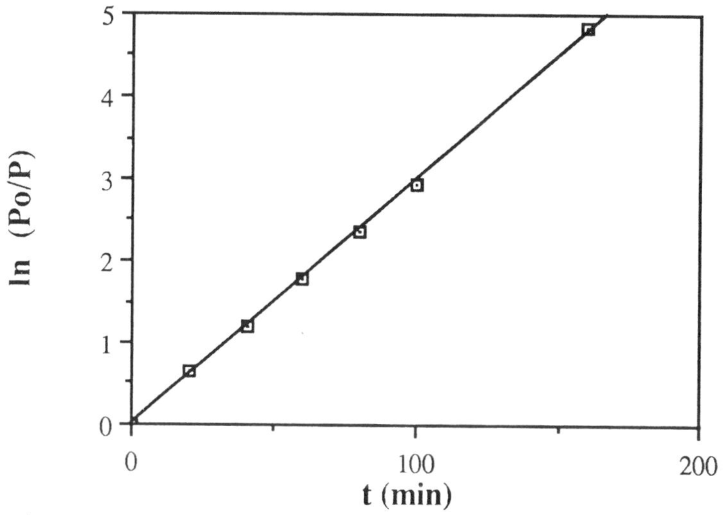

10.6 The reaction:

$$(CH_3)_3COOC(CH_3)_3 = 2CH_3COCH_3 + C_2H_6$$

was studied manometrically and found to be first-order. Use the data below to calculate the rate constant. (The measured pressures include 4.2 torr due to nitrogen that was present in the reaction container.)

t/min	P/torr	t/min	P/torr
0	173.5	12	244.4
2	187.3	14	254.4
3	193.4	15	259.2
5	205.3	17	268.7
6	211.3	18	273.9
8	222.9	20	282.0
9	228.6	21	286.8
11	239.8		

Introducing an extent of reaction x,

$P((CH_3)_3COOC(CH_3)_3) = P_0 - x$, $P(CH_3COCH_3) = 2x$ and $P(C_2H_6) = x$.

Then $P = P_0 + 2x$ and $x = \dfrac{(P - P_0)}{2}$. $\dfrac{dx}{dt} = k(P_0 - x)$ so that

$\displaystyle\int_0^x \frac{dx}{(P_0 - x)} = \int_0^t k\, dt$ and $\ln\left[\frac{(P_0 - x)}{P_0}\right] = -kt$ or

$\ln\left[\frac{3}{2} - \frac{P}{2P_0}\right] = -kt$. Subtracting 4.2 torr from the measured

pressure and regressing $\ln\left[\frac{3}{2} - \frac{P}{2P_0}\right]$ vs. t , we find

$k = 1.921 \times 10^{-2}\ min^{-1}$ with $\sigma = 5.6 \times 10^{-5}\ min^{-1}$ and $r = -0.99995$.

10.7 The first-order gas reaction:

$$SO_2Cl_2 = SO_2 + Cl_2$$

has $k = 2.20 \times 10^{-5}\ sec^{-1}$. What percentage of the SO_2Cl_2 would be decomposed after 5 hours?

Rearranging Eq. (10.11c) to $\dfrac{C}{C_0} = e^{-kt}$, then

$\dfrac{C}{C_0} = \exp(-[2.20 \times 10^{-5} s^{-1}][18{,}000\ s]) = 0.673$. The % decomposed

is $(1 - 0.673)100\% = 32.7\%$.

10.8 The data below represent instrument readings (R) vs. time for a first-order reaction. The readings vary linearly with extent of reaction. Analyze these data to calculate the rate constant.

t/s	R	t/s	R
.200	77.8	1.00	137.6
.400	98.4	1.20	145.3
.600	114.9	1.60	156
.800	127.7	2.00	162.7
		∞	173.0

If R varies linearly with the extent of reaction x, then:

$R = \alpha x + \beta$ where α and β are constants. $R(0) = R_0$ and $R(1) = R_\infty$, so that $R = (R_\infty - R_0)x + R_0$. With $x = \left(1 - \frac{C}{C_0}\right)$, for a first-order reaction: $\frac{dx}{dt} = k(1 - x)$.

Using $x = \left(\frac{R - R_0}{R_\infty - R_0}\right)$ and $\frac{dR}{dt} = k(R_\infty - R)$ we have

$\frac{d\ln(R_\infty - R)}{dt} = -k$ so that: $\ln\left(1 - \frac{R}{R_\infty}\right) = -kt$. Draw up the following table:

$\frac{R}{R_\infty}$	$\ln\left(1 - \frac{R}{R_\infty}\right)$	t (s)
0.450	-0.597	0.20
0.569	-0.841	0.40
0.664	-1.091	0.60
0.738	-1.340	0.80
0.795	-1.587	1.00
0.840	-1.832	1.20
0.902	-2.320	1.60
0.940	-2.821	2.00

Linear regression of $\ln\left(1 - \frac{R}{R_\infty}\right)$ vs. t gives $k = 1.234\ s^{-1}$ and $\sigma = 0.0018\ s^{-1}$.

10.9 A first-order reaction has a half-life of 26.2 minutes. At what time will the reaction be 90% complete?

From Eq. (10.16), $k = \frac{\ln 2}{t_{1/2}} = \frac{\ln 2}{1572\ s} = 4.41 \times 10^{-4}\ s^{-1}$.

Rearranging Eq. (10.11a),

$$t = \frac{1}{k} \ln\left(\frac{C_0}{C}\right) = \frac{1}{4.41 \times 10^{-4}\ s^{-1}} \ln\left(\frac{1}{0.1}\right) = 5221\ s = 87\ min\ .$$

10.10 If a first-order reaction is 20% complete in 20 minutes, at what time will it be 90% complete?

From Eq. (10.11a),

$$k = \frac{1}{t} \ln\left(\frac{C_0}{C}\right) = \frac{1}{1200\ s} \ln\left(\frac{1}{0.8}\right) = 1.86 \times 10^{-4}\ s^{-1}\ .$$

The reaction will be 90% complete at

$$t = \frac{1}{k} \ln\left(\frac{1}{0.1}\right) = 1.24 \times 10^{4}\ s = 206\ min\ .$$

10.11 A 0.0250-mol/dm^3 solution of oxalic acid in concentrated H_2SO_4 was studied by Lichty [*J. Phys. Chem.*, **11**, 225 (1907)] by titration with $KMnO_4$ (volume *V*, below). Assume first-order kinetics and calculate the rate constant.

t/min	V ($KMnO_4$)/cm^3	*t*/min	V ($KMnO_4$)/cm^3
0	11.45	600	4.79
120	9.63	900	2.97
240	8.11	1440	1.44
420	6.22		

$\ln V = \ln V_0 - kt$. We assume that the concentration of $KMnO_4$ is directly proportional to the concentration of oxalic acid. Regressing $\ln V_{KMnO_4}$ vs. t , we find

slope = $-k = -1.45 \times 10^{-3}\ min^{-1}$ or $k = 1.45 \times 10^{-3}$ min with

$\sigma = 2.07 \times 10^{-5}\ min^{-1}$ and $r = -0.9996$.

10.12   W. W. Heckert and E. Mack, Jr. [*J. Am. Chem. Sec.*, **51**, 2706 (1929)] measured the following for the decomposition of ethylene oxide:

$$CH_2-CH_2 = CH_4 + CO$$

(with O bridging the two CH_2 groups)

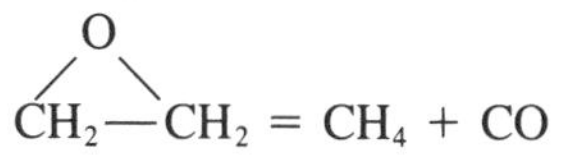

Assume that this reaction is first-order and calculate the rate constant. (If you use linear regression, compare the results with and without the $t = 0$ point. Can you explain the difference?)

t/min	P/torr	t/min	P/torr
0	115.30	10	129.10
6	122.91	11	130.57
7	124.51	12	132.02
8	126.18	13	133.49
9	127.53	18	140.16

Introducing an extent of reaction x: $\dfrac{d(P_0 - x)}{dt} = -k(P_0 - x)$.

Integrating and using x = P - P_0 and P_0 = 115.30 we find:

$\ln(2P_0 - P) = \ln P_0 - kt$.   **Draw up the following table:**

$2P_0$ - P	$\ln(2P_0 - P)$	t (min)
115.30	4.748	0
107.69	4.679	6
106.09	4.664	7
104.42	4.648	8
103.07	4.635	9
101.50	4.620	10
100.03	4.605	11
98.58	4.591	12
97.11	4.576	13
90.44	4.505	18

Including the point at t = 0: k = 1.37 x 10^{-2} min^{-1} ,

r^2 **= 0.9964 , and σ = 2.9 x 10^{-4} min^{-1} .   Excluding the**

point at t = 0: k = 1.45 x 10^{-2} min^{-1} , r^2 = 0.9998 ,

and σ = 7.2 x 10^{-5} min^{-1} .

10.13 F. G. Ciapetta and M. Kilpatrick [*J. Am. Chem. Soc.*, **70**, 639 (1948)] studied the hydration of isobutene in perchloric acid; the reaction was found to be pseudo-first-order. Use the dilatometer readings (h) below to calculate the rate constant.

t/min	h	t/min	h
0	18.84	25	16.86
5	18.34	30	16.56
10	17.91	35	16.27
15	17.53	40	16.00
20	17.19	∞	12.16

Letting $h = \lambda$ with $\lambda_0 = 18.84$ and $\lambda_\infty = 12.16$, and using Eq. (10.14), $\ln\left[\frac{\lambda_0 - \lambda_\infty}{\lambda - \lambda_\infty}\right] = kt$, we draw up the following table:

t (min)	$\ln\left[\frac{\lambda_0 - \lambda_\infty}{\lambda - \lambda_\infty}\right]$
5	0.0778
10	0.1499
15	0.2183
20	0.2837
25	0.3516
30	0.4175
35	0.4857
40	0.5536

From linear regression, we find $k = 1.35 \times 10^{-2}$ min^{-1} , with $\sigma = 5.47 \times 10^{-5}$ min^{-1} and $r = 0.99995$.

10.14 The HCl-catalyzed isomerization of *N*-chloroacetanilide to *p*-chloroacetanilide is pseudo-first-order. The reactant was destroyed with KI (to form I_2) followed by titration with sodium thiosulphate. Calculate the rate constant from the data below.

t/min	Titer/ml
0	24.5
15	18.1
30	13.2
45	9.7
60	7.1
75	5.2

From Eq. (10.11a), $\ln\left(\frac{C}{C_0}\right) = -kt$. Since C is proportional to the titer, a plot of $\ln\left(\frac{\text{Titer}}{(\text{Titer})_0}\right)$ vs. t should be linear with slope -k .

$\ln\left(\frac{\text{Titer}}{(\text{Titer})_0}\right)$	t (min)
-0.30	15
-0.62	30
-0.93	45
-1.24	60
-1.55	75

Regressing the data we find $k = 2.08 \times 10^{-2}\ \text{min}^{-1}$, with $\sigma = 7.70 \times 10^{-5}\ \text{min}^{-1}$ and $r = -0.99998$.

10.15 A second-order reaction, A + B $\longrightarrow$ . . ., with rate law $v = k[\text{A}][\text{B}]$, has $k = 5.21\ \text{dm}^3\ \text{mol}^{-1}\ \text{min}^{-1}$. If a reaction mixture has initial concentrations $a = 0.1$, $b = 0.2\ \text{mol/dm}^3$, what will be the concentrations of A and B after one minute?

From Eq. (10.25), $k = \frac{1}{t(b - a)} \ln\left[\frac{a(b - x)}{b(a - x)}\right]$ where a, b are the initial concentrations . Substituting,

$$5.21\ \text{dm}^3\ \text{mol}^{-1}\ \text{min}^{-1} = \frac{1}{1\ \text{min}(0.1\ \text{mol}\ \ \text{dm}^{-3})} \ln\left[\frac{0.100(0.200 - x)}{0.200(0.100 - x)}\right]$$

or $x = 0.059\ \text{mol dm}^{-3}$. After 1 min,

$[\text{A}] = a - x = 0.041\ \text{mol dm}^{-3}$ and $[\text{B}] = 0.141\ \text{mol dm}^{-3}$.

10.16 A second-order reaction, A + B $\rightarrow$ . . ., has a rate law $v = k[A][B]$ and $k = 1.23\ dm^3\ mol^{-1}\ sec^{-1}$. If A and B are mixed with equal initial concentrations of $0.365\ mol/dm^3$, at what time will the reaction be 90% complete?

Since [A] = [B] , we may use Eq. (10.18), $\frac{1}{C} = \frac{1}{C_0} + kt$. When the reaction is 90% complete,

$C = 0.1(0.365\ mol\ dm^{-3}) = 0.365\ mol\ dm^{-3}$. Substituting,

$$\frac{1}{0.0365\ mol\ dm^{-3}} = \frac{1}{0.365\ mol\ dm^{-3}} + t(1.23\ dm^3\ mol^{-1}\ s^{-1})$$

or $t = 20.0$ sec .

10.17 The data below represent instrument readings (R) vs. time for a second-order reaction (stoichiometry A + A or A + B with equal initial concentrations). The instrument reading varies linearly with extent of reaction. Analyze these data to calculate the rate constant, assuming an initial concentration of $0.1\ mol/dm^3$.

t/s	R	t/s	R
2.0	128.5	22.0	72.0
6.0	108.4	26.0	66.7
10.0	95.9	30.0	63.9
14.0	85.5	42.0	54.1
18.0	76.2	∞	24.5

Using Eq. (10.22) with $\lambda = R$: $\frac{1}{R - R_\infty} = \frac{1}{R_0 - R_\infty} + \frac{C_0 kt}{R_0 - R_\infty}$.

Regress $\frac{1}{R - R_\infty}$ vs. t to find slope = $\frac{C_0 k}{R_0 - R_\infty} = 5.962 \times 10^{-4}$

with $\sigma = 1.135 \times 10^{-5}$, intercept = $\frac{1}{R_0 - R_\infty} = 8.203 \times 10^{-3}$,

and $r = 0.9987$. With $C_0 = 0.1\ mol\ dm^{-3}$, we find:

$k = 0.727\ dm^3\ mol^{-1}\ s^{-1}$ and $\sigma(k) = 0.014\ dm^3\ mol^{-1}\ s^{-1}$.

10.18 The second-order reaction:

$$OH^- + CH_3COOC_2H_5 = CH_3COO^- + C_2H_5OH$$

was investigated by measuring solution conductance (L). Use the results below for initial concentrations of 0.01 mol/dm^3 (both reactants) to calculate the rate constant.

t/min	$\frac{L}{L_0 - L_\infty}$	t/min	$\frac{L}{L_0 - L_\infty}$
0	1.560	18	1.020
5	1.315	20	0.994
7	1.247	25	0.945
9	1.193	27	0.923
15	1.064	∞	0.560

Letting $\lambda = \frac{L}{L_0 - L_\infty}$ and using Eq. (10.22), $k = \frac{1}{C_0 t}\left\{\frac{\lambda_0 - \lambda}{\lambda - \lambda_\infty}\right\}$,

with $\lambda_0 = 1.560$ and $\lambda_\infty = 0.560$, we draw up the following table:

$\left(\frac{\lambda_0 - \lambda}{\lambda - \lambda_\infty}\right)$	t (min)
0.325	5
0.456	7
0.580	9
0.984	15
1.174	18
1.304	20
1.597	25
1.755	27

Regressing $\frac{1}{C_0}\left(\frac{\lambda_0 - \lambda}{\lambda - \lambda_\infty}\right)$ vs. t, we find

slope = k = 6.45 dm^3 mol^{-1} min^{-1} with

$\sigma = 5.30 \times 10^{-2}$ dm^3 mol^{-1} min^{-1} and $r = 0.99980$.

10.19 The dimerization of 1,3-butadiene at 326°C was followed by measuring the total pressure. Assume second-order, and calculate the rate constant.

t/min	P/torr
0	632.0
3.25	618.5
12.18	584.2
24.55	546.8
42.50	509.3
68.05	474.6

For $2A \rightarrow B$, we have $-\frac{dP_A}{dt} = kP_A^2$. Defining an extent of reaction x, $P_A = P_0 - 2x$. $P_B = x$ and $P = P_0 - x$. Then

$2\frac{dx}{dt} = k(P_0 - 2x)^2$. Integrating, $\int_0^x \frac{dx}{(P_0 - 2x)^2} = \int_0^t \frac{1}{2} k\, dt$ or

$\frac{1}{(P_0 - 2x)} - \frac{1}{P_0} = kt$. With $2x = 2(P_0 - P)$,

$\frac{1}{(2P - P_0)} - \frac{1}{P_0} = kt$. Regressing the l.h.s. vs. t, we find

slope = k = 2.32×10^{-5} torr^{-1} min^{-1} with

$\sigma = 2.06 \times 10^{-7}$ torr^{-1} min^{-1} and $r = 0.9998$.

10.20 Farkas, Lewin, and Bloch [*J. Am. Chem. Soc.*, **71**, 1988 (1949)] studied the reaction:

$$Br^- + ClO^- = BrO^- + Cl^-$$

in water at 25°C. With initial concentrations $[ClO^-] = 3.230 \times 10^{-3}$ mol/dm^3, $[Br^-] = 2.508 \times 10^{-3}$ mol/dm^3, the results were:

t/min	$[BrO^-]$/(mmol/dm^3)
0	0
3.65	0.560
7.65	0.953
15.05	1.420
26.00	1.800
47.60	2.117
90.60	2.367

Assume a second-order rate law and calculate the rate constant.

For a second order reaction: $kt = \frac{1}{b - a} \ln\left[\frac{a(b - x)}{b(a - x)}\right]$ where a and b are initial concentrations . A plot of the r.h.s. vs. t thus has slope k . With $[BrO^-] = x$, we may draw up the following table:

t (sec)	$\frac{1}{b - a} \ln\left[\frac{a(b - x)}{b(a - x)}\right]$
219	86.259
459	177.82
903	354.56
1560	623.25
2856	1098.5
5436	2158.8

Including the (0,0) point in a linear regression, one finds:

$k = 0.3956$ dm^3 mol^{-1} s^{-1} with $\sigma = 3.02 \times 10^{-3}$ dm^3 mol^{-1} s^{-1}

and $r^2 = 0.9997$.

10.21 F. M. Miller and M. L. Adams [*J. Am. Chem. Soc.*, **75**, 4599 (1953)] have measured the kinetics for the alkaline hydrolysis of *p*-nitrosodiumdimethylaniline (NSA). This is a second-order reaction. Use the data below to calculate the rate constant.

t/s	$\frac{[NSA]}{mol\ dm^{-3}}$	$\frac{[OH^-]}{mol\ dm^{-3}}$
0	0.0500	0.199
135	0.0413	0.190
380	0.0365	0.186
610	0.0325	0.182
945	0.0282	0.177
1880	0.0187	0.168

Eq. (10.25a) is applicable, with $[B] = [OH^-]$ and $[A] = [NSA]$:

$\ln \frac{[B]}{[A]} = \ln \frac{b}{a} + (b - a)kt$. Thus a plot of $\ln \frac{[B]}{[A]}$ vs. $(b - a)t$ should have slope = k .

t (sec)	(b - a)t (s mol dm^{-3})	$\ln \frac{[B]}{[A]}$
0	0	1.381
135	20.12	1.526
380	56.62	1.628
610	90.89	1.773
945	140.81	1.837
1880	280.12	2.195

Regression gives $k = 2.73 \times 10^{-3}\ dm^3\ mol^{-1}\ s^{-1}$ with $\sigma = 2.34 \times 10^{-4}\ dm^3\ mol^{-1}\ s^{-1}$ and $r = 0.9855$.

10.22 Derive the integrated rate law for the autocatalytic second-order reaction:

$$A \rightarrow P$$

$$\frac{-d[A]}{dt} = k[A][P]$$

with initial $[A] = a$, $[P] = p$.

Defining an extent of reaction x so that $[A] = a - x$ and $[P] = p + x$, then $\frac{dx}{dt} = k(a - x)(p + x)$. Integrating,

$$\int_0^x \frac{dx}{(a - x)(p + x)} = \int_0^t k\ dt \text{ or}$$

$$\frac{1}{(p + a)}\int_0^x\left[\frac{1}{(a - x)} + \frac{1}{(p + x)}\right] dx = \frac{1}{(p + a)}\left[-\ln(a - x) + \ln(p + x)\right]\Big|_0^x = kt$$

or $$\ln\left[\frac{a(p + x)}{p(a - x)}\right] = (p + a)kt \ .$$

10.23 If f is defined as the fraction of the reactant remaining in time t (for example, $f = \frac{1}{2}$ for the half-life), derive an equation for the "f-life" of a general nth-order reaction.

If f is the fraction of reactant remaining, the concentration at the f-life is $C = fC_0$. Substituting into Eq. (10.27),

$$\frac{1}{(fC_0)^{n-1}} = \frac{1}{C_0^{n-1}} + (n - 1)kt_f \text{ or } C_0^{n-1}(n - 1)kt_f = f^{(1-n)} - 1 \ .$$

10.24 Comparing two reactions with different activation energies, for which will the rate increase more rapidly with temperature?

$\frac{d \ln k}{dT} = \frac{E_a}{RT^2}$. At any given T, it is clear from inspection that $\frac{d \ln k}{dT}$ is proportional to E_a . Alternatively:

$\left(\frac{d \ln k(1)}{d \ln k(2)}\right) = \frac{E_a(1)}{E_a(2)}$. The reaction with the larger E_a will accelerate more rapidly with temperature .

10.25 It takes longer to cook foods at high altitude because water boils at a lower temperature. For example, at 8000 ft (2438 m) elevation, water boils at 92°C. The major reaction when eggs are boiled is the denaturization of the protein, which has an activation energy of about 40 kJ/mol. If a "three-minute egg" refers to a consistency obtained by boiling an egg for three minutes at sea level, how long would it take to make a three-minute egg at an elevation of 8000 ft?

The ratio of the rate constants for denaturization is:

$$\frac{k_1}{k_2} = \exp\left[-\frac{E_a}{R}\left(\frac{1}{T_1} - \frac{1}{T_2}\right)\right] .$$ Using T_1 = 92°C and T_2 = 100°C:

$$\frac{k(92°)}{k(100°)} = 0.754 .$$ Assuming the reaction is first order, we require that the quantity kt (termed the "severity") remain constant . Thus: $$\frac{t(92°)}{t(100°)} = \frac{k(100°)}{k(92°)} = 1.326 .$$

$$t(92°) = 1.326(3\text{ min}) = 4\text{ min} .$$

10.26 A commonly-used rule of thumb is that rate constants will double for each 10°C rise in temperature. Assuming it applies in the vicinity of room temperature, what does this rule suggest about typical activation energies?

Using the relation $$E_a = \frac{R\ln\left(\frac{k_1}{k_2}\right)}{\left(\frac{1}{T_2} - \frac{1}{T_1}\right)}$$ with $\frac{k_1}{k_2} = 2$, T_1 = 308 K and T_2 = 298 K , we find E_a = 53 kJ mol^{-1} .

10.27 Use the data in Table 10.2 to calculate the rate constant for the reaction:

$$C_2H_6 = 2\ CH_3$$

at 700 K.

From Table 10.2, A = 2.5 x 10^{17} s^{-1} and E_a = 384 kJ mol^{-1} .

From Eq. (10.41), $k = A\exp\left(-\frac{E_a}{RT}\right)$. At T = 700 K ,

$$k = 5.5 \times 10^{-12}\ s^{-1} .$$

10.28 Use the data (below) for the reaction:

$$N_2O_5 = N_2O_4 + \frac{1}{2}O_2$$

to calculate the Arrhenius parameters.

T/K	$k/(s^{-1})$	T/K	$k/(s^{-1})$
273.1	7.87×10^{-7}	313.1	2.47×10^{-4}
288.1	1.04×10^{-5}	318.1	4.98×10^{-4}
293.1	1.76×10^{-5}	323.1	7.59×10^{-4}
298.1	3.38×10^{-5}	328.1	1.50×10^{-3}
308.1	1.35×10^{-4}	338.1	4.87×10^{-3}

From Eq. (10.40), $\ln k = \ln A - \frac{E_a}{RT}$. A plot of $\ln k$ vs. $\frac{1}{T}$ should have slope = $-\frac{E_a}{R}$ and intercept = $\ln A$. Linear regression gives E_a = (101 ± 2) kJ mol^{-1} (90% confidence) and

$$A = 2.2 \times 10^{13} \text{ s}^{-1} .$$

10.29 Calculate the Arrhenius parameters for the reaction:

$$2\ NO + O_2 = 2\ NO_3$$

from the data:

T/K	$10^{-9}k/(cm^6\ mol^{-2}\ s^{-1})$
270	9.12
370	4.67
470	3.28
570	2.75
670	2.49

From Eq. (10.40), $\ln k = \ln A - \frac{E_a}{RT}$ Regressing $\ln k$ vs. $\frac{1}{T}$, we find E_a = (−4.96 ± 0.6) kJ mol^{-1} (90% confidence) and $A = 9.7 \times 10^{8}$ cm^{6} mol^{-2} s^{-2} with r = 0.99642 .

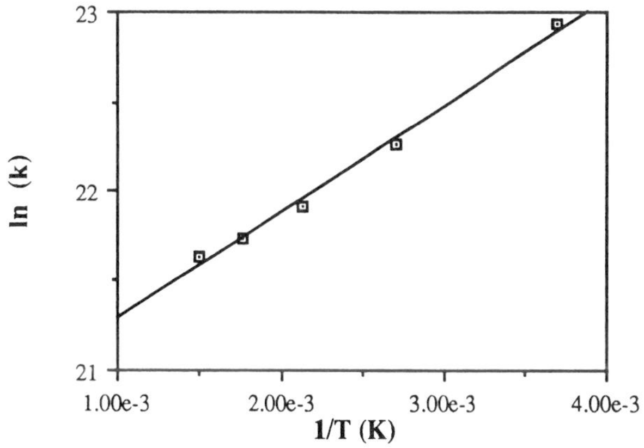

10.30 Use the rate constants (below) for the reaction:

$$2\ HI = H_2 + I_2$$

to calculate the Arrhenius parameters.

T/K	k/(dm^3 mol^{-1} s^{-1})	T/K	k/(dm^3 mol^{-1} s^{-1})
556	3.52×10^{-7}	683	5.12×10^{-4}
575	1.22×10^{-6}	700	1.16×10^{-3}
629	3.02×10^{-5}	716	2.50×10^{-3}
647	8.59×10^{-5}	781	3.95×10^{-2}
666	2.19×10^{-4}		

Using the same procedure as in problems 10.28 and 10.29,

slope $= -\frac{E_a}{R} = -2.23 \times 10^4$ with $\sigma = 206.7$ or

$E_a = (185.4 \pm 3.3)$ kJ mol^{-1} (90% confidence) and

intercept = ln A = 25.2 with $\sigma = 0.317$ or

$A = 8.8 \times 10^{10}$ dm^3 mol^{-1} s^{-1} . Also r = -0.9997 .

10.31 Use simple collision theory to calculate the rate constant of the reaction:

$$CH_3 + CH_3 = C_2H_6$$

assuming $p = 1$ and $E_{min} = 0$. Assume $\sigma = 4 \times 10^{-8}$ cm, $T = 500$ K. Compare your result to that given in Table 10.2.

$k = pLS_{AB}\left(\frac{8RT}{\pi L\mu}\right)^{1/2} \exp\left(-\frac{E_{min}}{RT}\right)$, where $S_{AB} = \pi\sigma_{AB}^2$ and

$L\mu = \frac{M_A M_B}{M_A + M_B}$. For this reaction, $\sigma_{AB} = \sigma = 4 \times 10^{-8}$ cm ,

$S_{AB} = 5.03 \times 10^{-15}$ cm^2 and $L\mu = \frac{(15\ g)^2}{30\ g} = 7.5$ g . Thus

$$k = (1)L(5.03 \times 10^{-15}\ cm^2)\left(\frac{8(8.3145 \times 10^7\ erg\ K^{-1})(500\ K)}{\pi(7.5\ g)}\right)^{1/2}$$

$$k = 3.59 \times 10^{14}\ mol^{-1}\ cm^3\ s^{-1}\ .$$

10.32 Estimate $\Delta H^{\ddagger}$ and $\Delta S^{\ddagger}$ for the reaction:

$$CH_3NC = CH_3CN$$

from the Arrhenius constants (Table 10.2) assuming $T = 300$ K.

From Table 10.2 , $A = 4 \times 10^{13}\ s^{-1}$ and $E_a = 160\ kJ\ mol^{-1}$. For a gas phase unimolecular reaction,

$$\Delta S^{\ddagger} = R \ln\left[\frac{Ah}{ek_bT}\right]$$

$$\Delta S^{\ddagger} = (8.3145\ J\ K^{-1}\ mol^{-1}) \times$$

$$\ln\left[\frac{(4 \times 10^{13}\ s^{-1})(6.63 \times 10^{-27}\ erg\ s)}{e(1.38 \times 10^{-16}\ erg\ K^{-1})(300\ K)}\right]$$

$\Delta S^{\ddagger} = 7.1\ J\ mol^{-1}\ K^{-1}$.

$\Delta H^{\ddagger} = E_a - RT$

$\Delta H^{\ddagger} = 160\ kJ\ mol^{-1} - (8.3143\ J\ K^{-1}\ mol^{-1})(300\ K) = 158\ kJ\ mol^{-1}$.

10.33 Estimate $\Delta H^{\ddagger}$ and $\Delta S^{\ddagger}$ for the reaction:

$$OH + H_2 \longrightarrow H_2O + H$$

from the Arrhenius constants (Table 10.2) assuming $T = 300$ K.

From Table 10.2, $A = 8 \times 10^{13}\ s^{-1}$ and $E_a = 42\ kJ\ mol^{-1}$. For a gas phase bimolecular reaction,

$$\Delta S^{\ddagger} = R \ln\left[\frac{AhC^{\ominus}}{e^2k_bT}\right]$$

$$\Delta S^{\ddagger} = (8.3145\ J\ K^{-1}\ mol^{-1}) \times$$

$$\ln\left[\frac{(8 \times 10^{13}\ s^{-1})(6.63 \times 10^{-27}\ erg\ s)(1\ mol\ cm^{-3})}{e^2(1.38 \times 10^{-16}\ erg\ K^{-1})(300\ K)}\right]$$

$\Delta S^{\ddagger} = 4.6\ J\ K^{-1}\ mol^{-1}$.

$$\Delta H^{\ddagger} = E_a - 2RT = 42\ \text{kJ mol}^{-1} - 2(8.3143\ \text{J K}^{-1}\ \text{mol}^{-1})(300\ \text{K})$$

$$\Delta H^{\ddagger} = 37\ \text{kJ mol}^{-1}\ .$$

10.34 Use Eq. (10.56) to analyze the data of Problem 10.28 (for the N_2O_5 reaction) and to determine $\Delta H^{\ddagger}$ and $\Delta S^{\ddagger}$ of this reaction.

$\ln\left[\frac{khc^{\ominus}}{k_bT}\right] = \frac{\Delta S^{\ddagger}}{R} - \frac{\Delta H^{\ddagger}}{RT}$. A plot of $\ln\left[\frac{khc^{\ominus}}{k_bT}\right]$ vs. $\frac{1}{T}$ will have slope $= -\frac{\Delta H^{\ddagger}}{R}$ and intercept $= \frac{\Delta S^{\ddagger}}{R}$. From linear regression we find $-\frac{\Delta H^{\ddagger}}{R} = -1.19 \times 10^4$ with $\sigma = 139.7$ or

$\Delta H^{\ddagger} = (99 \pm 2)\ \text{kJ mol}^{-1}$ (90% conf.) and $\Delta S^{\ddagger} = 2\ \text{J K}^{-1}\ \text{mol}^{-1}$ with $r = -0.99945$.

10.35 Analyze the data of Problem 10.30 (for the HI reaction) using Eq. (10.56) to determine $\Delta H^{\ddagger}$ and $\Delta S^{\ddagger}$ of the reaction.

Regress $\ln\left(\frac{k}{T}\right)$ vs. $\frac{1}{T}$ to find slope $-\frac{\Delta H^{\ddagger}}{R}$ and intercept $\left(\frac{\Delta S^{\ddagger}}{R} + \ln\left(\frac{k_b}{h}\right)\right)$. Draw up the following table:

$-\ln\left(\frac{k}{T}\right)$	$\frac{1}{T} \times 10^3$
-21.180	1.7986
-19.971	1.7931
-16.852	1.5898
-15.835	1.5456
-14.928	1.5015
-14.104	1.4641
-13.310	1.4286
-12.565	1.3966
- 9.892	1.2804

Regressing the data, we find:

slope $m = -21.687 \times 10^3$, $\sigma(m) = 0.200 \times 10^3$

intercept = 17.717 , $\sigma(\text{int}) = 0.308$

$\Delta H^\ddagger = 180.3$ kJ , $\sigma(\Delta H^\ddagger) = 1.7$ kJ

$\Delta S^\ddagger = -52.2$ J K^{-1} , $\sigma(\Delta S^\ddagger) = 2.65$ J K^{-1} .

10.36 The rate constant for the reaction:

$$\phi N(Me)_2 + EtI = \phi N(Me)_2Et^+ + I^-$$

is 3.18×10^{-5} dm^3 mol^{-1} sec^{-1} at 52.5°C, 1 atm, and 12×10^{-5} at 1500 atm, same temperature. Calculate $\Delta V^\ddagger$ for this reaction.

From Eq. (10.62), $\left(\frac{\partial \ln k}{\partial P}\right)_T = -\frac{\Delta V^\ddagger}{RT}$. Approximating $\left(\frac{\partial \ln k}{\partial P}\right) \cong \frac{\Delta \ln k}{\Delta P}$, then $\frac{\ln k_2 - \ln k_1}{P_2 - P_1} = -\frac{\Delta V^\ddagger}{RT}$. Substitution gives $\Delta V^\ddagger = -2.368 \times 10^{-5}$ m^3 mol^{-1} = -23.7 cm^3 mol^{-1} .

10.37 The concentration of the intermediate (B) for consecutive first-order reactions is:

$$[B] = \frac{k_1 a}{k_2 - k_1}(e^{-k_1 t} - e^{-k_2 t})$$

Find the value of this expression if $k_1 = k_2$.

Using l'Hôpital's rule, $\lim_{t\to a} \frac{f(x)}{g(x)} = \lim_{t\to a} \frac{f'(x)}{g'(x)}$ where $f'(x) = \frac{df}{dx}$ and $g'(x) = \frac{dg}{dx}$. Letting $x = k_2$, $a = k_1$, $f = k_1 a(e^{-k_1 t} - e^{-k_2 t})$ and $g = k_2 - k_1$, then

$$\lim_{k_2 \to k_1} \left\{ \frac{k_1 a}{k_2 - k_1} \left[e^{-k_1 t} - e^{-k_2 t} \right] \right\} = \lim_{k_2 \to k_1} \left\{ \frac{k_1 a(te^{-k_2 t})}{1} \right\} \quad \text{or}$$

$$\lim_{k_2 \to k_1} [B] = k_1 a t e^{-k_1 t} .$$

10.38 In consecutive first-order reactions with $k_1 = 0.25\ s^{-1}$ and $k_2 = 0.15\ s^{-1}$, at what time will the intermediate reach its maximum concentration, and what percent of the total material will be present as the intermediate at that time?

$\frac{d[B]}{dt} = k_1 a e^{-k_1 t} - k_2[B]$. [B] is a maximum when $\frac{d[B]}{dt} = 0$,

then $\frac{[B]}{a} = \frac{k_1 e^{-k_1 t}}{k_2}$. Rearranging Eq. (10.70b) we have

$\frac{[B]}{a} = \frac{k_1}{k_2 - k_1}\left(e^{-k_1 t} - e^{-k_2 t}\right)$. Substituting,

$\frac{k_1 e^{-k_1 t}}{k_2} = \frac{k_1}{k_2 - k_1}\left(e^{-k_1 t} - e^{-k_2 t}\right)$ or

$t = \ln\left(\frac{k_1}{k_2}\right)\left[\frac{1}{k_1 - k_2}\right] = \ln\left(\frac{0.25}{0.15}\right)\left[\frac{1}{0.10\ s}\right] = 5.11\ s$. The

fraction of intermediate present at this time is

$\frac{[B]}{a} = \frac{k_1 e^{-k_1 t}}{k_2} = 0.466$ or 46.6% .

10.39 Use the data below for the gas-phase isomerization of cyclopropane:

$$\begin{array}{c} CH_2 \\ \diagup \quad \diagdown \\ CH_2 - CH_2 \end{array} \rightarrow CH_3CH = CH_2$$

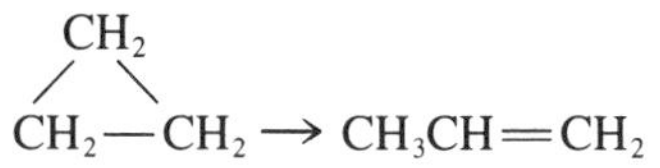

to test the Lindeman mechanism.

P/torr	$10^4k/(s^{-1})$	P/torr	$10^4k/(s^{-1})$
84.1	2.98	1.37	1.30
34.0	2.82	0.569	0.857
11.0	2.23	0.170	0.486
6.07	2.00	0.120	0.392
2.89	1.54	0.067	0.303

From Eq. (10.81), $k_{uni} = \dfrac{k_1 k_3 [M]}{k_3 + k_2[M]}$ or $\dfrac{1}{k_{uni}} = \dfrac{1}{k_1[M]} + \dfrac{k_2}{k_1 k_3}$.

Since $[M] = \dfrac{N}{V} = \dfrac{P}{RT}$, a plot of $\dfrac{1}{k_{uni}}$ vs. $\dfrac{1}{P}$ should be linear with

slope $= \dfrac{RT}{k_1}$ and intercept $= \dfrac{k_2}{k_1 k_3}$. There is considerable

curvature in the plot, indicating the shortcomings of the

mechanism.

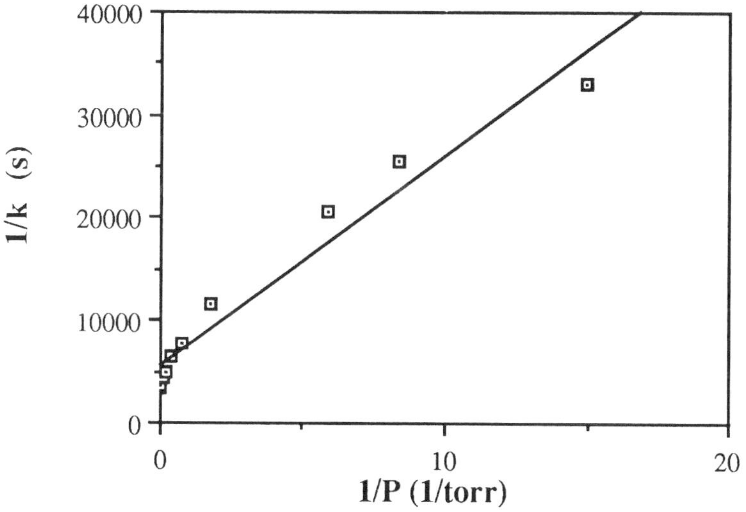

10.40 The chlorination of vinyl chloride (VC):

$$C_2H_3Cl + Cl_2 = C_2H_3Cl_3 \text{ (P)}$$

may be a chain reaction with an intermediate $R\cdot = C_2H_3Cl_2$. Derive the rate law for the following mechanism:

(1) $Cl_2 + h\nu \rightarrow 2\ Cl$

(2) $Cl + VC \rightarrow R\cdot$

(3) $R\cdot + Cl_2 \rightarrow P + Cl$

(4) $R\cdot + R\cdot \rightarrow$ stable molecules

Assigning rate constants as follows:

$$Cl_2 + h\nu \xrightarrow{k_1} 2\ Cl \qquad v_1 = \Phi I_a$$

$$Cl + VC \xrightarrow{k_2} R\cdot \qquad v_2 = k_2[Cl][VC]$$

$$R\cdot + Cl_2 \xrightarrow{k_3} P + Cl \qquad v_3 = k_3[R\cdot][Cl_2]$$

$$R\cdot + R\cdot \xrightarrow{k_4} \text{stable molecules} \qquad v_4 = k_4[R\cdot]^2$$

The overall velocity is $v = v_3 = k_3[R\cdot][Cl_2]$. Using the steady state approximation on $R\cdot$ and Cl,

$\frac{d[Cl]}{dt} = 0 = 2k_1I_a - k_2[Cl][VC] + k_3[R\cdot][Cl_2]$ or $-v_3 + v_2 = 2v_1$

and $\frac{d[R\cdot]}{dt} = 0 = k_2[Cl][VC] - k_3[R\cdot][Cl_2] - 2k_4[R\cdot]^2$ or $-v_3 + v_2 = 2v_4$. From the above, $v_1 = v_4$ and $k_1I_a = v_4$ or $\Phi I_a = k_4[R\cdot]^2$. Thus $[R\cdot]_{ss} = \sqrt{\frac{\Phi I_a}{k_4}}$. The overall velocity is

$$v = k_3[Cl_2]\sqrt{\frac{\Phi I_a}{k_4}} .$$

10.41 Derive the steady-state rate law for the photoinitiated reaction:

$$H_2 + Br_2 = 2\ HBr$$

assuming the mechanism:

(1) $Br_2 + h\nu \longrightarrow 2\ Br$

(2) $Br + H_2 \longrightarrow HBr + H$

(3) $H + Br_2 \longrightarrow HBr + Br$

(4) $H + HBr \longrightarrow H_2 + Br$

(5) $Br + Br \longrightarrow Br_2$

$Br_2 + h\nu \xrightarrow{k_1} 2\ BR \qquad v_1 = \Phi I_a$

$Br + H_2 \xrightarrow{k_2} HBr + H \qquad v_2 = k_2[Br][H_2]$

$H + Br_2 \xrightarrow{k_3} HBr + Br \qquad v_3 = k_3[H][Br_2\}$

$H + HBr \xrightarrow{k_4} H_2 + Br \qquad v_4 = k_4[H][HBr]$

$Br + Br \xrightarrow{k_5} Br_2 \qquad v_5 = k_5[Br]^2$

The overall velocity is $v = -\dfrac{d[Br_2]}{dt} = -v_1 - v_3 + v_5$. Using the steady-state approximation,

$\dfrac{d[Br]}{dt} = 0 = 2v_1 - v_2 + v_3 + v_4 - 2v_5$ and

$\dfrac{d[H]}{dt} = 0 = v_2 - v_3 - v_4 = -v_2 + v_3 + v_4$. Combining, $v_1 = v_5$ or $\Phi I_a = k_5[Br]^2$, thus $[Br]_{ss} = \sqrt{\dfrac{\Phi I_a}{k_5}}$. Then

$v = v_3 = k_3[H][Br_2]$. From $\dfrac{d[H]}{dt} = 0$, we have

$[H]_{ss} = \dfrac{k_2[Br][H_2]}{k_3[Br_2] + k_4[HBr]}$ and

$$v = \frac{k_3k_2[Br][H_2][Br_2]}{k_3[Br_2] + k_4[HBr]} = \frac{k_3k_2[H_2][Br_2]\sqrt{\dfrac{\Phi I_a}{k_5}}}{k_3[Br_2] + k_4[HBr]}.$$

10.42 The mechanism for the nitrogen-pentoxide-catalyzed decomposition of ozone ($2\ O_3 = 3\ O_2$) is given below. Derive a rate law by using the steady-state approximation for NO_2 and NO_3.

(1) $N_2O_5 \rightarrow NO_2 + NO_3$

(2) $NO_2 + NO_3 \rightarrow N_2O_5$

(3) $NO_2 + O_3 \rightarrow NO_3 + O_2$

(4) $NO_3 + NO_3 \rightarrow 2\ NO_2 + O_2$

$N_2O_5 \xrightarrow{k_1} NO_2 + NO_3 \qquad v_1 = k_1[N_2O_5]$

$NO_3 + NO_2 \xrightarrow{k_2} N_2O_5 \qquad v_2 = k_2[NO_2][NO_3]$

$NO_2 + O_3 \xrightarrow{k_3} NO_3 + O_2 \qquad v_3 = k_3[NO_2][O_3]$

$2\ NO_3 \xrightarrow{k_4} 2\ NO_2 + O_2 \qquad v_4 = k_4[NO_3]^2$

Using the steady-state approximation,

$\frac{d[NO_3]}{dt} = 0 = v_1 - v_2 + v_3 - 2v_4$ and

$\frac{d[NO_2]}{dt} = 0 = v_1 - v_2 - v_3 + 2v_4$. This gives $v_3 = 2v_4$ or

$[NO_3]^2_{ss} = \frac{k_3[NO_2]_{ss}[O_3]}{2k_4}$. Using $v_3 = 2v_4$ in $\frac{d[NO_2]}{dt}$, we find

$v_1 = v_2$ or $[NO_2] = \left(\frac{k_1[N_2O_5]\sqrt{2k_4}}{k_2(k_3[O_3])^{1/2}}\right)^{2/3}$. The overall velocity

$$v = \frac{1}{2}\frac{d[O_2]}{dt} = \frac{1}{3}(v_3 + v_4) = \frac{1}{2} v_3 = \frac{1}{2} k_3[NO_2][O_3]$$

$$v = \frac{1}{2} k_3[O_3]\left(\frac{k_1[N_2O_5]}{k_2}\right)^{2/3}\left(\frac{2k_4}{k_3[O_3]}\right)^{1/3}$$

$$v = \left(\frac{k_4 k_1^2 k_3^2}{4k_2^2}\right)^{1/3} [O_3]^{2/3}[N_2O_5]^{2/3} .$$

10.43 The autoxidation of hydrocarbons to form peroxides:

$$RH + O_2 = ROOH$$

is an important reaction involved in the deterioration of oils, fats, and gasoline and the drying of oil-based paints. At high oxygen concentrations, the mechanism in solution appears to be:

(1) $2\ ROOH \longrightarrow ROO\cdot + RO\cdot + H_2O$

(2) $ROO\cdot + RH \longrightarrow ROOH + R\cdot$

(3) $R\cdot + O_2 \longrightarrow ROO\cdot$

(4) $2\ ROO\cdot + ROOR + O_2$

Derive the rate law for $-d[O_2]/dt$.

$$2\ ROOH \xrightarrow{k_1} ROO\cdot + RO\cdot + H_2O \qquad v_1 = k_1[ROOH]^2$$

$$ROO\cdot + RH \xrightarrow{k_2} ROOH + R\cdot \qquad v_2 = k_2[ROO\cdot][RH]$$

$$R\cdot + O_2 \xrightarrow{k_3} ROO\cdot \qquad v_3 = k_3[R\cdot][O_2]$$

$$2\ ROO\cdot \xrightarrow{k_4} ROOR + O_2 \qquad v_4 = k_4[ROO\cdot]^2$$

The rate law is $-\frac{d[O_2]}{dt} = -v_4 + v_3$. Using the steady-state approximation for $R\cdot$ and $ROO\cdot$, $\frac{d[R\cdot]}{dt} = 0 = v_2 - v_3$ or

$$[R\cdot]_{ss} = \frac{k_2[ROO\cdot][RH]}{k_3[O_2]}$$ and

$$\frac{d[ROO\cdot]}{dt} = 0 = -2v_4 + v_3 - v_2 + v_1 = v_1 - 2v_4 \quad \text{or}$$

$$[ROO\cdot]_{ss} = \sqrt{\frac{k_1}{2k_4}}\,[ROOH]$$. The overall velocity is

$$v = -v_4 + v_3 = -k_4[ROO\cdot]^2 + k_3[R\cdot][O_2]$$. Substituting,

$$v = -\frac{k_1}{2}[ROOH]^2 + k_2[RH][ROOH]\sqrt{\frac{k_1}{2k_4}}$$. Using the long chain approximation, we then have $v = k_2\sqrt{\frac{k_1}{2k_4}}\,[RH][ROOH]$.

10.44 The halogenation of a hydrocarbon (RH):

$$RH + X_2 = RX + HX$$

may proceed by the mechanism below. Derive the rate law for this mechanism using the long-chain approximation.

(1) $X_2 \rightarrow 2X$

(2) $X + RH \rightarrow R + HX$

(3) $R + X_2 \rightarrow RX + X$

(4) $X + R \rightarrow RX$

$$X_2 \xrightarrow{k_1} 2X \qquad v_1 = k_1[X_2]$$

$$X + RH \xrightarrow{k_2} R + RX \qquad v_2 = k_2[X][RH]$$

$$R + X_2 \xrightarrow{k_3} RX + X \qquad v_3 = k_3[R][X_2]$$

$$X + R \xrightarrow{k_4} RX \qquad v_4 = k_4[X][R]$$

The reaction velocity is the rate at which RH disappears (v_2).

Because rate of initiation = rate of termination, $v_1 = v_4$ so that $[R] = \frac{k_1[X_2]}{k_4[X]}$. In the long chain approximation, $v_2 = v_3$ so that $[R] = \frac{k_2[X][RH]}{k_3[X_2]} = \frac{k_1[X_2]}{k_4[X]}$. Thus $[X] = \left(\frac{k_1k_3}{k_2k_4}\right)^{1/2} \frac{[X_2]}{[RH]^{1/2}}$

and $v = v_2 = \left(\frac{k_1k_2k_3}{k_4}\right)^{1/2} [X_2][RH]^{1/2}$.

10.45 Tetraethyl lead was once added to gasoline to prevent engine "knock." Explain in chemical terms what this material does.

Tetraethyl lead is a radical scavenger, dissociating in the piston to form relatively unreactive $C_2H_5\cdot$. This species terminates combustion chains by combining with radical ends, thereby limiting pre-ignition ("dieseling" or "knock").

10.46 Derive a relationship between the rate, kinetic chain length, and the light absorbed (I_a) for a photochemically initiated vinyl polymerization. Assume bimolecular termination.

The photochemical initiation may be modelled as

$\mathrm{In} + h\nu \xrightarrow{k_1} \mathrm{R}\cdot$ with $v_i = k_1 I_a = \Phi I_a$. The rate of propagation is $-\frac{d[M]}{dt} = v_p = \sum_n v_{pn} = \sum_{n=0}^{\infty} k_{pn}[M][RM_n\cdot]$. Assuming k_p is independent of n, then $v_p = k_p[M] \sum_{n=0}^{\infty} [RM_n\cdot] = k_p[M][R_x\cdot]$. For bimolecular termination, $v_t = k_t[R_x\cdot]^2$. If the rate of initiation is equal to the rate of termination, $\Phi I_a = k_t[R_x\cdot]^2$ and $[R_x\cdot] = \sqrt{\frac{\Phi I_a}{k_t}}$. Then $v_p = k_p[M]\sqrt{\frac{\Phi I_a}{k_t}}$. The kinetic chain length is then $\nu = \frac{v_p}{v_i} = \frac{k_p[M]\sqrt{\frac{\Phi I_a}{k_t}}}{\Phi I_a} = \frac{k_p[M]}{\sqrt{\Phi I_a k_t}}$.

10.47 Derive expressions for the rate of polymerization and kinetic chain length for a vinyl polymerization with a transfer termination:

$$R_x\cdot + S \longrightarrow P + S\cdot \qquad (k_{tr})$$

Assume that S· does not react further, and that initiation is via an added initiator (In).

$v_i = fk_i[In]$, $v_p = k_p[M][R_x\cdot]$ and $v_t = k_{tr}[R_x\cdot][S]$. In the steady state, $v_i = v_t$ so that $[R_x\cdot] = \frac{fk_i[In\}}{k_{tr}[S]}$. Then $v_p = \frac{k_p k_i f[M][In]}{k_{tr}[S]}$. The kinetic chain length is

$$\nu = \frac{v_p}{v_i} = \left(\frac{k_p[M]fk_i[In]}{k_{tr}[S]}\right)\left(\frac{1}{k_{tr}[S][R_x\cdot]}\right) = \frac{k_p[M]}{k_{tr}[S]} .$$

10.48 The rate constants for the polymerization of vinyl acetate at 60°C are:

$$k_p = 2.3 \times 10^3 \text{ dm}^3 \text{ mol}^{-1} \text{ s}^{-1} \qquad (E_a = 26 \text{ kJ/mol})$$

$$k_t = 2.9 \times 10^2 \text{ dm}^3 \text{ mol}^{-1} \text{ s}^{-1} \qquad (E_a = 13 \text{ kJ/mol})$$

The initiator azobisisobutyronitrile has (at the same T):

$$k_i = 1.07 \times 10^{-5} \text{ s}^{-1} \qquad (E_a = 130 \text{ kJ/mol})$$

Assume $f = 1$ and calculate the rate of polymerization when [In] = 0.001, [M] = 1 mol/dm³. Calculate the activation energy for the rate of polymerization. Will (1) the rate, and (2) the average chain length, increase or decrease with temperature?

From Eq. (10.95),

$$v_p = k_p\sqrt{\frac{k_i f}{k_t}}[M][In]^{1/2}$$

$$v_p = \frac{(2.3 \text{ x } 10^3 \text{ dm}^3 \text{ mol}^{-1} \text{ s}^{-1})(1.07 \text{ x } 10^{-5} \text{ s}^{-1})^{1/2}(1)}{(2.9 \text{ x } 10^3 \text{ dm}^3 \text{ mol}^{-1} \text{ s}^{-1})^{1/2}} \text{ x}$$

$$\left[1 \frac{\text{mol}}{\text{dm}^3}\right]\left[0.001 \frac{\text{mol}}{\text{dm}_3}\right]^{1/2}$$

$$v_p = 0.014 \text{ mol dm}^{-3} \text{ s}^{-1}.$$

E_a for the rate of polymerization is

$$E_a = E_a(\text{prop}) + \frac{E_a(\text{init})}{2} - \frac{E_a(\text{term})}{2}\ .$$ Then $E_a = 84.5 \text{ kJ mol}^{-1}$ and the overall rate will increase with increasing T. The expression for the chain length is $\nu = \frac{k_p[M]}{\sqrt{fk_ik_t}[In]^{1/2}}$. Hence

$$\nu \propto \exp\left[\frac{-\left(E_a(\text{prop}) - \frac{E_a(\text{init})}{2} - \frac{E_a(\text{term})}{2}\right)}{RT}\right]$$

$$\nu \propto \exp\left[\frac{45.5 \text{ kJ mol}^{-1}}{RT}\right]$$

and ν will decrease with increasing T.

10.49 Use the data below for the adsorption of nitrogen on mica to determine the Langmuir adsorption parameters.

$V_{ads}/(cm^3/g)$	$P/torr$
0.494	2.1×10^{-3}
0.782	4.6×10^{-3}
1.16	1.3×10^{-2}

From Eq. (10.99b), $\frac{P}{V_{ads}} = \frac{1}{bV_{max}} + \left(\frac{1}{V_{max}}\right)P$. Thus a plot of $\frac{P}{V_{ads}}$ vs. P should be linear with slope $\frac{1}{V_{max}}$. Using linear regression, slope = 6.37×10^{-1} g cm^{-3} or $V_{max} = 1.57\ cm^3\ g^{-1}$. Also, intercept = $\frac{1}{bV_{max}} = 2.93 \times 10^{-3}$ g torr cm^{-3} or b = 217 $torr^{-1}$ with r = 0.999985 .

10.50 The data for the adsorption of krypton on charcoal at 193.5 K is given below. Find if these data fit Langmuir's isotherm and calculate the constants.

$V_{ads}/(cm^3/g)$	$P/torr$	$V_{ads}/(cm^3/g)$	$P/torr$
5.98	2.45	16.45	11.2
7.76	3.5	18.05	12.8
10.10	5.2	19.72	14.6
12.35	7.2	21.10	16.1

As in problem 10.49, we regress $\frac{P}{V_{ads}}$ vs. P to find

slope = $\frac{1}{V_{max}} = 2.58 \times 10^{-2}$ g cm^{-3} with $\sigma = 1.5 \times 10^{-3}$ g cm^{-3} or

$V_{max} = 38.8\ cm^3\ g^{-1}$, and

intercept = $\frac{1}{bV_{max}} = 3.71 \times 10^{-1}$ g torr cm^{-3} with $\sigma = 1.5 \times 10^{-2}$

or b = 0.069 $torr^{-1}$. r = 0.9900 .

10.51 Use a graph of P/V vs. P to determine the Langmuir parameters for the adsorption of nitrous oxide on barium fluoride using the data below (−40°C).

P/torr	V/cm^3
35.9	3.70
64.5	5.09
120	6.70
232	8.48
357	9.92

As in problem 10.49, we use linear regression to find

V_{max} = 12.2 cm^3 and b = 0.011 torr^{-1} with r = 0.99763 .

10.52 The decomposition of ammonia:

$$NH_3 = \tfrac{1}{2}N_2 + \tfrac{3}{2}H_2$$

on a tungsten wire was investigated by Hinshelwood and Burk at 856°C. Use the results (below) to show that the reaction is approximately zero-order and determine the rate constant. Make a graph of $P(NH_3)$ vs. t and compare to Figure 10.21. Explain these results assuming Langmuir adsorption.

t/s	P/torr	t/s	P/torr
0	200	800	292
100	214	1000	312
200	227	1200	332
300	238	1400	349
400	248.5	1800	378
500	259	2000	387
600	270		

Defining an extent of reaction, x, then $P_{NH_3} = P_0 - x$,

$P_{H_2} = \frac{3}{2}x$, $P_{N_2} = \frac{1}{2}x$ and $P = P_0 + x$. Thus we have

$P_{NH_3} = 2P_0 - P$. Plotting P_{NH_3} vs. t:

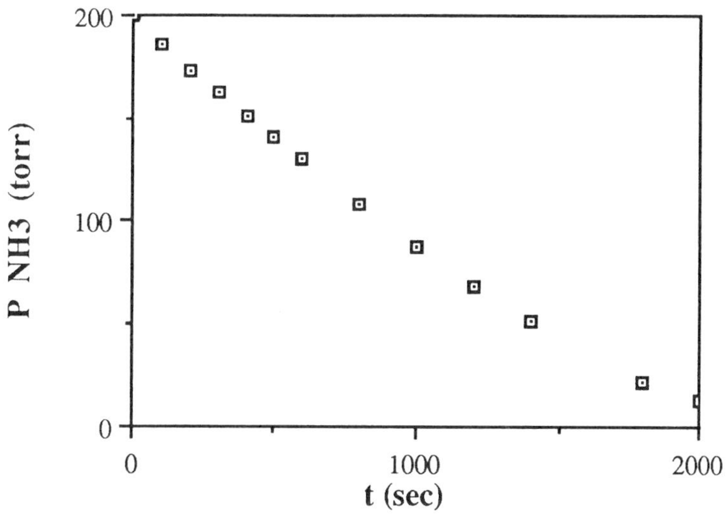

This is a good straight line down to $P_{NH_3} \cong 50$ torr . Above 50 torr, $P_{NH_3} = P_0 - k_0 t$ (zero order behavior). Linear regression of these points gives $k_0 = (0.107 \pm 0.02)\text{torr s}^{-1}$ (90% conf.) with r = -0.9996 .

10.53 The Pt-catalyzed decomposition of NO (into $N_2 + O_2$) is found to have a rate law:

$$v = \frac{kP_{NO}}{P_{O_2}}$$

Show how this rate law could result from Langmuir adsorption and surface catalysis.

Assuming that the RDS is the unimolecular decomposition of NO, then Eq. (10.102) is applicable:

$$v = \frac{kS_0 b_{NO} P_{NO}}{1 + b_{NO}P_{NO} + b_{N_2}P_{N_2} + b_{O_2}P_{O_2}}$$. If $b_{O_2}P_{O_2} >> 1$, $b_{NO}P_{NO}$, and $b_{N_2}P_{N_2}$, then $v = \dfrac{kS_0 b_{NO} P_{NO}}{b_{O_2}P_{O_2}} = k' \dfrac{P_{NO}}{P_{O_2}}$.

10.54 Two gas-phase reactions are studied in a small vessel and then in a large vessel. One reacts faster in the large vessel and the other reacts slower. Explain each case.

The one which reacts faster in the larger vessel is apparently undergoing surface catalysis. The one which reacts slower in the larger vessel is exhibiting wall termination of radical species.

10.55 The adsorption of hydrogen on some surfaces has an adsorption isotherm of the form:

$$\theta = \frac{bP^{1/2}}{1 + bP^{1/2}}$$

Propose a mechanism and derive this isotherm; state assumptions clearly.

Supposing that dissociation occurs upon adsorption,

$$H_2 + 2\ S \xrightarrow{k_a} 2\ H{\cdot}S$$

$$2\ H{\cdot}S \xrightarrow{k_d} H_2 + 2\ S \qquad (S = \text{surface site})$$

Rate adsorption $= k_a P_{H_2}(1 - \theta)^2$, rate desorption $= k_d\theta^2$.

At equilibrium, the rates are equal, thus

$k_a^{1/2} P_{H_2}^{1/2}(1 - \theta) = k_d^{1/2}\theta$ or

$$\theta = \frac{\left(\frac{k_a}{k_d}\right)^{1/2} P_{H_2}^{1/2}}{1 + \left(\frac{k_a}{k_d}\right)^{1/2} P_{H_2}^{1/2}} \equiv \frac{bP_{H_2}^{1/2}}{1 + bP_{H_2}^{1/2}} \quad \text{where } b = \left(\frac{k_a}{k_d}\right)^{1/2} .$$

10.56 H. DeVoe and G. B. Kistiakowsky [*J. Am. Chem. Soc.*, **83**, 274 (1961)] studied the kinetics of the reaction:

$$CO_2 + H_2O = HCO_3^- + H^+$$

as catalyzed by the enzyme bovine carbonic anhydrase at 0.5°C, $pH = 7.1$, $E_0 + 2.8 \times 10^{-9}$ mol dm^{-3}. Use the data below to calculate the kinetic parameters of this reaction.

$[CO_2]/(mol/dm^3)$	$v/(mol\ dm^{-3}\ s^{-1})$
1.25×10^{-3}	2.8×10^{-5}
2.5×10^{-3}	5.0×10^{-5}
5×10^{-3}	8.3×10^{-5}
20×10^{-3}	17×10^{-5}

From Eq. (10.111), we expect a plot of $\frac{1}{v}$ vs. $\frac{1}{[CO_2]}$ to be linear. Regressing the data, we find $\frac{1}{v_{max}} = 4.00 \times 10^3$ dm^3 mol^{-1} with $\sigma = 104$ dm^3 s mol^{-1} and $\frac{K_m}{v_{max}} = 39.7$ s with $\sigma = 0.23$ s .

Thus $v_{max} = 2.50 \times 10^{-4}$ mol dm^{-3} s^{-1} and

$K_m = 9.92 \times 10^{-3}$ mol^{-1} dm^3 . From Eq. (10.110),

$$k_2 = \frac{v_{max}}{E_0} = \frac{2.50 \times 10^{-4}}{2.8 \times 10^{-9}}\ s^{-1} = 8.93 \times 10^4\ s^{-1}\ .$$

10.57 Use the data (below) for the hydrolysis of *N*-glutamyl-L-phenylalanine catalyzed by α-chymotrypsin to determine the kinetic constants for the Michaelis-Menten mechanism [*J. Chem. Ed.*, **50**, 149 (1973)].

$[S]/(mol/dm^3)$	$v/(mol\ dm^{-3}\ min^{-1})$
2.5×10^{-4}	2.2×10^{-6}
5.0×10^{-4}	3.8×10^{-6}
1×10^{-3}	5.9×10^{-6}
1.5×10^{-3}	7.1×10^{-6}

From Eq. (10.111), $\frac{1}{v} = \frac{1}{v_{max}} + \frac{K_m}{v_{max}}\frac{1}{[S]}$. Plotting $\frac{1}{v}$ vs. $\frac{1}{[S]}$, we find $\frac{1}{v_{max}} = 7.56 \times 10^4$ min dm^3 mol^{-1} with

$\sigma = 2 \times 10^3$ min dm^3 mol^{-1} and $\frac{K_m}{v_{max}} = 94.6$ min with $\sigma = 0.9$ min .

Then $v_{max} = 1.32 \times 10^{-5}$ mol dm^{-3} min^{-1} and

$$K_m = 1.25 \times 10^{-3}\ dm^3\ mol^{-1}\ .$$

10.58 Integrate the Michaelis-Menten rate law to obtain an equation for [S] (initial value S_0) as a function of t and S_0.

From Eq. (10.109), $v = -\frac{d[S]}{dt} = \frac{d[P]}{dt} = \frac{k_2E_0[S]}{K_m + [S]}$ or

$$\frac{(K_m + [S])d[S]}{[S]} = -\,k_2E_0dt \;.\quad \text{Then}$$

$$(K_m \ln[S] + [S])\Big|_{S_0}^{[S]} = -k_2E_0t\Big|_0^t \text{ or } K_m\ln\left(\frac{[S]}{S_0}\right) + [S] = S_0 - k_2E_0t \;.$$

10.59 In analyzing enzyme data, the Hanes plot, $[S]/v$ vs. [S], is considered to be more reliable than the Lineweaver-Burk plot, $1/v$ vs. $1/[S]$, for obtaining kinetic constants from the data. How are the slope and intercepts of this plot related to v_{max} and K_m for the Michaelis-Menten mechanism?

Multiply Eq. (10.111) by [S] to get $\frac{[S]}{v} = \frac{K_m}{v_{max}} + \frac{[S]}{v_{max}}$. A plot of $\frac{[S]}{v}$ vs. [S] thus has slope $= \frac{1}{v_{max}}$ and intercept $= \frac{K_m}{v_{max}}$.

10.60 Derive Eq. (10.116) for the velocity of an enzyme-catalyzed reaction with noncompetitive inhibition.

For noncompetitive inhibition, $K_I = K_I'$ or

$K_I = \frac{[E][I]}{[EI]} = \frac{[ES][I]}{[ESI]}$. From Eq. (10.108), $[ES]_{ss} = \frac{[E][S]}{K_m}$.

The material balance is

$$E_0 = [E] + [ES] + [EI] + [EIS]$$

$$E_0 = [E] + \frac{[E][S]}{K_m} + \frac{[E][I]}{K_I} + \frac{[E][S][I]}{K_mK_I} \;.$$

Thus $[E] = \dfrac{E_0}{\left(1 + \frac{[S]}{K_m} + \frac{[I]}{K_I} + \frac{[S][I]}{K_mK_I}\right)}$. The reaction velocity is

$v = k_2[ES]$, so that $v = \dfrac{k_2E_0[S]}{\left(K_m + [S] + \left(\frac{K_m}{K_I}\right)[I] + \frac{[S][I]}{K_I}\right)}$.

With Eq. (10.110), $v_{max} = k_2E_0$, so that

$$v = \frac{v_{max}[S]}{\left(K_m + [S] + \left(\frac{K_m}{K_I}\right)[I] + \frac{[S][I]}{K_I}\right)} .$$

10.61 Derive the rate law for the enzyme mechanism:

$$E + S \overset{1}{\rightleftarrows} ES$$

$$ES \overset{2}{\rightarrow} P$$

$$ES + I \rightleftarrows ESI$$

This is uncompetitive inhibition.

This is uncompetitive inhibition. The material balance is

$E_0 = [E] + [ES] + [ESI] = [E] + \frac{[E][S]}{K_m} + \frac{[E][S][I]}{K_mK_I'}$, so that

$[E] = \frac{E_0}{\left(1 + \frac{[S]}{K_m} + \frac{[S][I]}{K_mK_I'}\right)}$ and $v = \frac{k_2E_0[S]}{\left(K_m + [S] + \frac{[S][I]}{K_I'}\right)}$. With

Eq. (10.110), $v_{max} = k_2E_0$, then $v = \frac{v_{max}[S]}{K_m + [S]\left(1 + \frac{[I]}{K_I'}\right)}$.

10.62 A molecule that absorbs light (I_a) may reemit the light in a process called fluorescence or phosphorescence (depending on the time scale, cf. Chapter 13) or lose its energy by collision with another molecule (Q); this is called *quenching* of fluorescence. Show that the intensity of fluorescence (I_f) is related to the intensity of the light absorbed (I_a) by the Stern-Volmer equation:

$$\frac{1}{I_f} = \frac{1}{I_a}\left(1 + \frac{k_q[\text{Q}]}{k_f}\right)$$

where k_q is the rate constant for quenching and k_f is the rate constant for fluorescent emission.

$$A + h\nu \rightarrow A^* \qquad k_1$$

$$A^* + Q \rightarrow A + Q \qquad k_q$$

$$A^* \rightarrow A + h\nu' \qquad k_f$$

At steady state, $k_1[A] = k_q[A^*][Q] + k_f[A^*]$. The ratio of absorbed to emitted light is

$$\frac{I_a}{I_f} = \frac{\text{rate light absorbed}}{\text{rate light emitted}} = \frac{k_1[A]}{k_f[A^*]} = \frac{k_q[A^*][Q] + k_f[A^*]}{k_f[A^*]}$$

$$\frac{I_a}{I_f} = \left(\frac{k_q}{k_f}[Q] + 1\right)$$

so that $\frac{1}{I_f} = \frac{1}{I_a}\left\{1 + \frac{k_q}{k_f}[Q]\right\}$.

10.63 Two molecules have, respectively, diffusion constants 2×10^{-5} and 3×10^{-5} cm^2/s and radius 3×10^{-8} and 2×10^{-8} cm. Estimate the maximum rate constant for their reaction in solution.

The diffusion controlled rate constant is: $k = 4\pi L(D_A + D_B)\sigma_{AB}$ where $\sigma_{AB} = r_a + r_B$. With $D_A = 2 \times 10^{-5}\ cm^2\ s^{-1}$, $D_B = 3 \times 10^{-5}\ cm^2\ s^{-1}$, and $\sigma_{AB} = 5 \times 10^{-8}$ cm we find

$$k = 1.89 \times 10^{13}\ cm^3\ mol^{-1}\ s^{-1} .$$

10.64 Use Eq. (10.119) to estimate the rate of a diffusion-controlled reaction in heptane at 40°C. Assume the molecules are of equal size.

If $r_A = r_B$, then $k = \frac{8RT}{3\eta}$. For heptane at 40°C (Table 9.2),

$$\eta = 3.410 \times 10^{-3}\ \text{g cm}^{-1}\ \text{s}^{-1} = 3.410 \times 10^{-4}\ \text{kg m}^{-1}\ \text{s}^{-1}$$

$$k = 2.036 \times 10^{7}\ \text{m}^3\ \text{mol}^{-1}\ \text{s}^{-1}\ .$$

10.65 Equation (10.119) demonstrates how the size of molecules may affect their diffusion-controlled rates rate constants. What would be the rate constants for molecules with radius-ratios of 2, 5 and 10, relative to the rate for equal-sized molecules under the same conditions?

In general: $k = \frac{2RT}{3\eta} \frac{\left(\frac{r_A}{r_B} + 1\right)^2}{\left(\frac{r_A}{r_B}\right)}$. Thus $k(1) = \frac{8RT}{3\eta}$,

$\frac{k(2)}{k(1)} = 1.125$, $\frac{k(5)}{k(1)} = 1.800$, and $\frac{k(10)}{k(1)} = 3.025$.

10.66 Use Eq. (10.119) to estimate the rate constant for a diffusion-controlled reaction in water at 50°C relative to the rate at 20°C.

The ratio of rate constants will be:

$\frac{k(50^\circ C)}{k(20^\circ C)} = \left(\frac{323.15}{\eta(50^\circ C)}\right)\left(\frac{\eta(20^\circ C)}{293.15}\right)$. Using $\eta(50^\circ C) = 5.494$ mp and

$\eta(20^\circ C) = 10.050$ mp we find $\frac{k(50^\circ C)}{k(20^\circ C)} = 2.016$.

10.67 Other things being equal, what would you expect the rate of a diffusion-controlled reaction in acetone to be relative to the same reaction (at the same temperature) in water?

The relative rates would be related to the viscosities through the relation: $\frac{k(\text{acetone})}{k(H_2O)} = \frac{\eta(H_2O)}{\eta(\text{acetone})}$. At 20°C, $\eta(H_2O)$ = 10.050 mp and η(acetone) = 3.311 mp so that

$$\frac{k(\text{acetone})}{k(H_2O)} = 3.035 \ .$$

10.68 The relaxation time for:

$$H^+ + OH^- = H_2O$$

with pH = 7.00 is 36 μs. Calculate the rate constants.

Rearranging Eq. (10.124), $k_1 = \frac{1}{\tau\left[1 + \frac{k_2}{k_1}(A_{eq} + B_{eq})\right]}$. With

A = $[H^+]$ and B = $[OH^-]$, $A_{eq} = B_{eq} = 10^{-7}$ mol dm^{-3} and

$$\frac{k_2}{k_1} = \left(\frac{[H_2O]}{[H^+][OH^-]}\right)_{eq} = \frac{55.6}{(10^{-7})^2} = 5.56 \times 10^{15} \text{ dm}^3 \text{ mol}^{-1} .$$ Then

$$k_1 = \frac{1}{(36 \times 10^{-6} \text{ s})\{1 + (5.56 \times 10^{15} \text{ dm}^3 \text{ mol}^{-1})(2 \times 10^{-7} \text{ mol dm}^{-3})\}}$$

$$k_1 = 2.5 \times 10^{-5} \text{ s}^{-1}$$

and $k_2 = 1.4 \times 10^{11}$ dm^3 mol^{-1} s^{-1} .

10.69 Calculate the relaxation time for:

$$H^+ + OH^- = H_2O$$

in water (25°C) for pH = 5.

Using data from Table 10.4, $\tau = \{k_1 + k_2([H^+]_{eq} + [OH^-]_{eq})\}^{-1}$ or

$$\tau = \{2.5 \times 10^{-5} + 1.4 \times 10^{11}(10^{-5} + 10^{-9})\}^{-1} = 7.1 \times 10^{-7} \text{ s}$$

$$\tau = 0.71 \ \mu\text{s} .$$

10.70 Derive a formula for the relaxation time of reversible first-order reactions:

$$A \underset{-1}{\overset{1}{\rightleftarrows}} B$$

$\frac{d[A]}{dt} = -k_1[A] + k_{-1}[B]$. If $[A] = [A]_{eq} - x$ and $[B] = [B]_{eq} + x$, then

$$\frac{dx}{dt} = k_1([A]_{eq} - x) - k_{-1}([B]_{eq} + x)$$

$$\frac{dx}{dt} = -(k_1 + k_{-1})x + (k_1[A]_{eq} - k_{-1}[B]_{eq}) .$$

Because of the equilibrium condition, the 2nd term above is zero, then $\frac{dx}{dt} = -(k_1 + k_{-1})x$. From Eqs. (10.123) and (10.124),

$$\tau \equiv -\frac{x}{\left(\frac{dx}{dt}\right)} = \frac{1}{(k_1 + k_{-1})} .$$

10.71 Derive a formula for the relaxation time of

$$A + B \underset{-2}{\overset{2}{\rightleftarrows}} C + D$$

$\frac{d[A]}{dt} = -k_2[A][B] + k_{-2}[C][D]$. If $[A] = [A]_{eq} - x$, $[B] = [B]_{eq} - x$, $[C] = [C]_{eq} + x$ and $[D] = [D]_{eq} + x$, then

$$\frac{dx}{dt} = k_2([A]_{eq} - x)([B]_{eq} - x) - k_{-2}([C]_{eq} + x)([D]_{eq} + x)$$

$$\frac{dx}{dt} = (k_2[A]_{eq}[B]_{eq} - k_{-2}[C]_{eq}[D]_{eq}) - \{k_2([A]_{eq} + [B]_{eq}) + k_{-2}([C]_{eq} + [D]_{eq})\}x - (k_2 + k_{-2})x^2 .$$

The first term above is zero by the equilibrium condition. If x is small then $x^2 \cong 0$ and

$\frac{dx}{dt} = -[k_2([A]_{eq} + [B]_{eq}) + k_{-2}([C]_{eq} + [D_{eq})]x$. From the definition of τ,

$$\tau = -\frac{x}{\left(\frac{dx}{dt}\right)} = [k_2([A]_{eq} + [B]_{eq}) + k_{-2}([C]_{eq} + [D]_{eq})]^{-1} .$$

11
Quantum Theory

11.1 (a) Calculate the energy in joules for a mole of photons with wavelengths: 420 nm (violet), 30 nm (ultraviolet), 0.1 nm (X-ray).
(b) If a mole of 420 nm photons is absorbed by 1 kg of water, how much would the temperature rise?

$E = h\nu = \frac{hc}{\lambda}$. Using $h = 6.6261 \times 10^{-34}$ J s and

$c = 2.9979 \times 10^{8}$ m s^{-1} we find:

$$\lambda = 420 \times 10^{-9} \text{ m}, \; E = 284.8 \text{ kJ mol}^{-1} .$$

$$\lambda = 30 \times 10^{-9} \text{ m}, \; E = 3.99 \times 10^{3} \text{ kJ} = 3.99 \text{ MJ} .$$

$$\lambda = 0.1 \times 10^{-9} \text{ m}, \; E = 1.20 \times 10^{6} \text{ kJ} = 1.20 \text{ GJ} .$$

With 4.184 J K^{-1} g^{-1} as the heat capacity of water, we find

$$\Delta T = \frac{E}{C_p} = 68.1^\circ\text{C} .$$

11.2 The dissociation of nitrogen, $N_2 \rightarrow 2N$, requires 941.74 kJ/mol. What would be the wavelength of a photon with sufficient energy to cause this process?

$$\lambda = \frac{hc}{E}$$

$$\lambda = \frac{(6.022 \times 10^{23} \text{ mol}^{-1})(6.6261 \times 10^{-34} \text{ J s})(3.0 \times 10^{8} \text{ m s}^{-1})}{(941.74 \times 10^{3} \text{ J mol}^{-1})}$$

$$\lambda = 1.27 \times 10^{-7} \text{ m} = 127 \text{ nm} .$$

11.3 Calculate the Bohr radius as defined [Eq. (11.6)] and confirm the numerical value given. (Use all cgs units.)

$$a_0 = \frac{\hbar^2}{me^2} = \frac{(1.05457 \times 10^{-27} \text{ erg s})^2}{(9.10939 \times 10^{-28} \text{ g})(4.80321 \times 10^{-10} \text{ esu})^2}$$

$$a_0 = 5.2917 \times 10^{-9} \text{ cm} = 0.52917 \text{ Å}$$

11.4 Coulomb's law for the potential between a charge $+Ze$ and a charge $-e$ is:

$$V = -\frac{Ze^2}{r}$$

For the first Bohr orbit ($N = 1$) of the hydrogen atom ($Z = 1$), calculate the total (E), potential (V), and kinetic (T) energies of the electron. You will note that $E = -T = \frac{1}{2}V$—an example of the *virial theorem*.

$$E_1 = -Z^2\left(\frac{e^2}{2a_0}\right)\frac{1}{N^2} = -(1)^2\left(\frac{(4.80321 \times 10^{-10} \text{ esu})^2}{2(0.52918 \times 10^{-8})}\right)\frac{1}{(1)^2}$$

$$E_1 = -2.18 \times 10^{-11} \text{ erg} .$$

$$V = -\frac{Ze^2}{r} = -\frac{e^2}{a_0} = 2 E_1 = -4.36 \times 10^{-11} \text{ erg} .$$ Then

$$T = E - V = 2.18 \times 10^{-11} \text{ erg} .$$

11.5 In the Compton effect, the change in wavelength of the scattered photon is related to the angle of scattering by:

$$\Delta\lambda = (h/mc)(1 - \cos\theta)$$

Calculate the wavelength of photons scattered at 90° if the incident photon has $\lambda = 3.00$ Å. What will be the velocity of the scattered electron?

$\Delta\lambda = \left(\frac{h}{mc}\right)(1 - \cos\theta)$. With $\theta = 90°$, $\cos\theta = 0$, and

$m = m_e = 9.1091 \times 10^{-31}$ kg . Thus $\Delta\lambda = 2.4 \times 10^{-12}$ m $= 0.024$ Å .

The energy of the scattered electron will be:

$$E = hc\left(\frac{1}{\lambda_1} - \frac{1}{\lambda_2}\right) .$$ With $\lambda_1 = 3.00$ Å and $\lambda_2 = 3.024$ Å :

$E = 5.25 \times 10^{-18}$ J . This energy appears as the kinetic energy of the electron, so that $v = \left(\frac{2E}{m}\right)^{1/2} = 3.4 \times 10^6 \text{ m s}^{-1}$.

11.6 (a) Calculate the wavelength of the line of the hydrogen atom spectrum corresponding to $N_1 = 2$, $N_2 = 4$.
(b) Repeat the calculation for $N_2 = 9, 10, 11, \ldots$, until it is obvious that you are approaching a *series limit*. What is that limit for $N_1 = 2$?

a) $$\tilde{\nu} = \mathcal{R}\left(\frac{1}{N_1^2} - \frac{1}{N_2^2}\right) = 109{,}667.6 \text{ cm}^{-1}\left(\frac{1}{4} - \frac{1}{16}\right) = 20{,}562.7 \text{ cm}^{-1} .$$

$$\lambda = 1/\tilde{\nu} = 4.86 \times 10^{-5} \text{ cm} = 486 \text{ nm} .$$

b) With $N_1 = 2$, we draw up the following table:

N_2	$\lambda = 1/\tilde{\nu}$ (nm)
9	383.7
10	379.9
11	377.2
.	.
.	.
.	.
∞	364.7

11.7 The hydrogen atom spectrum, given by the Rydberg formula [Eq. (11.9)], falls into series that have been named for their discoverers. Calculate the range (in cm^{-1}) for the following series: $N_1 = 1$ (Lyman series); $N_1 = 2$ (Balmer series); $N_1 = 3$ (Paschen series); $N_1 = 4$ (Brackett series); $N_1 = 5$ (Pfund series). What region of the spectrum are these series found (see Table 11.9)?

$$\tilde{\nu} = \mathcal{R}\left(\frac{1}{N_1^2} - \frac{1}{N_2^2}\right) .$$

Lyman Series: Using $N_1 = 1$, $N_2 = 2$ and $\mathcal{R} = 109{,}667.6\ cm^{-1}$, we find $\tilde{\nu}_1 = 82{,}251\ cm^{-1}$. Using $N_2 = \infty$, $\tilde{\nu}_2 = 109{,}668\ cm^{-1}$. This series is found in the ultraviolet region.

Balmer Series: $N_1 = 2$, $N_2 = 3$ $\quad \tilde{\nu}_1 = 15{,}232\ cm^{-1}$

$N_1 = 2$, $N_2 = \infty$ $\quad \tilde{\nu}_2 = 27{,}417\ cm^{-1}$

Visible region.

Paschen Series: $N_1 = 3$, $N_2 = 4$ $\quad \tilde{\nu}_1 = 5331\ cm^{-1}$

$N_1 = 3$, $N_2 = \infty$ $\quad \tilde{\nu}_2 = 12{,}185\ cm^{-1}$

Infrared region.

Bracket Series: $N_1 = 4$, $N_2 = 5$ $\quad \tilde{\nu}_1 = 2467\ cm^{-1}$

$N_1 = 4$, $N_2 = \infty$ $\quad \tilde{\nu}_2 = 6854\ cm^{-1}$

Infrared region.

Pfund Series: $N_1 = 5$, $N_2 = 6$ $\quad \tilde{\nu}_1 = 1340\ cm^{-1}$

$N_1 = 5$, $N_2 = \infty$ $\quad \tilde{\nu}_2 = 4387\ cm^{-1}$

Infrared region.

11.8 Calculate the velocity of the electron in the first Bohr orbit of a hydrogen atom. (Remember that angular momentum = mvr.) Repeat the calculation for Hg (Z = 80).

From Eq. (11.13), $v = \frac{h}{m\lambda}$. In the first Bohr orbit,

$\lambda = 2\pi r = 2\pi a_0$, thus

$$v = \frac{h}{2\pi m a_0} = \frac{(6.6261 \times 10^{-27}\ \text{erg s})}{2\pi(9.1094 \times 10^{-28}\ \text{g})(5.2918 \times 10^{-9}\ \text{cm})}$$

$$v = 2.2 \times 10^{8}\ \text{cm s}^{-1} .$$

For Z = 80 , $r = \frac{a_0}{80}$ so that $v = \frac{80\hbar}{m a_0} = 1.75 \times 10^{10}\ \text{cm s}^{-1}$. v is 58% of the speed of light.

11.9 Find the result of operating with $\hat{A} = y - (d/dy)$ and $\hat{B} = y + (d/dy)$ on the function $f(y) = e^{-y^2/2}$.

a) $\hat{A}f(y) = ye^{-y^2/2} - \frac{d}{dy}\left(e^{-y^2/2}\right) = 2ye^{-y^2/2}$.

b) $\hat{B}f(y) = ye^{-y^2/2} + \frac{d}{dy}\left(e^{-y^2/2}\right) = 0$.

11.10 Find the result of operating with:

$$\hat{O} = \frac{d}{d\theta} \sin\theta \frac{d}{d\theta}$$

on the function $e^{i\theta}$. Is this an eigenfunction of $\hat{O}$?

$$\frac{d}{d\theta}\left(\sin\theta \frac{d}{d\theta}(e^{i\theta})\right) = \frac{d}{d\theta}(i \sin\theta\, e^{i\theta}) = i\cos\theta\, e^{i\theta} - \sin\theta\, e^{i\theta}$$

$$\frac{d}{d\theta}\left(\sin\theta \frac{d}{d\theta}(e^{i\theta})\right) = ie^{2i\theta} .$$

This is not an eigenfunction, because the operator does not just multiply by a constant (see Eq. 11.17).

11.11 Find the commutator $[d/dx, \sin x]$.

$\left[\frac{d}{dx}, \sin x\right] = \frac{d}{dx}(\sin x) - (\sin x)\frac{d}{dx}$. Operators act on everything that follows them, including the still unspecified function f(x), so that $\frac{d}{dx}(\sin x) = \cos x + (\sin x)\frac{d}{dx}$ by the chain rule. Thus $\left[\frac{d}{dx}, \sin x\right] = \cos x$.

11.12 Derive the commutator:

$$\left[\frac{d}{dx} - x, \frac{d}{dx} + x\right]$$

We examine the result of operating on f(x):

$$\left[\frac{d}{dx} - x, \frac{d}{dx} + x\right]f(x) = \left(\frac{d}{dx} - x\right)\left(\frac{d}{dx} + x\right)f - \left(\frac{d}{dx} + x\right)\left(\frac{d}{dx} - x\right)f$$

$$\left[\frac{d}{dx} - x, \frac{d}{dx} + x\right]f(x) = \left(\frac{d}{dx} - x\right)\left(\frac{df}{dx} + xf\right) - \left(\frac{d}{dx} + x\right)\left(\frac{df}{dx} - xf\right)$$

$$\left[\frac{d}{dx} - x, \frac{d}{dx} + x\right]f(x) = \frac{d^2f}{dx^2} + f + \frac{xdf}{dx} - \frac{xdf}{dx} - x^2f - \frac{d^2f}{dx^2} + f + \frac{xdf}{dx} - \frac{xdf}{dx} + x^2f$$

$$\left[\frac{d}{dx} - x, \frac{d}{dx} + x\right]f(x) = 2f$$

Thus: $\left[\frac{d}{dx} - x, \frac{d}{dx} + x\right] = 2$.

11.13 Derive the commutator:

$$\left[\frac{d}{dr}, \frac{1}{r}\right]$$

Examine the result of operating on f(r):

$$\left[\frac{d}{dr}, \frac{1}{r}\right]f(r) = \frac{d}{dr}\left(\frac{f}{r}\right) - \frac{1}{r}\frac{df}{dr} = \frac{1}{r}\frac{df}{dr} - \frac{1}{r^2}f - \frac{1}{r}\frac{df}{dr} = -\frac{1}{r^2}f$$

Thus: $\left[\frac{d}{dr}, \frac{1}{r}\right] = -\frac{1}{r^2}$.

11.14 Find the commutators:

$$\text{(a)} \quad \left[\frac{d}{dx}, x^2\right] \qquad \text{(b)} \quad \left[\frac{d^2}{dx^2}, x\right]$$

a) If f = f(x):

$$\left[\frac{d}{dx}, x^2\right]f = \frac{d}{dx}(x^2 f) - x^2\frac{df}{dx} = 2fx + x^2\frac{df}{dx} - x^2\frac{df}{dx} = 2fx .$$

Thus: $\left[\frac{d}{dx}, x^2\right] = 2x$.

b) $$\left[\frac{d^2}{dx^2}, x\right]f = \frac{d^2}{dx^2}(xf) - x\frac{d^2f}{dx^2} = \frac{d}{dx}\left(f + x\frac{df}{dx}\right) - x\frac{d^2f}{dx^2}$$

$$\left[\frac{d^2}{dx^2}, x\right]f = \frac{df}{dx} + \frac{df}{dx} + x\frac{d^2f}{dx^2} - x\frac{d^2f}{dx^2} = 2\frac{df}{dx} .$$

Thus: $\left[\frac{d^2}{dx^2}, x\right] = 2\frac{d}{dx}$.

11.15 Find the result of operating with:

$$\hat{O} = i\frac{d}{d\phi} \quad \text{on} \quad f(\phi) = 3e^{i\phi}$$

Is it an eigenfunction? What is the eigenvalue?

$\hat{O}f(\Phi) = i\frac{d}{d\Phi}(3e^{i\Phi}) = -3e^{i\Phi}$. Thus $f(\Phi)$ is an eigenfunction with eigenvalue = -1 .

11.16 Find the result of operating with:

$$\hat{O} = \frac{d^2}{dx^2} - 4x^2 \quad \text{on the function} \quad \psi = e^{-ax^2}$$

What must be the value of a if ψ is to be an eigenfunction of this operator?

$\hat{O}\psi = \left(\frac{d^2}{dx^2} - 4x^2\right)e^{-ax^2} = (4a^2x^2 - 2a - 4x^2)e^{-ax^2}$. For ψ to be an eigenfunction of $\hat{O}$, we require $\hat{O}\psi = b\psi$, where b is a constant. Thus: $4a^2x^2 = 4x^2$ and $a = \pm 1$.

11.17 Find the result of operating with the operator:

$$\hat{O} = \frac{1}{r^2}\frac{d}{dr}r^2\frac{d}{dr} + \frac{2}{r}$$

on the function $\psi = Ae^{-br}$. What values must the constants have for ψ to be an eigenfunction of $\hat{O}$?

$$\hat{O}\psi = \frac{1}{r^2}\frac{d}{dr}\left[r^2\frac{d}{dr}(Ae^{-br})\right] + \frac{2A}{r}e^{-br} = \frac{1}{r^2}\frac{d}{dr}[-Abr^2e^{-br}] + \frac{2A}{r}e^{-br}$$

$$\hat{O}\psi = \left(Ab^2 - \frac{2Ab}{r} + \frac{2A}{r}\right)e^{-br} .$$

For ψ to be an eigenfunction of $\hat{O}$, $\left(Ab^2 - \frac{2Ab}{r} + \frac{2A}{r}\right)$ = constant .

Thus $\frac{2Ab}{r} = \frac{2A}{r}$ or b = 1 and A is arbitrary. With b = 1 , the eigenvalue is 1.

11.18 Show that the Legendre polynomials $P_1 = \cos\theta$ and $P_2 = 3\cos^2\theta - 1$ are eigenfunctions of:

$$\hat{O} = \frac{1}{\sin\theta}\frac{d}{d\theta}\left(\sin\theta\frac{d}{d\theta}\right)$$

What are the eigenvalues?

$$\hat{O}P_1 = \frac{1}{\sin\theta}\frac{d}{d\theta}\left(\sin\theta\frac{d}{d\theta}(\cos\theta)\right) = \frac{1}{\sin\theta}\frac{d}{d\theta}(-\sin^2\theta)$$

$$\hat{O}P_1 = -\frac{2\sin\theta\cos\theta}{\sin\theta} = -2\cos\theta .$$

Thus P_1 is an eigenfunction of $\hat{O}$ with eigenvalue -2. For P_2:

$$\hat{O}P_2 = \frac{1}{\sin\theta}\frac{d}{d\theta}\left(\sin\theta\frac{d}{d\theta}(3\cos^2\theta - 1)\right) = \frac{1}{\sin\theta}\frac{d}{d\theta}(-6\cos\theta\sin^2\theta)$$

$$\hat{O}P_2 = 6\sin^2\theta - 12\cos^2\theta .$$

Since $6\sin^2\theta = 6 - 6\cos^2\theta$, $\hat{O}P_2 = 6 - 18\cos^2\theta = -6P_2$.

Thus P_2 is an eigenfunction with eigenvalue -6.

11.19 Find the result of operating ∇^2 on the function $(x^2 + y^2 + z^2)$. Is it an eigenfunction? Try the same problem in polar coordinates; you should get the same answer.

$$\nabla^2(x^2 + y^2 + z^2) = \frac{\partial}{\partial x^2}(x^2) + \frac{\partial}{\partial y^2}(y^2) + \frac{\partial}{\partial z^2}(z^2)$$

$$\nabla^2(x^2 + y^2 + z^2) = \frac{\partial}{\partial x}(2x) + \frac{\partial}{\partial y}(2y) + \frac{\partial}{\partial z}(2z) = 6 .$$

In polar coordinates, $x^2 + y^2 + z^2 = r^2$. Then

$$\nabla^2(r^2) = \frac{1}{r^2}\frac{\partial}{\partial r}\left\{r^2\frac{\partial}{\partial r}(r^2)\right] = \frac{1}{r^2}\frac{\partial}{\partial r}[2r^3] = 6 .$$

$(x^2 + y^2 + z^2)$ is not an eigenfunction of ∇^2 since

$\nabla^2(x^2 + y^2 + z^2) \neq a(x^2 + y^2 + z^2)$ where a is a constant.

11.20 Operate with ∇^2 (in Cartesian coordinates) on the function $\psi = \exp(ax + by + cz)$. Is it an eigenfunction?

$\nabla^2\psi = \frac{\partial}{\partial x}\left(\frac{\partial\psi}{\partial x}\right) + \frac{\partial}{\partial y}\left(\frac{\partial\psi}{\partial y}\right) + \frac{\partial}{\partial z}\left(\frac{\partial\psi}{\partial z}\right)$. $\frac{\partial\psi}{\partial x} = a\psi$, $\frac{\partial\psi}{\partial y} = b\psi$, and $\frac{\partial\psi}{\partial z} = c\psi$. Also, $\frac{\partial^2\psi}{\partial x^2} = a^2\psi$, $\frac{\partial^2\psi}{\partial y^2} = b^2\psi$ and $\frac{\partial^2\psi}{\partial z^2} = c^2\psi$. Thus

Thus $\nabla^2\psi = (a^2 + b^2 + c^2)\psi$. ψ is an eigenfunction of ∇^2 with eigenvalue $(a^2 + b^2 + c^2)$.

11.21 Show that the momentum operator $\hat{p}_x$ has eigenfunctions of the form $\psi = e^{ikx}$. What is the physical significance of the constant k?

$\hat{p}_x\psi = -i\hbar \frac{d}{dx}(e^{ikx}) = k\hbar(e^{ikx})$. Thus ψ is an eigenfunction of $\hat{p}_x$ with eigenvalue $k\hbar$. k is the momentum, in units of $\hbar$.

11.22 Calculate $\langle x\rangle$ and $\langle x^2\rangle$ for the one-dimensional particle in a box.

From Eqs. (11.33), (11.43) and (11.46), $\langle x\rangle = \frac{2}{a}\int_0^a x \sin^2\left(\frac{n\pi x}{a}\right)dx$.

Using $\sin^2 \alpha = \frac{1}{2}(1 - \cos 2\alpha)$,

$\langle x\rangle = \frac{1}{a}\int_0^a x\, dx - \frac{1}{a}\int_0^a x \cos\left(\frac{2n\pi x}{a}\right)dx = \frac{1}{a}\int_0^a x\, dx = \frac{a}{2}$, where we have evaluated the cosine integral by parts to show that it is zero.

From Eq. (11.33), $\langle x^2\rangle = \frac{2}{a}\int_0^a x^2\sin^2\left(\frac{n\pi x}{a}\right)dx$. Using an integral table, $\int x^2\sin^2(\alpha x)dx = \frac{x^3}{6} - \left(\frac{x^2}{4\alpha} - \frac{1}{8\alpha^3}\right)\sin 2\alpha x - \frac{x\cos 2\alpha x}{4\alpha^2}$

and with $\alpha = \frac{n\pi}{2}$, $\langle x^2\rangle = \frac{a^3}{3} - \frac{a^2}{2n^2\pi^2}$.

11.23 Derive an equation for the probability that a particle in a one-dimensional box is in the first quarter of the box. Show that this probability approaches the classical limit as $n \to \infty$.

Using Eqs. (11.27), (11.43) and (11.46),

$P = \int_0^{0.25a} \frac{2}{a}\sin^2\left(\frac{n\pi x}{a}\right)dx$. Since $\sin^2 \alpha = \frac{1}{2}(1 - \cos 2\alpha)$,

$$P = \int_0^{0.25a}\frac{1}{a}\left(1 - \cos\left(\frac{2n\pi x}{a}\right)\right)dx = \left\{\frac{x}{a} - \frac{1}{2n\pi}\sin\left(\frac{2n\pi x}{a}\right)\right\}\Bigg|_0^{0.25a}$$

$$P = 0.25 - \frac{1}{2n\pi}\sin\left(\frac{n\pi}{2}\right) .$$

In the limit $n \to \infty$, $P = 0.25$.

11.24 Prove that the functions $\psi_1 = A\sin(\pi x/a)$ and $\psi_2 = A\sin(2\pi x/a)$ are orthogonal.

$$\int_{-\infty}^{\infty} \psi_1\psi_2 dx = \int_0^a A^2 \sin\left(\frac{\pi x}{a}\right) \sin\left(\frac{2\pi x}{a}\right)dx$$

$$\int_{-\infty}^{\infty} \psi_1\psi_2 dx = \frac{A^2 a}{\pi}\left[\frac{\sin\left\{(1-2)\frac{\pi x}{a}\right\}}{2(1-2)} - \frac{\sin\left\{(1+2)\frac{\pi x}{a}\right\}}{2(1+2)}\right]\Bigg|_0^a$$

$$\int_{-\infty}^{\infty} \psi_1\psi_2 dx = \frac{A^2 a}{\pi}\left[\frac{1}{2}\sin\left(\frac{\pi x}{a}\right) - \frac{1}{6}\sin\left(\frac{3\pi x}{a}\right)\right]\Bigg|_0^a = 0 .$$

11.25 Calculate the value of A so that $\psi_n = A\sin(n\pi x/a)$ is normalized in the region $0 < x < a$.

From Eq. (11.35), $\int_0^a A^2 \sin^2\left(\frac{n\pi x}{a}\right)dx = 1$. Using

$\sin^2 \alpha = \frac{1}{2}(1 - \cos 2\alpha)$,

$$\int_0^a \frac{A^2}{2}\left(1 - \cos\left(\frac{2n\pi x}{a}\right)\right)dx = \frac{A^2}{2}\left(x - \frac{a}{2n\pi}\sin\left(\frac{2n\pi x}{a}\right)\right)\Bigg|_0^a = \frac{A^2 a}{2} = 1$$

or $A = \sqrt{\frac{2}{a}}$.

11.26 Demonstrate that the $n = 1$ state of the one-dimensional particle in a box conforms to the Heisenberg uncertainty principle. To do this, calculate $\langle x\rangle$, $\langle x^2\rangle$, $\langle p\rangle$ and $\langle p^2\rangle$ and, from these, calculate the uncertainty product $\delta x\, \delta p$.

From problem 11.22, with n = 1: $\langle x\rangle = \frac{a}{2}$, $\langle x^2\rangle = \frac{a^3}{3} - \frac{a^2}{2\pi^2}$.

With $\hat{p}_x = \frac{\hbar}{i}\frac{\partial}{\partial x}$ and $\hat{p}_x^2 = -\hbar^2\frac{\partial^2}{\partial x^2}$:

$$\langle p\rangle = \frac{2\hbar}{ai}\int_0^a \sin\left(\frac{n\pi x}{a}\right)\frac{d}{dx}\left(\sin\left(\frac{n\pi x}{a}\right)\right)dx = 0 \quad \text{and}$$

$$\langle p^2\rangle = -\frac{2\hbar^2}{a}\int_0^a \sin\left(\frac{n\pi x}{a}\right)\frac{d^2}{dx^2}\left(\sin\left(\frac{n\pi x}{a}\right)\right)dx$$

$$\langle p^2\rangle = \frac{2\hbar^2}{a}\left(\frac{n^2\pi^2}{a^2}\right)\int_0^a \sin^2\!\left(\frac{n\pi x}{a}\right) dx = \frac{n^2h^2}{4a^2} .$$

Thus: $\delta x = [\langle x^2\rangle - \langle x\rangle^2]^{1/2} = \left[\frac{a^2}{3} - \frac{a^2}{2\pi^2} - \frac{a^2}{4}\right]^{1/2} = 0.18a$.

$\delta p = \left[\frac{n^2h^2}{4a^2}\right]^{1/2} = \frac{h}{2a}$ so that $\delta p\delta x = 0.09h > \frac{\hbar}{2}$.

11.27 Derive a formula for the energy of a particle in a two-dimensional square box. List the energies (as multiples of h^2/ma^2) and degeneracies of the ten lowest energy levels.

In two dimensions: $-\frac{\hbar^2}{2m}\left(\frac{\partial^2\psi}{\partial x^2} + \frac{\partial^2\psi}{\partial y^2}\right) = E\psi$. Assuming $\psi = \psi_x(x)\psi_y(y)$ then: $-\frac{\hbar^2}{2m}\left[\frac{\psi_x''}{\psi_x} + \frac{\psi_y''}{\psi_y}\right] = E$. With $E = E_x + E_y$, we have, $-\frac{\hbar^2}{2m}\frac{\psi_x''}{\psi_x} = E_x$, $\frac{d^2\psi_x}{dx^2} = -k_x^2\psi_x$, and $k_x = \frac{n_x\pi}{a}$, with similar results for the y dimension. Thus

$E_{n_xn_y} = \frac{h^2}{8ma^2}(n_x^2 + n_y^2)$. The ten lowest levels and degeneracies are as follows with $\alpha \equiv \frac{h^2}{8ma^2}$:

n_x	n_y	$E_{n_xn_y}$	g
1	1	α	1
1	2	5α	2
2	1	5α	
2	2	8α	1
1	3	10α	2
3	1	10α	
2	3	13α	2
3	2	13α	

n_x	n_y	$E_{n_x n_y}$	g
1	4	17α	2
4	1	17α	
3	3	18α	1
2	4	20α	2
4	2	20α	
3	4	25α	2
4	3	25α	
1	5	26α	2
5	1	26α	

11.28 Generally, the quantization of translational motion is not significant for objects as massive as an atom. However, this conclusion could change if the atom were restricted to a very small region of space. Zeolites (Chapter 16) are minerals with small pores into which small molecules readily penetrate; chambers with diameter 10 Å are typical. In such restricted regions one may wonder whether the quantization of translational motion is important. Calculate the energy of the $n_x = 10, n_y = 10, n_z = 10$ state of an H_2 molecule in a 10-Å cubic box. Compare this number to kT at 300 K. (Look at Figure 11.9—this will give you a feeling for how many states are occupied at this temperature.)

With $n_x = n_y = n_z = 10$, $E = E_x + E_y + E_z = \dfrac{3(10)^2 h^2}{8ma^2}$. Using

$a = 10 \times 10^{-10}$ m and $m = 2.016(1.6725 \times 10^{-27}$ kg) we find

$E = 4.88 \times 10^{-21}$ J . $kT = 4.14 \times 10^{-21}$ J .

11.29 Calculate the zero-point translational energy of (a) an H_2 molecule in a 1-mm cubic box, (b) an electron in a 1-Å cubic box.

a) $E = (n_x^2 + n_y^2 + n_z^2)\dfrac{h^2}{8ma^2} = \dfrac{3(6.626 \times 10^{-34}\ \text{J s})^2}{8(3.3468 \times 10^{-27}\ \text{kg})(10^{-3}\ \text{m})^2}$

$E = 4.92 \times 10^{-35}$ J $= 4.92 \times 10^{-28}$ erg .

b) E(e- , 1 Å box) $= 1.81 \times 10^{-17}$ J $= 1.81 \times 10^{-10}$ erg .

11.30 You recently found a 10 g bar of gold in a 1 dm^3 cubic box, placed there by your ancestor 500 years ago. How far has the bar moved since it was placed in the box?

If we consider the bar to be a particle in a box, then:

$E = \frac{h^2}{8ma^2}(n_x^2 + n_y^2 + n_z^2)$. The minimum energy is:

$E_{min} = \frac{3h^2}{8ma^2}$. Using m = 10 g and a = 10 cm:

$E_{min} = 1.646 \times 10^{-56}$ ergs . Also, $E_{min} = \frac{1}{2} mv_{min}^2$ where v_{min} is the minimum velocity. Thus: $v_{min} = 5.74 \times 10^{-29}$ cm s^{-1} .

$t = (500 \text{ years})(365 \text{ days year}^{-1})(24 \text{ hrs day}^{-1})(3600 \text{ s hr}^{-1})$

$t = 1.577 \times 10^{10}$ s .

Thus, $\Delta x = vt = 9 \times 10^{-19}$ cm = 0.009 am .

11.31 Calculate the average translational quantum number for a H_2 molecule in a cubic box 1 mm on a side when T = 10 K.

$E = \frac{3}{2} kT = \frac{3}{2}(1.38 \times 10^{-23} \text{ J K}^{-1})(10 \text{ K}) = 2.07 \times 10^{-22}$ J .

Defining $\bar{n}$ as the average translational quantum number, then

$E = \frac{3\bar{n}^2 h^2}{8ma^2}$ or

$\bar{n} = \frac{a}{h}\left(\frac{8mE}{3}\right)^{1/2}$

$$\bar{n} = \frac{10^{-3} \text{ m}}{6.626 \times 10^{-34} \text{ J s}}\left(\frac{8(3.3468 \times 10^{-27} \text{ kg})(2.07 \times 10^{-22} \text{ J})}{3}\right)^{1/2}$$

$\bar{n} = 2 \times 10^6$.

11.32 Derive a formula for the energy of a particle in a box with nonequal sides — that is, $0 < x < a$, $0 < y < b$, $0 < z < c$.

$\frac{d^2\psi}{dx^2} = -\left(\frac{2mE_x}{\hbar^2}\right)\psi$ with analogous equations for the y and z directions. Solving each equation separately with appropriate boundary conditions, we find $E_x = \frac{n_x^2 h^2}{8ma^2}$, $E_y = \frac{n_y^2 h^2}{8mb^2}$ and $E_2 = \frac{n_z^2 h^2}{8mc^2}$. The total energy is

$$E = E_x + E_y + E_z = \left(\frac{n_x^2}{a^2} + \frac{n_y^2}{b^2} + \frac{n_z^2}{c^2}\right)\frac{h^2}{8m} .$$

11.33 Calculate the value for the constant A_v required to normalize the $v = 2$ harmonic-oscillator wave function.

From Eq. (11.62), $\int_{-\infty}^{\infty} \psi_v^2\, dx = 1 = \alpha A_2^2 \int_{-\infty}^{\infty} (4y^2 - 2)e^{-y^2} dy$ where α is given by Eq. (11.55) and $dx = \alpha dy$. Then

$1 = \alpha A_2^2 \int_{-\infty}^{\infty} (16y^4 - 16y^2 + 4)e^{-y^2} dy$. Using Table 11.3,

$1 = \alpha A_2^2(12\sqrt{\pi} - 8\sqrt{\pi} + 4\sqrt{\pi})$ or $A_2^2 = \frac{1}{8\sqrt{\pi}\alpha}$.

11.34 In the harmonic-oscillator problem, what are the units of the following quantities in the cgs system? k, μ, α, ψ.

a) $k \; [=] \; \dfrac{\text{force}}{\text{displacement}} \; [=] \; \dfrac{\text{g cm s}^{-2}}{\text{cm}} \; [=] \; \text{g s}^{-2}$.

b) $\mu = \dfrac{m_1 m_2}{m_1 + m_2} \; [=] \; \text{g}$ (mass) .

c) $\alpha = \left(\dfrac{k^2}{k\mu}\right)^{1/4} = \left(\dfrac{\text{g}^2\ \text{cm}^4\ \text{s}^{-2}}{\text{g}^2\ \text{s}^{-2}}\right)^{1/4} \; [=] \; \text{cm}$.

d) $\int_{-\infty}^{\infty} \psi_v^2\, dx = 1$, with $x \; [=] \; \text{cm}$, then $\psi_v \; [=] \; \text{cm}^{-1/2}$.

11.35 Prove that the harmonic-oscillator wave function for $v = 0$ is orthogonal to those for $v = 1$ and $v = 2$.

Using Eq. (11.62) and Table 11.2,

$\int_{-\infty}^{\infty} \psi_0\psi_1\, dy = A_0A_1\int_{-\infty}^{\infty} 2ye^{-y^2} dy = -A_0A_1e^{-y^2}\Big|_{-\infty}^{\infty} = 0$. Thus ψ_1 and ψ_0 are orthogonal. Also, $\int_{-\infty}^{\infty} \psi_0\psi_2\, dy = A_0A_2\int_{-\infty}^{\infty} (4y^2 - 2)e^{-y^2} dy$.

Using Table 11.3, $\int_{-\infty}^{\infty} \psi_0\psi_2\, dy = A_0A_2\left(\frac{4\sqrt{\pi}}{2} - 2\sqrt{\pi}\right) = 0$. Thus ψ_0 and ψ_2 are also orthogonal.

11.36 Calculate the probability that a harmonic oscillator in the $v = 0$ state will be found outside its classical turning points.

At the classical turning point, $E = V = \frac{1}{2} kx_0^2$ or $x_0 = \left(\frac{2E}{k}\right)^{1/2}$.

The probability that the particle will be found at $x > x_0$ is

$P = 2\int_{x_0}^{\infty} \psi^*\psi \, dx = 2\int_{1}^{\infty} \psi^*\psi \, dy$, where $dx = \alpha \, dy$. For the $v = 0$ state, $\psi_0 = \frac{1}{\pi^{1/4}} e^{-y^2/2}$, so that $P = \frac{2}{\sqrt{\pi}}\int_{1}^{\infty} e^{-y^2} dy$. The integral is equal to $\frac{2}{\sqrt{\pi}}\int_{0}^{\infty} e^{-y^2} dy - \frac{2}{\sqrt{\pi}}\int_{0}^{1} e^{-y^2} dy$. Using the example of AI.4 (Simpson's Rule), $P = 1 - \frac{2}{\sqrt{\pi}}(0.747) = 15.73\%$.

11.37 (a) For the harmonic oscillator, calculate:

$$\langle V \rangle = \tfrac{1}{2}k\langle x^2 \rangle$$

for the $v = 0$ state.
(b) Using $T = p^2/2\mu = E - V$, calculate $\langle p^2 \rangle$ for the harmonic oscillator.
(c) Show that $\delta p \, \delta x = \hbar/2$ for the harmonic-oscillator $v = 0$ state.

a) $x = \alpha y$, so that using Eq. (11.33) and Tables 11.2 and 11.3,

$\langle x^2 \rangle = \frac{\alpha^2}{\pi^{1/2}}\int_{-\infty}^{\infty} y^2 e^{-y^2} dy = \frac{\alpha^2}{2} = \frac{\hbar}{2(k\mu)^{1/2}}$. Then $\langle v \rangle = \frac{k\alpha^2}{4}$.

b) $\langle p^2 \rangle = 2\mu\langle E - V \rangle = 2\mu\left(E_0 - \frac{k\alpha^2}{4}\right)$ where $E_0 = \frac{\hbar}{2}\left(\frac{k}{\mu}\right)^{1/2}$. Thus

$$\langle p^2 \rangle = \hbar(k\mu)^{1/2} - \frac{k\mu\alpha^2}{2} = \frac{\hbar}{2}(k\mu)^{1/2}.$$

c) If we take $\delta x = \langle x^2 \rangle^{1/2} = \left(\frac{\hbar^2}{4k\mu}\right)^{1/4}$ and

$\delta p = \langle p^2 \rangle^{1/2} = \left(\frac{\hbar^2 k\mu}{4}\right)^{1/4}$, then $\delta p \delta x = \frac{\hbar}{2}$.

11.38 (a) Prove that the product of the operators $\hat{A}$ and $\hat{B}$ [defined by Eq. (11.59)] is equal to $\hat{h} - 1$ [$\hat{h}$ is defined by Eq. (11.56)].
(b) For the lowest harmonic oscillator function, $\hat{B}\psi_0 = 0$, therefore $\hat{A}\hat{B}\psi = 0$. Use the result of part (a) to prove that the lowest eigenvalue of the operator $\hat{h}$ [Eq. (11.56)] is 1 *without* assuming any specific form for the function ψ_0.

a) We wish to calculate:

$$\hat{A}\hat{B}f(y) = \left(y - \frac{d}{dy}\right)\left(y + \frac{d}{dy}\right)f = y^2 f + y\frac{df}{dy} - f - y\frac{df}{dy} - \frac{d^2 f}{dy^2}$$

$$\hat{A}\hat{B}f(y) = y^2 f - \frac{d^2 f}{dy^2} - f$$

so that $\hat{A}\hat{B} = y^2 - \frac{d^2}{dy^2} - 1 = \hat{h} - 1$.

b) Given $\hat{B}\psi_0 = 0$ and $\hat{A}\hat{B}\psi_0 = 0$ we must have $\hat{A}\hat{B}\psi_0 = (\hat{h} - 1)\psi_0 = 0$

so that $\hat{h}\psi_0 = \psi_0$. Clearly, 1 is the lowest eigenvalue for $\hat{h}$.

11.39 Given the harmonic oscillator eigenvalue equation:

$$\hat{h}\psi_n = (2n + 1)\psi_n$$

Find the result $\hat{A}\hat{B}\psi_n$. Is this an eigenvalue relationship?

$\hat{h}\psi_n = (2n + 1)\psi_n$. From the previous problem, $\hat{h} = \hat{A}\hat{B} + 1$ so

that $(\hat{A}\hat{B} + 1)\psi_n = (2n + 1)\psi_n$ and $\hat{A}\hat{B}\psi_n = 2n\psi_n$. 2n is a

constant, so that the eigenvalue of $\hat{A}\hat{B}$ is 2n .

11.40 (a) Derive the commutator for the harmonic oscillator operators $\hat{A}$ and $\hat{B}$ [Eq. (11.59)].
(b) Given that $\hat{A}\psi_n = \psi_{n+1}$, show that $\hat{B}\psi_n = (\text{const})\psi_{n-1}$. What is the value of the constant?

a) We wish to find $[\hat{A}, \hat{B}]f(y) = (\hat{A}\hat{B} - \hat{B}\hat{A})f(y)$. From problem 11.38, $\hat{A}\hat{B} = \hat{h} - 1$.

$$\hat{B}\hat{A}f = \left(y + \frac{d}{dy}\right)\left(y - \frac{d}{dy}\right)f = y^2 f + f + y\frac{df}{dy} - y\frac{df}{dy} - \frac{d^2f}{dy^2}$$

$$\hat{B}\hat{A}f = (\hat{h} + 1)f \ .$$

Thus: $[\hat{A}, \hat{B}] = (\hat{h} - 1) - (\hat{h} + 1) = -2$.

b) $\hat{A}\psi_n = \psi_{n+1}$. From the text: $\hat{h}\psi_n = (\epsilon_0 + 2n)\psi_n$ so that:

$\hat{B}\hat{A}\psi_n = (\hat{h} + 1)\psi_n = (\epsilon_0 + 2n + 1)\psi_n$. But $\hat{A}\psi_n = \psi_{n+1}$, thus:

$\hat{B}\psi_{n+1} = (\epsilon_0 + 2n + 1)\psi_n$. Letting n = n - 1 gives

$\hat{B}\psi_n = (\epsilon_0 + 2n - 1)\psi_{n-1}$ with $\hat{B}\psi_0 = 0$, $\hat{A}\hat{B}\psi_0 = (\hat{h} - 1)\psi_0 = 0$

and $\hat{h}\psi_0 = \psi_0$. But $\hat{h}\psi_0 = \epsilon_0\psi_0$ so that $\epsilon_0 = 1$ and $\hat{B}\psi_n = 2n\psi_{n-1}$.

11.41 The vibrational constant for H_2 is $\nu_0 = 132$ THz. Calculate the force constant. If you had a spring with this force constant, how much mass would be required to stretch the spring one centimeter?

$k = 4\mu(\pi\nu_0)^2$. With $\mu = \frac{1}{2}(1.67 \times 10^{-27}\ \text{kg})$ and $\nu_0 = 132 \times 10^{12}\ \text{s}^{-1}$ we find: $k = 574\ \text{kg s}^{-2}$. The force of the spring must balance the force due to gravity: $kx = mg$.

$$m = \frac{kx}{g} = 0.586\ \text{kg} = 586\ \text{g} \ .$$

11.42 Show that the functions:

$$\psi_m = \frac{1}{\sqrt{2\pi}} e^{im\phi}$$

where m is an integer, are orthonormal—that is:

$$\int \psi_m^* \psi_{m'}\, d\phi \begin{cases} = 0 & \text{if } m \neq m' \\ = 1 & \text{if } m = m' \end{cases}$$

If m ≠ m' , then

$$\int_{\text{all space}} \psi_m^* \psi_{m'}\, d\phi = \frac{1}{2\pi}\int_0^{2\pi} e^{i(m+m')\phi} d\phi$$

$$\int_{\text{all space}} \psi_m^* \psi_{m'}\, d\phi = \frac{1}{2\pi}\int_0^{2\pi} [\cos(m + m')\phi + i \sin(m + m')\phi] d\phi$$

$$\int_{\text{all space}} \psi_m^* \psi_{m'}\, d\phi = \frac{1}{2\pi(m + m')}[\sin(m + m')\phi - i \cos(m + m')\phi] \Big|_0^{2\pi} .$$

If m and m' are integers, then $\sin[2\pi(m + m')] = \sin 0 = 0$.

Also $\cos [(m + m')2\pi] = \cos 0$, so $\frac{1}{2\pi}\int_{\text{all space}} e^{i(m+m')\phi} d\phi = 0$ if

m ≠ m' . If m = m' ,

$$\int_{\text{all space}} \psi_m^* \psi_{m'}\, d\phi = \frac{1}{2\pi}\int_0^{2\pi} e^{-im\phi} e^{im\phi} d\phi = \frac{1}{2\pi}\int_0^{2\pi} d\phi = 1 .$$ Thus the

functions ψ_m are orthonormal.

11.43 Use the commutators $[\hat{L}_x, \hat{L}_y]$ and so on to prove $[\hat{L}^2, \hat{L}_x] = 0$.

Using Eq. (11.74a),

$$[\hat{L}^2, \hat{L}_x] = \hat{L}^2\hat{L}_x - \hat{L}_x\hat{L}^2$$

$$[\hat{L}^2, \hat{L}_x] = \hat{L}_x^2\hat{L}_x + \hat{L}_y^2\hat{L}_x + \hat{L}_z^2\hat{L}_x - \hat{L}_x\hat{L}_x^2 - \hat{L}_x\hat{L}_y^2 - \hat{L}_x\hat{L}_z^2$$

From Eq. (11.75), $\hat{L}_x^2\hat{L}_x - \hat{L}_x\hat{L}_x^2 = 0$, so

$$[\hat{L}^2, \hat{L}_x] = \hat{L}_y^2\hat{L}_x + \hat{L}_z^2\hat{L}_x - \hat{L}_x\hat{L}_z^2 - \hat{L}_x\hat{L}_y^2$$

$$[\hat{L}^2, \hat{L}_x] = \hat{L}_y[\hat{L}_y, \hat{L}_x] - [\hat{L}_x, \hat{L}_y]\hat{L}_y + \hat{L}_z[\hat{L}_z, \hat{L}_x] - [\hat{L}_x, \hat{L}_z]\hat{L}_z .$$

Using Eq. (11.72), $[\hat{L}_x, \hat{L}_y] = i\hbar\hat{L}_z$, etc., then

$$[\hat{L}^2, \hat{L}_x] = i\hbar[-\hat{L}_y\hat{L}_z - \hat{L}_z\hat{L}_y + \hat{L}_z\hat{L}_y + \hat{L}_y\hat{L}_z] = 0$$

11.44 (a) Prove that, in spherical polar coordinates:

$$\hat{L}_+ = \hbar\left(e^{i\phi}\frac{\partial}{\partial\theta} + i \cot\theta\, e^{i\phi}\frac{\partial}{\partial\phi}\right)$$

(b) Find the result $\hat{L}_+ \cos\theta$ and $\hat{L}_+^2 \cos\theta$. Explain these results.

a) Using Eqs. (11.73a) and (11.73b),

$$\hat{L}_+ = \hat{L}_x + i\hat{L}_y$$

$$\hat{L}_+ = \hbar(\cos\Phi + i\sin\Phi)\frac{\partial}{\partial\theta} + \hbar\cot\theta(i\cos\Phi - \sin\Phi)\frac{\partial}{\partial\Phi}.$$

$e^{i\Phi} = \cos\Phi + i\sin\Phi$, so $\hat{L}_+ = \hbar e^{i\Phi}\frac{\partial}{\partial\theta} + i\hbar\cot\theta\, e^{i\Phi}\frac{\partial}{\partial\Phi}$.

b) $\hat{L}_+\cos\theta = \hbar e^{i\Phi}\frac{\partial}{\partial\theta}(\cos\theta) = -\hbar e^{i\Phi}\sin\theta$.

$$\hat{L}_+^2\cos\theta = \hat{L}_+\left(-\hbar e^{i\Phi}\sin\theta\right) = \hbar\left(e^{i\Phi}\frac{\partial}{\partial\theta} + i\cot\theta\, e^{i\Phi}\frac{\partial}{\partial\Phi}\right)\left(-\hbar e^{i\Phi}\sin\theta\right)$$

$$\hat{L}_+^2\cos\theta = -\hbar^2\left(e^{2i\Phi}\cos\theta - e^{2i\Phi}\cos\theta\right) = 0 .$$

11.45 Show that a state function that is radially symmetric, such as $\psi(r) = Ae^{-cr}$, has no angular momentum.

$\psi = \psi(r)$. By comparison with Eq. (11.74c),

$$\hat{L}^2 = -\hbar^2\left[\frac{\partial^2}{\partial\theta^2} + \cot\theta\,\frac{\partial}{\partial\theta} + \frac{1}{\sin^2\theta}\,\frac{\partial^2}{\partial\phi^2}\right]$$. Thus $\hat{L}^2\psi(r) = 0$.

Similarly, comparison with Eqs. (11.73a) - (11.73c) shows that

$\hat{L}_x\psi(r) = 0$, $\hat{L}_y\psi(r) = 0$ and $\hat{L}_z\psi(r) = 0$.

11.46 The effect of the raising operator $\hat{L}_+$ on an angular momentum eigenfunction is:

$$\hat{L}_+\psi_{l,m} = C\psi_{l,l+1}$$

where C is a constant. This can be reversed with the lowering operator:

$$\hat{L}_-\psi_{l,m+1} = C'\psi_{l,m}$$

where C' is a constant. Assuming $C = C'$, determine the value of C in terms of the quantum numbers l and m. (Hint: Operate on the first equation with $\hat{L}_-$; then use the second equation on the right-hand side.) Take special note of the case $m = l$.

$\hat{L}_+\psi_{l,m} = C\psi_{l,m+1}$, $\hat{L}_-\psi_{l,m+1} = C\psi_{l,m}$. Thus:

$\hat{L}_-(\hat{L}_+\psi_{l,m}) = \hat{L}_-(C\psi_{l,m+1}) = C^2\psi_{l,m}$. Also,

$\hat{L}_-\hat{L}_+ = \hat{L}^2 - \hat{L}_z^{\,2} - \hbar\hat{L}_z$, $\hat{L}^2\psi_{l,m} = l(l + 1)\hbar^2\psi_{l,m}$ and

$\hat{L}_z\psi_{l,m} = m\hbar\psi_{l,m}$. Thus $C^2\psi_{l,m} = (l(l + 1) - m^2 - m)\hbar^2\psi_{l,m}$ and

$$C = \hbar[l(l + 1) - m(m + 1)]^{1/2} .$$

11.47 Show that the angular momentum eigenfunctions ($\psi_{l,m}$) are eigenfunctions of the operator $\hat{L}_+\hat{L}_-$. What is the eigenvalue? Take special note of the case $m = -l$.

$\hat{L}_+\hat{L}_-\psi_{l,m} = (\hat{L}^2 - \hat{L}_z^{\,2} + \hbar\hat{L}_z)\psi_{l,m}$, $\hat{L}^2\psi_{l,m} = l(l + 1)\hbar^2$ and

$\hat{L}_z\psi_{l,m} = m\hbar\psi_{l,m}$. Thus:

$$\hat{L}_+\hat{L}_-\psi_{l,m} = \hbar^2[l(l + 1) - m^2 + m]\psi_{l,m}$$

$$\hat{L}_+\hat{L}_-\psi_{l,m} = \hbar^2[l(l + 1) - m(m - 1)]\psi_{l,m} .$$

11.48 For an angular momentum quantum number $l = 3/2$, what is the magnitude of the angular momentum? How many orientations are permitted? What are the angles of these orientations with respect to the z axis?

Magnitude: $\sqrt{\frac{3}{2}\left(\frac{3}{2} + 1\right)}\ \hbar = 1.9365\ \hbar$.

Orientations: $4 \left(m = \frac{3}{2}, \frac{1}{2}, -\frac{1}{2}, -\frac{3}{2}\right)$

Angles: $\theta = \cos^{-1}\left[\frac{m}{\sqrt{l(l + 1)}}\right]$

$$m = \frac{3}{2},\ \theta = 39^\circ;\ m = \frac{1}{2},\ \theta = 75^\circ;$$

$$m = -\frac{1}{2},\ \theta = 105^\circ;\ m = -\frac{3}{2},\ \theta = 141^\circ$$

11.49 (a) Calculate the moment of inertia of HCl^{35}; use $R = 0.1275$ nm.
(b) Assuming R to be the same, calculate I for the other isotopes: HCl^{37}, DCl^{35}, DCl^{37}.

a) The moment of inertia is

$$I = \mu R^2 = \frac{m_1 m_2}{m_1 + m_2} R^2 = \frac{(1.0079)(34.969)(0.1275 \times 10^{-7}\ cm)^2}{(1.0079 + 34.969)(6.022 \times 10^{23})g^{-1}}$$

$$I = 2.64 \times 10^{-40}\ g\ cm^2 .$$

b) Using $m_D = \frac{2.0140\ g}{6.022 \times 10^{23}}$ and $m_{Cl^{37}} = \frac{36.966\ g}{6.022 \times 10^{23}}$,

$I(HCl^{37}) = 2.65 \times 10^{-40}\ g\ cm^2$, $I(DCl^{35}) = 5.14 \times 10^{-40}\ g\ cm^2$ and

$$I(DCl^{37}) = 5.16 \times 10^{-4}\ g\ cm^2 .$$

11.50 (a) Calculate the average l of a small gyroscope that has $I = 1$ g cm^2 and is rotating with an angular velocity $\omega = 159$ rad/sec. What is the minimum amount by which the velocity may change for this gyroscope? Is the orientation "quantized"?
(b) Calculate the average l of CO molecules ($I = 14.48 \times 10^{-40}$ g cm^2) with an average rotational energy of kT at $T = 300$ K.

a) From Eq. (11.91), $L = \sqrt{l(l+1)}\,\hbar$. The classical angular momentum is $L = I\omega$. Thus for $l \gg 1$,

$$l \cong \frac{I\omega}{\hbar} = \frac{(1\ \text{g cm}^2)(159\ \text{s}^{-1})}{(1.0544 \times 10^{-27}\ \text{erg s})} = 1.51 \times 10^{29}$$

. The minimum change in angular velocity corresponds to $\Delta l = \pm 1$, thus

$$\Delta\omega = \frac{I\hbar}{I} = \pm 1.05 \times 10^{-27}\ \text{s}^{-1}$$

. The orientation is not quantized.

b) From Eq. (11.97), $l(l+1) = \dfrac{8\pi^2 I E_l}{h^2}$. Using

$E_l = kT = 4.1415 \times 10^{-14}$ erg , $l = 9.9 \cong 10$.

11.51 Calculate the commutator: $[\hat{L}_+, \hat{L}_-]$, starting with $[\hat{L}_x, \hat{L}_y] = i\hbar\hat{L}_z$, etc.

Using Eq. (11.81),

$$[\hat{L}_+, \hat{L}_-] = (\hat{L}_x + i\hat{L}_y)(\hat{L}_x - i\hat{L}_y) - (\hat{L}_x - i\hat{L}_y)(\hat{L}_x + i\hat{L}_y)$$

$$[\hat{L}_+, \hat{L}_-] = \hat{L}_x^2 + i\hat{L}_y\hat{L}_x - i\hat{L}_x\hat{L}_y + \hat{L}_y^2 - \hat{L}_x^2 + i\hat{L}_y\hat{L}_x - i\hat{L}_x\hat{L}_y - \hat{L}_y^2$$

$$[\hat{L}_+, \hat{L}_-] = 2i(\hat{L}_y\hat{L}_x - \hat{L}_x\hat{L}_y) = 2i[\hat{L}_y, \hat{L}_x]\ .$$

Since $[\hat{L}_y, \hat{L}_x] = -i\hbar\hat{L}_z$, $[\hat{L}_+, \hat{L}_-] = 2\hbar\hat{L}_z$.

11.52 Prove, by direct operation, that the function $(3\cos^2\theta - 1)$ is an eigenfunction of $\hat{L}^2$. What must the quantum numbers (l, m) be for this function?

Using Eq. (11.74b),

$$\hat{L}^2\psi = -\hbar^2\left[\frac{1}{\sin\theta}\left(\frac{\partial}{\partial\theta}\left[\sin\theta\,\frac{\partial}{\partial\theta}(3\cos^2\theta - 1)\right]\right)\right]$$

$$\hat{L}^2\psi = -\hbar^2\left[\frac{1}{\sin\theta}\left(\frac{\partial}{\partial\theta}[-6\cos\theta\,\sin^2\theta]\right)\right] = -\hbar^2(6\sin^2\theta - 12\cos^2\theta)\ .$$

Since $6\sin^2\theta + 6\cos^2\theta = 6$, $\hat{L}^2\psi = -\hbar^2(6 - 18\cos^2\theta) = 6\hbar^2\psi$.

The eigenvalue is $6\hbar^2$. From Eq. (11.91),

$\hat{L}^2\psi_{l,m} = l(l + 1)\hbar^2\psi_{l,m}$, thus $l(l + 1) = 6$ and $l = 2$. Also,

$\hat{L}_z\psi_{l,m} = m\hbar\psi_{l,m} = -i\hbar\,\frac{\partial}{\partial\phi}(3\cos^2\theta - 1) = 0$, so that $m = 0$.

11.53 From Table 11.8, what is the spherical harmonic for $l = 2, m = -2$? Show by direct operation that this function is an eigenfunction of $\hat{L}^2$ and $\hat{L}_z$ with the appropriate eigenvalues.

From Table 11.8 with $l = 2$ and $|m| = 2$: $\psi_{2,-2} = \sin^2\theta\, e^{-2i\phi}$,

$\hat{L}_z = -i\hbar\,\frac{\partial}{\partial\phi}$, $\hat{L}_z\psi_{2,-2} = -2\hbar\psi_{2,-2}$ so that the eigenvalue of $\hat{L}_z$

is $-2\hbar$. $\hat{L}^2 = -\hbar^2\left(\frac{\partial^2}{\partial\theta^2} + \cot\theta\,\frac{\partial}{\partial\theta} + \frac{1}{\sin^2\theta}\,\frac{\partial^2}{\partial\phi^2}\right)$,

$$\frac{\partial^2}{\partial\theta^2}(\psi_{2,-2}) = (2\cos^2\theta - 2\sin^2\theta)e^{-2i\phi}\ ,$$

$\cot\theta\,\frac{\partial}{\partial\theta}(\psi_{2,-2}) = 2\cos^2\theta\, e^{-2i\phi}$, and $\frac{1}{\sin^2\theta}\,\frac{\partial^2}{\partial\phi^2}(\psi_{2,-2}) = -4e^{-2i\phi}$.

Thus:

$$\hat{L}^2(\psi_{2,-2}) = -\hbar^2(4\cos^2\theta - 2\sin^2\theta - 4)e^{-2i\phi} = 6\hbar^2\sin^2\theta\, e^{-2i\phi}$$

so that the eigenvalue of $\hat{L}^2$ is $6\hbar^2$.

11.54 According to the equipartition principle, the average rotational energy of a linear molecule is kT. Calculate the average rotational quantum number for carbon monoxide ($I = 1.45 \times 10^{-39}$ g cm^2) at $T = 300$ K.

We have $kT = E_l = \dfrac{l(l+1)h^2}{8\pi^2 I}$. Using $T = 300$ K ,

$I = 1.45 \times 10^{-39}$ g cm^2 , $h = 6.626 \times 10^{-27}$ erg s , and

$k = 1.38 \times 10^{-16}$ erg K^{-1} we find: $\underline{l} = 10$.

11.55 Calculate the energy of light with a wavelength of 600 nm (which is near the center of the visible part of the spectrum) in ergs, eV, Hz, cm^{-1} and kJ/mol.

With $\lambda = 600 \times 10^{-7}$ cm : $E = \dfrac{hc}{\lambda} = 3.31 \times 10^{-12}$ erg . Also:

$E(\text{eV}) = 300\,\dfrac{E}{e} = 2.07$ eV , $E(\text{Hz}) = \dfrac{c}{\lambda} = 5.0 \times 10^{14}$ Hz ,

$E(\text{cm}^{-1}) = \dfrac{1}{\lambda} = 16{,}667$ cm^{-1} , $E(\text{kJ mol}^{-1}) = 10^{-10}\,EL = 199$ kJ mol^{-1}.

11.56 (a) Assuming that a harmonic oscillator is capable of absorbing radiation, show that the transition $v = 0 \rightarrow 1$ is allowed.
(b) Show that the transitions $v = 0 \rightarrow 2$ and $v = 0 \rightarrow 3$ are not allowed.

a) From Eq. (11.100), $I_y \equiv \int_{-\infty}^{\infty} \psi_0 y \psi_1 \, dy$. From Tables 11.2 and 11.3, $I_y = \int_{-\infty}^{\infty} \left(\dfrac{8}{\pi}\right)^{1/2} y^2 e^{-y^2} dy = \sqrt{2}$. Since $I_y \neq 0$,the transition is allowed.

b) $I_y = \int_{-\infty}^{\infty} \psi_o y \psi_2 \, dy = \int_{-\infty}^{\infty} \frac{2}{\sqrt{3\pi}} (4y^3 - 2y)e^{-y^2} dy$

$$I_y = \int_{-\infty}^{\infty} \frac{2}{\sqrt{3\pi}} (4y^3 e^{-y^2}) dy - \int_{-\infty}^{\infty} \frac{4}{\sqrt{3\pi}} y e^{-y^2} dy \; .$$

The second integral is $\int_{-\infty}^{\infty} \frac{4}{\sqrt{3\pi}} y e^{-y^2} dy = - \frac{2}{\sqrt{3\pi}} e^{-y^2} \Big|_{-\infty}^{\infty} = 0$. We do the first integral by parts,

$\int_{-\infty}^{\infty} \frac{2}{\sqrt{3\pi}} 4y^3 e^{-y^2} dy = - \frac{4}{\sqrt{3\pi}} y^2 e^{-y^2} \Big|_{-\infty}^{\infty} + \int_{-\infty}^{\infty} \frac{8}{\sqrt{3\pi}} y e^{-y^2} dy$. Both of the above terms are zero. Thus $I_y = 0$ and the transition is forbidden. For the $\nu = 0 \rightarrow 3$ transition:

$$I_y = \int_{-\infty}^{\infty} \psi_0 y \psi_3 \, dy = \int_{-\infty}^{\infty} A_0 A_3 y(8y^3 - 12y)e^{-y^2} dy$$

$$I_y = A_0 A_3 \int_{-\infty}^{\infty} (8y^4 - 12y^2)e^{-y^2} dy \; .$$

From Table 11.3, $\int_{-\infty}^{\infty} y^4 e^{-y^2} dy = \frac{3\sqrt{\pi}}{4}$ and $\int_{-\infty}^{\infty} y^2 e^{-y^2} dy = \frac{\sqrt{\pi}}{2}$. Thus $I_y(0 \rightarrow 3) = A_0 A_3 [6\sqrt{\pi} - 6\sqrt{\pi}] = 0$ and the transition is forbidden.

11.57 Determine the electric dipole selection rules for a particle on a ring assuming that the particle has a charge q and there is a charge $+q$ at the center of the ring.

For a particle on a ring, $\psi_m = \frac{1}{\sqrt{2\pi}} e^{im\phi}$. A transition $\psi_i \rightarrow \psi_j$ is electric dipole allowed if $\int_{\text{all space}} \psi_i \mu \psi_j \, d\tau$ is nonzero.

From Eq. (11.99), $\mu_x = qr\sin\theta\cos\phi$, $\mu_y = qr\sin\theta\sin\phi$ and $\mu_z = qr\cos\theta$. Since r and θ are constant for a particle on a ring, $\int \psi_m^* \mu_x \psi_n \, d\tau \propto \int_0^{2\pi} e^{i(n-m)\phi} \cos\phi \, d\phi$ and

$\int \psi_m^* \mu_y \psi_n \, d\tau \propto \int_0^{2\pi} e^{i(n-m)\phi} \sin\phi \, d\phi$. Using Euler's formulas,

$\int \psi_m^* \mu_x \psi_n \, d\tau \propto \int_0^{2\pi} \left(e^{i(n-m+1)\phi} + e^{i(n-m-1)\phi}\right) d\phi$ and

$\int \psi_m^* \mu_y \psi_n \, d\tau \propto \int_0^{2\pi} \left(e^{i(n-m+1)\phi} - e^{i(n-m-1)\phi}\right) d\phi$. The integrals above are nonzero only if n - m = 1 or n - m = -1 . Thus $\Delta m = \pm 1$.

11.58 Calculate the wavelength of light that an electron in a (1×10^{-7})-cm box (one dimension) must absorb to change its quantum number from $n = 1 \rightarrow 2$. In what region of the spectrum will this be found? What will be the wavelength of the $n = 1 \rightarrow 3$ transition? Will it be a strong absorption?

$\lambda = \frac{c}{\nu} = \frac{hc}{\Delta E}$. Since $\Delta E = \frac{h^2}{8ma^2}(n_2^2 - n_1^2)$, then

$$\lambda = \frac{8mca^2}{h(n_2^2 - n_1^2)}$$

$$\lambda = \frac{8(9.1094 \times 10^{-31}\ \text{kg})(2.998 \times 10^{8}\ \text{m s}^{-1})(1 \times 10^{-9}\ \text{m})^2}{(6.626 \times 10^{-34}\ \text{J s})(2^2 - 1^2)}$$

$$\lambda = 1.1 \times 10^{-6}\ \text{m} = 1100\ \text{nm} .$$

This is in the uv region. The n = 1 → n = 3 transition will have λ = 412.5 nm . It will not be a strong absorption since it is a forbidden transition.

11.59 F-centers occur in crystals when an anion vacancy is occupied by an electron. These electrons often absorb light in the visible region of the spectrum giving color to the crystal (the "F" in the term is from *Farben*—the German word for color). This can be treated roughly as a particle in a box problem. For example, the chloride ion has a diameter of 3.62 Å, and we could approximate its vacancy as a cubic box of this size. Calculate the energy of the lowest transition of an electron in a 3.62 Å cubic box. The observed F-center absorption in NaCl is 3.6 eV (29000 cm^{-1}); your answer will be significantly in error, but, at least, in the right ball park.

For the particle-in-a-box, the energy of the lowest transition, in wavenumbers, is: $\frac{\Delta E}{hc} = \frac{3h}{8cma^2}$. Using m = 9.109×10^{-28} kg and a = 3.62×10^{-8} cm we find: $\frac{\Delta E}{hc}$ = 69,400 cm^{-1} .

11.60 The formulas for the one-dimensional particle-in-a-box have been used to approximate the energies of the pi electrons in linear conjugated molecules. For example, butadiene:

$$CH_2{=}CH{-}CH{=}CH_2$$

is approximated as a linear "box" with a length equal to the sum of the bond lengths—4.24 Å in this case. The resulting energy levels are "filled" with the available pi electrons (4 in this case) with two per level (spin-up and spin-down). Estimate the absorption frequency of butadiene with this model. Your answer will be quite close to the observed value: 46100 cm^{-1}; the agreement, considering the crudeness of the model, can only be considered fortuitous.

For the one dimensional particle-in-a-box, the lowest energy transition (in wavenumbers) is: $\frac{\Delta E}{hc} = \frac{3h}{8cma^2}$. Using m = 9.109×10^{-28} g and a = 4.24×10^{-8} cm we find:

$$\frac{\Delta E}{hc} = 50578 \text{ cm}^{-1} .$$

11.61 Assuming that a diatomic rotor can absorb radiation and has $I = 10^{-38}$ g cm^2, calculate the frequency of the radiation that will cause a transition from the $l = 1$ to the $l = 2$ state. In what region of the spectrum is this?

From Eqs. (11.97) and (11.98),

$$\nu = [l_2(l_2 + 1) - l_1(l_1 + 1)] \frac{h}{8\pi^2 I}$$

$$\nu = [6 - 2] \frac{(6.626 \times 10^{-27} \text{ erg s})}{8\pi^2(10^{-38} \text{ g cm}^2)} = 3.36 \times 10^{10} \text{ Hz} = 33.6 \text{ GHz}$$

(microwave region).

11.62 (a) If a harmonic oscillator is capable of absorbing energy, the selection rule is $\Delta v = \pm 1$. Show that the frequency absorbed is identical to the *vibrational constant*, ν_0.
(b) What will be the wavelength of a photon absorbed by HCl ($\nu_0 = 8.97 \times 10^{13}$ s^{-1}). In what region of the spectrum will this absorption be found?

a) The energy of the v state is $E_v = \left(v + \frac{1}{2}\right)h\nu_0$. The transitional energy is $\Delta E = (v_2 - v_1)h\nu_0$. With $(v_2 - v_1) = \pm 1$, $\Delta E = \pm h\nu_0 = h\nu$. The frequency of absorption is thus $\nu = \nu_0$.

b) $\lambda = \frac{c}{\nu_0} = 3.34 \times 10^{-4}$ cm = 3.34 μm , IR region of spectrum.

11.63 The $v = 0$ to $v = 1$ transition of CO is found to absorb at $\lambda = 4.6$ μm. In what region of the spectrum is this? Calculate the force constant of this molecule.

$\lambda = 4.6 \times 10^{-6}$ m . $\nu = \frac{c}{\lambda} = 6.52 \times 10^{13}$ s^{-1} . This is in the infrared region. From Eq. (11.63): $k = \mu(2\pi\nu_0)^2$. With $\mu = 1.14 \times 10^{-23}$ g we find $k = 1.91 \times 10^6$ g s^{-1} .

11.64 The orthogonality relationship for the harmonic oscillator wave functions can be written:

$$\int H_v(y)H_{v'}(y)e^{-y^2}dy = 0 \quad \text{unless } v = v'$$

Use this with the recursion relationship for Hermite polynomials (Table 11.2) to prove that the selection rule for absorption of radiation by the harmonic oscillator is $v = v' \pm 1$.

From Table 11.2: $H_{v+1} = 2yH_v - 2vH_{v-1}$ (Recursion Formula). The selection rule is: $\int H_v y H_{v'} e^{-y^2} dy = 0$ unless $v = v' \pm 1$.

With $yH_v = \frac{1}{2} H_{v+1} + vH_{v-1}$,

$\int H_v y H_{v'} e^{-y^2} dy = \frac{1}{2}\int H_{v+1}H_{v'}e^{-y^2}dy + v\int H_{v-1}H_{v'}e^{-y^2}dy$. Because of the orthogonality of the wave functions, the first integral on the r.h.s. above is zero unless $v' = v + 1$, and the second integral is zero unless $v' = v - 1$. Thus the selection rule is proven.

12

Atoms

12.1 Prove, by direct substitution, that the function

$$R = \sigma e^{-\sigma/2}$$

is an eigenfunction of the hydrogen-atom radial equation if $l = 1$. What is the eigenvalue? What is the principle quantum number (n)?

Using Eq. (12.5) with l = 1 ,

$$\left\{\frac{1}{\sigma^2}\frac{\partial}{\partial\sigma}\left(\sigma^2 \frac{\partial}{\partial\sigma}\right) + \frac{2}{\sigma} - \frac{2}{\sigma^2}\right\}\sigma e^{-\sigma/2} =$$

$$\left\{\frac{1}{\sigma^2} \frac{\partial}{\partial\sigma}\left(\sigma^2 e^{-\sigma/2} - \frac{\sigma^3}{2} e^{-\sigma/2}\right) + 2e^{-\sigma/2} - \frac{2}{\sigma} e^{-\sigma/2}\right\} =$$

$$\left\{\frac{1}{\sigma^2}\left(2\sigma e^{-\sigma/2} - \frac{3\sigma^2}{2} e^{-\sigma/2} - \frac{\sigma^2}{2} e^{-\sigma/2} + \frac{\sigma^3}{4} e^{-\sigma/2}\right) + 2e^{-\sigma/2} - \frac{2}{\sigma}e^{-\sigma/2}\right\} =$$

$$\left\{\frac{2}{\sigma} - \frac{3}{2} - \frac{1}{2} + \frac{\sigma}{4} + 2 - \frac{2}{\sigma}\right\}e^{-\sigma/2} = \frac{\sigma}{4} e^{-\sigma/2} = \frac{1}{4} R .$$

Thus R is an eigenfunction of the H atom radial eq. with eigenvalue $\frac{1}{4}$.

12.2 Find the number and location of the radial nodes of the hydrogen 3*s* wave function.

From Table 12.1, $R_{30} = L_{30}e^{-\sigma/3} = \left(1 - \frac{2\sigma}{3} + \frac{2\sigma^2}{27}\right)e^{-\sigma/3}$. The radial wavefunction has nodes at $L_{30} = 0$, or

$$\sigma = \frac{\frac{2}{3} \pm \sqrt{\frac{4}{9} - \frac{8}{27}}}{\frac{4}{27}} = \frac{9}{2} \pm \frac{\sqrt{27}}{2} .$$

The roots are $\sigma_1 = 7.098$ and $\sigma_2 = 1.902$ or using $r = \sigma a_0$, $r_1 = 1.006$ Å and $r_2 = 3.756$ Å .

12.3 Find the constant that will normalize $\psi_{2p_z} = A\sigma e^{-\sigma/2} \cos \theta$.

The normalization condition is

$$\int_0^{2\pi}\int_0^{\pi}\int_0^{\infty} \psi^*_{nlm}\psi_{nlm}\, r^2 dr \sin\theta\, d\theta\, d\Phi = 1$$

or, with $r = a_0\sigma$,

$$A^2 a_0^3 2\pi \int_0^{\pi}\int_0^{\infty} \sigma^4 e^{-\sigma} \cos^2\theta \sin\theta\, d\sigma\, d\theta = A^2 a_0^3 \frac{4\pi}{3}\int_0^{\infty} \sigma^4 e^{-\sigma} d\sigma = 1 .$$

From Eq. (12.9), $\int_0^{\infty} \sigma^4 e^{-\sigma} d\sigma = 4! = 24$, thus $A^2 = \frac{1}{32\pi a_0^3}$ or

$$A = (32\pi a_0^3)^{-1/2} .$$

12.4 Which of the hydrogen-atom states, 2*s* or 2*p*, has the lower energy?

Because $E_n = -\frac{Z^2 e^2}{2a_0 n^2}$ is dependent only on n, and n = 2 for both the 2s and 2p states, these states are degenerate.

12.5 Calculate the probability that a $1s$ electron is outside the Bohr radius.

From Eq. (12.11), $P(r > a_0) = \dfrac{\int_{a_0}^{\infty} f(r)dr}{\int_0^{\infty} f(r)dr}$ where $f(r) = R^2r^2$.

For the 1s electron, $R_{10} = e^{-\sigma}$. Using $r = a_0\sigma$,

$P(r > a_0) = \dfrac{\int_1^{\infty} \sigma^2 e^{-2\sigma} d\sigma}{\int_0^{\infty} \sigma^2 e^{-2\sigma} d\sigma}$. From Eq. (12.9), the denominator is

$\frac{1}{4}$. Defining $\alpha = 2\sigma$, then

$$P(r > a_0) = \frac{1}{2}\int_2^{\infty} \alpha^2 e^{-\alpha} d\alpha = \frac{1}{2}\left[-\alpha^2 e^{-\alpha} \Big|_2^{\infty} + 2\int_2^{\infty} \alpha e^{-\alpha} d\alpha \right]$$

$$P(r > a_0) = \frac{1}{2}\left[\left(-\alpha^2 e^{-\alpha} - 2\alpha e^{-\alpha}\right) \Big|_2^{\infty} + 2\int_2^{\infty} e^{-\alpha} d\alpha \right]$$

$$P(r > a_0) = \frac{1}{2}[-\alpha^2 e^{-\alpha} - 2\alpha e^{-\alpha} - 2e^{-\alpha}] \Big|_2^{\infty} = 5e^{-2} = 0.6767 .$$

12.6 Calculate $\langle r \rangle$ and $\langle r^2 \rangle$ for the $1s$ state of hydrogen.

$\langle r \rangle = \dfrac{\int_0^{\infty} r^3 e^{-2r/a_0} dr}{\int_0^{\infty} r^2 e^{-2r/a_0} dr}$. From the text, $\int_0^{\infty} x^n e^{-ax} dx = \dfrac{n!}{a^{n+1}}$. Thus:

$\langle r \rangle = \dfrac{(3!)(a_0^4)(2^3)}{(2!)(a_0^3)(2^4)} = \dfrac{3}{2} a_0$. Similarly,

$$\langle r^2 \rangle = \frac{\int_0^{\infty} r^4 e^{-2r/a_0} dr}{\int_0^{\infty} r^2 e^{-2r/a_0} dr} = \frac{(4!)(a_0^5(2^3)}{(2!)(a_0^3)(2^5)} = 3a_0^2 .$$

12.7 Find the maximum of the radial distribution function [$f(r) = R^2r^2$] for a 2s function.

With $\sigma = \frac{Zr}{a_0}$, for a 2s function:

$f(r) = R^2r^2 = \left(\frac{a_0}{Z}\right)^2\left(1 - \frac{\sigma}{2}\right)^2\sigma^2e^{-\sigma}$. Dropping the constant and differentiating: $\frac{df}{d\sigma} = \left[2\sigma\left(1 - \frac{\sigma}{2}\right)^2 - \sigma^2\left(1 - \frac{\sigma}{2}\right) - \sigma^2\left(1 - \frac{\sigma}{2}\right)^2\right]e^{-\sigma}$.

f is at an extrema when $\frac{df}{d\sigma} = 0$, or $\sigma^2 - 6\sigma + 4 = 0$. The solutions are $\sigma = 5.236$ and 0.764 . Plug these into f(r) to find the maximum: $f(0.764) = 0.104\left(\frac{a_0}{Z}\right)^2$,

$f(5.236) = 0.382\left(\frac{a_0}{Z}\right)^2$. Thus $\sigma(\max) = 5.236$.

12.8 Calculate $\langle 1/r\rangle$ for the 1s hydrogen state.

Using Eqs. (12.10) and (12.11) with Table 12.1,

$\langle\frac{1}{r}\rangle = \frac{\int_0^\infty re^{-2r/a_0}dr}{\int_0^\infty r^2e^{-2r/a_0}dr}$. From Eq. (12.9), $\int_0^\infty re^{-2r/a_0}dr = \frac{a_0^2}{4}$ and

$\int_0^\infty r^2e^{-2r/a_0}dr = \frac{a_0^3}{4}$ Thus $\langle\frac{1}{r}\rangle = \frac{1}{a_0}$.

12.9 Derive a formula for the average potential energy of an electron in the $1s$ state of the hydrogen atom. Then calculate the average kinetic energy of the electron in this state. The result: $\langle V \rangle = 2E$, $\langle T \rangle = -E$ (E is the total energy) is an aspect of the *virial theorem* (cf. Problem 11.4, where this was done using Bohr's theory).

$V(r) = -\frac{Ze^2}{r}$ so that, with Z = 1 , $\langle V \rangle = -e^2\langle\frac{1}{r}\rangle$. From problem 12.8, $\langle\frac{1}{r}\rangle = \frac{1}{a_0}$, so that $\langle V \rangle = -\frac{e^2}{a_0}$. With n = 1 , Eq. (12.7) becomes: $E = -\frac{e^2}{2a_0}$. Thus $\langle V \rangle = 2E$.

12.10 What are the units of $R(r)$ (assumed normalized)? What are the units of R^2 and R^2r^2? (Use the cgs system.)

Since $\int_0^\infty R^2r^2\,dr = 1$, R^2 has units of $(\text{length})^{-3}$. In cgs units R^2 [=] cm^{-3} or R [=] $cm^{-3/2}$. Then r^2R^2 [=] cm^{-1} .

12.11 What linear combinations of the $3d_2$, $3d_1$, $3d_0$, $3d_{-1}$ and $3d_{-2}$ H-atom eigenfunctions will produce the Cartesian functions:

$$d_{xz} = xzF(r) \quad \text{and} \quad d_{xy} = xyF(r)$$

($F(r)$ is some function of r alone, not the same in each case, which you will discover when you do the problem.)

Angular components of the wavefunctions, from Table 11.8, are as follows:

Orbital	Angular Component
$d_{\pm 2}$	$\sin^2\theta\, e^{\pm 2i\phi}$
$d_{\pm 1}$	$\sin\theta \cos\theta\, e^{\pm i\phi}$
d_0	$3\cos^2\theta - 1$

We also know that: $x = r\sin\theta\cos\Phi$, $y = r\sin\theta\sin\Phi$,

$z = r\cos\theta$, $e^{i\Phi} = \cos\Phi + i\sin\Phi$, and $e^{-i\Phi} = \cos\Phi - i\sin\Phi$.

Thus: $xz = r^2\sin\theta\cos\theta\cos\Phi = \frac{1}{2} r^2(3d_1 + 3d_{-1})$ and

$d_{xz} = (3d_1 + 3d_{-1})F(r)$. Similarly, $xy = r^2\sin^2\theta\cos\Phi\sin\Phi$.

Because $\sin 2\Phi = 2\sin\Phi\cos\Phi$:

$xy = \frac{1}{2} r^2\sin^2\theta\sin 2\Phi = \frac{1}{2} r^2 i(3d_2 - 3d_{-2})$ and

$$d_{xy} = (3d_2 - 3d_{-2})F(r) .$$

12.12 What linear combinations of the $3d_2$, $3d_1$, $3d_0$, $3d_{-1}$ and $3d_{-2}$ H-atom eigenfunctions will produce the Cartesian functions:

$$d_{yz} = yzF(r) \quad \text{and} \quad d_{x^2-y^2} = (x^2 - y^2)F(r)$$

($F(r)$ is some function of r alone, not the same in each case, which you will discover when you do the problem.)

As in problem 12.11:

$yz = r^2\sin\theta\cos\theta\sin\Phi = -\frac{1}{2} r^2 i(3d_1 - 3d_{-1}) = (3d_1 - 3d_{-1})F(r)$.

$x^2 - y^2 = r^2(\sin^2\theta\cos^2\Phi - \sin^2\theta\sin^2\Phi) = r^2\sin^2\theta\cos 2\Phi$

$x^2 - y^2 = (3d_2 + 3d_{-2})F(r)$.

12.13 Prove that:

$$\hat{L}_x(2p_x) = 0$$

where:

$$(2p_x) = \left(\frac{x}{a_0}\right) e^{-r/2a_0}$$

(This may be easier to do in Cartesian coordinates.)

$\hat{L}_x = \frac{\hbar}{i}\left(y \frac{\partial}{\partial z} - z \frac{\partial}{\partial y}\right)$. With $r = (x^2 + y^2 + z^2)^{1/2}$,

$$(2p_x) = \left(\frac{x}{a_0}\right) \exp\left[- \frac{(x^2 + y^2 + z^2)^{1/2}}{2a_0} \right] .$$

$$\frac{\partial}{\partial z}(2p_x) = - \frac{zx}{2a_0^2 r} \exp\left(- \frac{r}{2a_0}\right) \quad \text{and}$$

$$\frac{\partial}{\partial y}(2p_x) = - \frac{yx}{2a_0^2 r} \exp\left(- \frac{r}{2a_0}\right) . \quad \text{Then}$$

$$\hat{L}_x(2p_x) = \frac{\hbar}{i}(-yzx + zyx) \frac{e^{-r/2a_0}}{2a_0^2 r} = 0 .$$

12.14 A p electron, with three degenerate states available, (p_x, p_y, p_z or p_1, p_0, p_{-1}) would share its time among those states. Its state would then be described as an equal mixture of these with:

$$\psi = p_x + p_y + p_z$$

The electron density would then be:

$$\psi^*\psi = p_x^2 + p_y^2 + p_z^2$$

The cross terms, $p_x p_y$ for example, have been omitted because their integral, by orthogonality, will be zero. Show that this sum is identical to:

$$\psi^*\psi = p_1 p_1^* + p_0 p_0 + p_{-1} p_{-1}^*$$

Do these sums (the functions are on Table 11.8) to show that the electron density in such a case is spherically symmetric—that is, it depends only on r and not the angles. This proof is a special case of the *spherical harmonic addition theorem* and will apply to the summation of all products $Y_{l,m}^* Y_{l,m}$ over $m = -l$ to l—for example, the d and f orbitals.

If $\psi = p_x + p_y + p_z$ and $\psi = p_1 + p_0 + p_{-1}$, then

$\psi^*\psi = (p_x + p_y + p_z)^2 = (p_1 + p_0 + p_{-1})^*(p_1 + p_0 + p_{-1})$. All of the wave functions are orthogonal, and p_0 is real, so that:

$p_x^2 + p_y^2 + p_z^2 = p_1{}^*p_1 + p_0p_0 + p_{-1}{}^*p_{-1}$. For a 2p electron,

$p_0 = \psi_{210} = \left(\frac{3}{4\pi}\right)^{1/2} \sigma e^{-\sigma/2} \cos\theta$, $p_1 = \psi_{211} = \left(\frac{3}{8\pi}\right)^{1/2} \sigma e^{-\sigma/2} \sin\theta\, e^{i\phi}$

and $p_{-1} = \psi_{21-1} = \left(\frac{3}{8\pi}\right)^{1/2} \sigma e^{-\sigma/2} \sin\theta\, e^{-i\phi}$.

$\psi^*\psi = \psi_{211}^*\psi_{211} + \psi_{210}^*\psi_{210} + \psi_{21-1}^*\psi_{21-1}$

$\psi^*\psi = \frac{3}{4\pi}\sigma^2 e^{-\sigma}\left(\frac{\sin^2\theta}{2} + \cos^2\theta + \frac{\sin^2\theta}{2}\right) = \frac{3}{4\pi}\sigma^2 e^{-\sigma}$. Since $\psi^*\psi$ has no angular dependence, it is radially symmetric.

12.15 Show that the one-electron spin function:

$$\chi = \alpha + \beta$$

is an eigenfunction of $\hat{S}_x$ and not an eigenfunction of $\hat{S}_z$. Can you find another such function?

$\hat{S}_x\chi = \hat{S}_x\alpha + \hat{S}_x\beta$. From Eq. (12.15), $\hat{S}_x\alpha = \frac{\hbar}{2}\beta$ and $\hat{S}_x\beta = \frac{\hbar}{2}\alpha$.

Then $\hat{S}_x\chi = \frac{\hbar}{2}(\alpha + \beta) = \frac{\hbar}{2}\chi$. χ is an eigenfunction of $\hat{S}_x$ with eigenvalue $\frac{\hbar}{2}$. $\hat{S}_z\chi = \hat{S}_z\alpha + \hat{S}_z\beta$. From Eq. (12.13),

$\hat{S}_z\chi = \frac{1}{2}\hbar(\alpha - \beta)$. Thus χ is not an eigenfunction of $\hat{S}_z$.

Another function with similar properties is $\chi' = \alpha - \beta$.

12.16 Consider a particle in a box with a rounded bottom. That is, the potential is infinite for $x < 0$ and $x > a$, as before, but inside the box, $V = 4V_0x(a - x)$. Sketch this potential. Where is it a maximum, and what is its value at the maximum? Use first-order perturbation theory to estimate the energy of a particle in such a box.

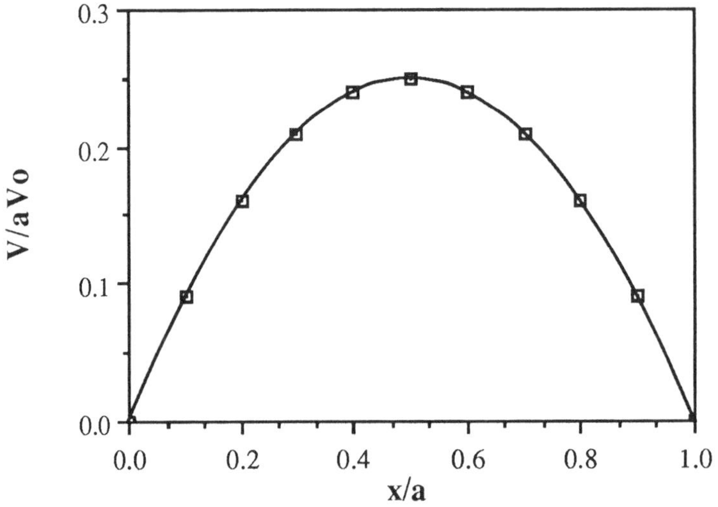

The first-order perturbation energy is: $E^{(1)} = E^{(0)} + \langle V \rangle$ with $\langle V \rangle = 4V_0(a\langle x \rangle - \langle x^2 \rangle)$. From problem 11.22: $\langle x \rangle = \frac{a}{2}$, $\langle x^2 \rangle = \frac{a^2}{3} - \frac{a^2}{2n^2\pi^2}$. Thus:

$$\langle V \rangle = V_0\left(2a^2 - \frac{4}{3}a^2 + \frac{2a^2}{n^2\pi^2} \right) = \frac{2}{3}V_0a^2\left(1 + \frac{3}{n^2\pi^2} \right) .$$

With $E^{(0)} = \frac{n^2h^2}{8ma^2}$, $E^{(1)} = \frac{n^2h^2}{8ma^2} + \frac{2}{3}V_0a^2\left(1 + \frac{3}{n^2\pi^2} \right)$.

12.17 The particle in a box potential (Chapter 11) is perturbed by a square barrier, so $V = V_0$ for $x = a/4$ to $x = 3a/4$, and is zero elsewhere. Use first-order perturbation theory to estimate the energy of a particle in such a box.

The first-order perturbation energy is: $E^{(1)} = E^{(0)} + \langle V \rangle$, where

$$\langle V \rangle = \int_{a/4}^{3a/4} V_0\psi_n^2\, dx \ .$$ With $\psi_n = \sqrt{\frac{2}{a}}\sin\frac{n\pi x}{a}$,

$$\langle V\rangle = \int_{a/4}^{3a/4} \frac{2V_0}{a}\left(\sin^2 \frac{n\pi x}{a}\right)dx = \int_{a/4}^{3a/4} \frac{V_0}{a}\left(1 - \cos \frac{2n\pi x}{a}\right)dx$$

$$\langle V\rangle = V_0\left(\frac{x}{a} - \frac{1}{2n\pi} \sin \frac{2n\pi x}{a}\right)\Bigg|_{a/4}^{3a/4} = V_0\left(\frac{1}{2} + \frac{1}{n\pi} \sin \frac{n\pi}{2}\right) .$$

Thus, with $E_n^{(0)} = \frac{n^2h^2}{8ma^2}$:

$$E_n^{(1)} = \frac{n^2h^2}{8ma^2} + V_0\left[\frac{1}{2} + \left(\frac{1}{n\pi}\right) \sin \left(\frac{n\pi}{2}\right)\right]$$

12.18 Find linear combinations of the electron spin functions (α and β) that will be eigenfunctions of $\hat{S}_y$.

If $\chi = \alpha + i\beta$, then $\hat{S}_y\chi = \hat{S}_y\alpha + \hat{S}_y i\beta = \frac{i\hbar}{2} \beta + \frac{\hbar}{2}\alpha = \frac{\hbar}{2}(\alpha + i\beta)$.

Thus χ is an eigenfunction of $\hat{S}_y$ with eigenvalue $\frac{\hbar}{2}$. Similarly, with $\chi' = \alpha - i\beta$,

$$\hat{S}_y\chi' = \hat{S}_y\alpha - \hat{S}_y i\beta = \frac{i\hbar}{2} \beta - \frac{\hbar}{2} \alpha = -\frac{\hbar}{2}(\alpha - i\beta) = -\frac{\hbar}{2}\chi' .$$

Thus χ' is an eigenfunction of $\hat{S}_y$ with eigenvalue $-\frac{\hbar}{2}$.

12.19 Estimate the second and third IP's of the lithium atom using formulas in this chapter. The observed values are 75.6 and 122.4 eV, respectively.

The energy of Li^+ is given by Eqs. (12.28) and (12.29),

$E_{var} = -2(Z')^2Ry = -2\left(\frac{43}{16}\right)^2(13.6 \text{ eV}) = -196.46$ eV . For Li^{+2},

$E(Li^{+2}) = -Z^2Ry = -(3)^2(13.6 \text{ eV}) = -122.4$ eV . For the process $Li^+ = Li^{+2} + e^-$, $\Delta E = E(Li^{+2}) - E(Li^+) = 74.06$ eV (2nd IP) . For $Li^{+2} = Li^{+3} + e^-$, $\Delta E = -E(Li^{+2}) = 122.4$ eV (3rd IP) .

12.20 The variation-theory formula for the energy of a two-electron atom or ion should apply to the hydride ion, H^-. Test this by calculating the electron affinity of the hydrogen atom. The electron affinity (EA) is the negative of the energy of the process:

$$H(1s) + e \longrightarrow H^-(1s^2)$$

The experimental value is 0.754 eV. Your answer should be close to the *negative* of this number; in other words, the error is about 1.5 eV.

$E_{var} = -2\left(Z - \frac{5}{16}\right)^2 Ry$. With Z = 1 and Ry = 13.606 eV ,

E_{var} = 12.862 eV . The electron affinity is:

$$E_a = E(H^-) - E(H) = E_{var} - Ry = -0.744 \text{ eV} .$$

12.21 (a) Prove that the function:

$$\chi_s = \frac{1}{\sqrt{2}}[\alpha(1)\beta(2) + \beta(1)\alpha(2)]$$

is normalized if the functions α and β are normalized and orthogonal.
(b) Prove that:

$$\chi_a = \frac{1}{\sqrt{2}}[\alpha(1)\beta(2) - \beta(1)\alpha(2)]$$

is normalized and is orthogonal to χ_s.

a) $$\int_{\text{all space}} \chi_s^*\chi_s \, d\tau = \int_{\text{all space}} \frac{1}{2}[\alpha(1)^2\beta(2)^2 + 2\alpha(1)\beta(2)\alpha(2)\beta(1) + \beta(1)^2\alpha(2)^2]d\tau(1)d\tau(2)$$

$$\int_{\text{all space}} \chi_s^*\chi_s \, d\tau = \frac{1}{2}\int\alpha(1)^2 d\tau_1\int\beta(2)^2 d\tau_2 + \int\alpha(1)\beta(1)d\tau_1 \int\alpha(2)\beta(2)d\tau_2 + \frac{1}{2}\int\beta(1)^2 d\tau_1 \int\alpha(2)^2 d\tau_2$$

$$\int_{\text{all space}} \chi_s^*\chi_s \, d\tau = \frac{1}{2} + 0 + \frac{1}{2} = 1 .$$

b) $\int \chi_a^* \chi_a \, d\tau = \frac{1}{2}\int \alpha(1)^2 d\tau_1 \int \beta(2)^2 d\tau_2 - \int \alpha(1)\beta(1) d\tau_1 \int \alpha(2)\beta(2) d\tau_2 +$

$\frac{1}{2}\int \beta(1)^2 d\tau_1 \int \alpha(2)^2 d\tau_2$.

With orthonormal $\alpha(i)$ and $\beta(i)$, $\int \chi_a^* \chi_a \, d\tau = \frac{1}{2} + 0 + \frac{1}{2} = 1$.

Finally, $\int \chi_a^* \chi_s \, \delta\tau = \frac{1}{2}\int \alpha(1)^2 d\tau_1 \int \beta(2)^2 d\tau_2 - \frac{1}{2}\int \beta(1)^2 d\tau_1 \int \alpha(2)^2 d\tau_2 = 0.$

Thus χ_a and χ_s are orthonormal.

12.22 The first ionization potential of He is 24.6 eV (from the ground state). The transition $1\,^1S \longrightarrow 2^1P$ absorbs energy at λ = 584.4 Å. Calculate the IP of He(2^1P) atoms.

$He\ (1^1S) \rightarrow He^+ + e^-$	IP (He(1^1S))
$He\ (2^1P) \rightarrow He^+ + e^-$	IP (He(2^1P))
$He\ (1^1S) \rightarrow He\ (2^1P)$	ΔE

We then have IP (He(2^1P)) = IP(He(1^1S)) - ΔE .

$$\Delta E = \frac{hc}{\lambda} = \frac{(6.6261 \times 10^{-34}\ J\ s)(2.998 \times 10^8\ m\ s^{-1})}{584.4 \times 10^{-10}\ m}$$

$\Delta E = 3.401 \times 10^{-18}$ J = 21.23 eV .

Then IP(He(2^1P)) = 24.6 - 21.23 = 3.4 eV .

12.23 In the He spectrum, the wavelengths of the transitions are:

$$1^1S - 2^1P: \quad 584.4\ \text{Å}$$

$$2^1S - 2^1P: \quad 20{,}582\ \text{Å}$$

Calculate $E(2^1S) - E(1^1S)$ from these numbers.

$1^1S \rightarrow 2^1P$	ΔE_1
$2^1S \rightarrow 2^1P$	ΔE_2
$1^1S \rightarrow 2^1S$	ΔE_3

Thus $\Delta E_3 = \Delta E_1 - \Delta E_2$.

$$\Delta E_1 = h\nu_1 = \frac{hc}{\lambda_1} = \frac{(6.626 \times 10^{-34}\ \text{J s})(2.998 \times 10^8\ \text{m s}^{-1})}{584.4 \times 10^{-10}\ \text{m}}$$

$$\Delta E_1 = 3.401 \times 10^{-18}\ \text{J} = 21.23\ \text{eV} .$$

Similarly, $\Delta E_2 = 9.657 \times 10^{-20}\ \text{J} = 0.60\ \text{eV}$. Then

$$\Delta E_3 = E(2^1S) - E(1^1S) = 20.63\ \text{eV} .$$

12.24 If two angular momenta, $j_1 = \frac{3}{2}$, $j_2 = \frac{5}{2}$, are added, what are the quantum numbers (J) of the total angular-momentum states? What are the degeneracies? How many states are there in all?

The quantum numbers J are given by Eq. (12.41), the degeneracies by the number of (J, M) states:

J = 4	M = ±4, ±3, ±2, ±1, 0	(9 states)
J = 3	M = ±3, ±2, ±1, 0	(7 states)
J = 2	M = ±2, ±1, 0	(5 states)
J = 1	M = ±1, 0	(3 states)

There are $(2j_1 + 1)(2j_2 + 1) = 24$ states in all.

12.25 What are the quantum numbers L and S of a state ^4G? What is the total degeneracy of this state?

For the ^4G state, $L = 4$, $g_S = 4 = 2S + 1$ or $S = \frac{3}{2}$. The degeneracy is $g = (2L + 1)(2S + 1) = 9(4) = 36$.

12.26 Derive the ground-state term symbols of the following atoms or ions: H, F, F^-, Na, Na^+, P, Sc, Sc^{2+}[Ar]$(3d)^1$.

Species	Quantum Nos.	Term Symbol
H(1s)	$S = \frac{1}{2}$, $L = 0$	^2S
F[He]$(2s)^2(2p)^5$	$S = \frac{1}{2}$, $L = 1$	^2P
F^-[Ne]	$S = 0$, $L = 0$	^1S
Na[Ne]$(3s)^1$	$S = \frac{1}{2}$, $L = 0$	^2S
Na^+[Ne]	$S = 0$, $L = 0$	^1S
P[Ne]$(3s)^2(3p)^3$	$S = \frac{3}{2}$, $L = 0$	^4S
Sc[Ar]$(4s)^2(3d)^1$	$S = \frac{1}{2}$, $L = 2$	^2D
Sc^{+2}[Ar]$(3d)^1$	$S = \frac{1}{2}$, $L = 2$	^2D

12.27 Contrast and compare the notations *spdf* with *SPDF*. In what circumstances would an *f*-electron give an *F*-state?

s, p, d and f refer to one electron states or orbitals, whereas S, P, D and F refer to many-electron atomic states. An f electron would correspond to an F state if it was a single electron outside a closed shell.

12.28 Derive all of the terms possible for a p^3 configuration. Do this by writing out all possible values of M_L and M_S as on Table 12.5 (but without the wave functions) and assigning the terms by elimination.

	p_1 (m=1)	p_0 (m=0)	p_{-1} (m=-1)	M_L	M_S	^2D	^2P	^4S
1	↑↓	↑	-	2	1/2	√		
2	↑↓	↓	-	2	-1/2	√		
3	↑	↑↓	-	1	1/2	√		
4	↓	↑↓	-	1	-1/2	√		
5	↑↓	-	↑	1	1/2		√	
6	↑↓	-	↓	1	-1/2		√	
7	↑	-	↑↓	-1	1/2	√		
8	↓	-	↑↓	-1	-1/2	√		
9	-	↑↓	↑	-1	1/2		√	
10	-	↑↓	↓	-1	-1/2		√	
11	-	↑	↑↓	-2	1/2	√		
12	-	↓	↑↓	-2	-1/2	√		
13	↑	↑	↑	0	3/2			√
14	↑	↑	↓	0	1/2			√
15	↑	↓	↑	0	1/2		√	
16	↓	↑	↑	0	1/2	√		
17	↓	↓	↑	0	-1/2			√
18	↓	↑	↓	0	-1/2		√	
19	↑	↓	↓	0	-1/2	√		
20	↓	↓	↓	0	-3/2			√

Possible states for 3 electrons: $\frac{(6)(5)(4)}{3!} = 20$.

^2D: 10 states, ^2P: 6 states, ^4S: 4 states. Note: States with the same quantum numbers are indistinguishable, so that assignment of states may be arbitrary.

12.29 (a) Calculate the number of ways to place 5 electrons into a *d* orbital.
(b) From Table 12.6, how many term-groups will there be for this configuration?
(c) List all of the terms with their degeneracies and show that the sum is equal to the number of combinations you calculated in (a).

a) 5 electrons in 5 orbitals: $\left(\frac{(10)(9)(8)(7)(6)}{5!}\right) = 252$.

b) 16.

c)

Term	(2S + 1)(2L + 1)	=	degeneracy
^2S	(2)(1)	=	2
^2P	(2)(3)	=	6
^2D (thrice)	(3)(2)(5)	=	30
^2F (twice)	(2)(2)(7)	=	28
^2G (twice)	(2)(2)(9)	=	36
^2H	(2)(11)	=	22
^2I	(2)(13)	=	26
^4P	(4)(3)	=	12
^4D	(4)(5)	=	20
^4F	(4)(7)	=	28
^4G	(4)(9)	=	36
^6S	(6)(1)	=	6
Totals: 16 terms			252 .

12.30 What would be the term designation of the ground state for the configurations d^2, f^9, f^{14}, s^1d^5, f^3, g^2? (Neglect spin-orbit coupling.)

Electronic Configuration	M_S(max)	M_L(max)	Ground State Term Symbol
d^2	1	3	^3F
f^9	5/2	5	^6H
f^{14}	0	0	^1S
s^1d^5	3	0	^7S
f^3	3/2	6	^4I
g^2	1	7	^3K

12.31 (a) How many ways are there to place 3 electrons into an *f*-orbital?
(b) What is the ground state term of this configuration? How many of the possible states of this configuration are part of this term?
(c) What are the *J*-values possible in the ground state? List the degeneracies of each *J*-state and show that their sum is equal to the number calculated in (b).

a) 3 electrons in 7 orbitals: $\frac{(14)(13)(12)}{3!} = 364$.

b) $M_S(\max) = \frac{3}{2}$, $M_L(\max) = 6$. Ground state term: ^4I . The degeneracy is $(2S + 1)(2L + 1) = 52$.

c) $J = (L + S), (L + S - 1) \ldots (L - S)$. With $L = 6$, $S = \frac{3}{2}$:

J	$g_j = (2J + 1)$
15/2	16
13/2	14
11/2	12
9/2	10
	Total = 52

12.32 Given that the operator form of the spin-orbit Hamiltonian is:

$$\hat{H}_{SO} = hcA\hat{\mathbf{L}} \cdot \hat{\mathbf{S}}$$

derive Eq. (12.45). (Hint: Square the vector **J**.)

$\hat{J} = \hat{L} + \hat{S}$, $\hat{J}^2 = (\hat{L} + \hat{S})^2 = \hat{L}^2 + \hat{S}^2 + 2\hat{L} \cdot \hat{S}$. Thus

$\hat{H}_{SO} = \frac{hcA}{2}(\hat{J}^2 - \hat{L}^2 - \hat{S}^2)$ and

$\hat{H}_{SO}\psi = \frac{hcA}{2}(J(J + 1) - L(L + 1) - S(S + 1))\psi$. Since $\hat{H}\psi = E\psi$, then $E_{SO} = \frac{hcA}{2}[J(J + 1) - L(L + 1) - S(S + 1)]$.

12.33 (a) Show that the spacing of a spin-orbit multiplet should be [by Eq. (12.45)]:

$$\frac{E_J - E_{J-1}}{hc} = AJ$$

(b) Test this formula on the data for oxygen 2^3P ground state:

$$J = 2: \quad E/hc = 0 \text{ (ground state)}$$
$$J = 1: \quad E/hc = 158.265 \text{ cm}^{-1}$$
$$J = 0: \quad E/hc = 226.997 \text{ cm}^{-1}$$

a) From Eq. (12.45),

$$E_J - E_{(J-1)} = \frac{hcA}{2}\{[J(J + 1) - L(L + 1) - S(S + 1)] - [J(J - 1) - L(L + 1) - S(S + 1)]\}$$

$$E_J - E_{(J-1)} = \frac{hcAJ}{2}[J + 1 - (J - 1)] = hcAJ$$

and $\dfrac{E_J - E_{(J-1)}}{hc} = AJ$.

b) For J = 2 , $A_{21} = \left(\dfrac{E_2 - E_1}{hc}\right)\dfrac{1}{2} = -79.133 \text{ cm}^{-1}$. For J = 1 , $A_{10} = \left(\dfrac{E_1 - E_0}{hc}\right) = -68.732 \text{ cm}^{-1}$.

12.34 The energies of the Ca 4^3P excited state are:

$$J = 0: \quad E/hc = 15{,}157.9 \text{ cm}^{-1}$$
$$J = 1: \quad E/hc = 15{,}210.0 \text{ cm}^{-1}$$
$$J = 2: \quad E/hc = 15{,}315.9 \text{ cm}^{-1}$$

Calculate the spin-orbit coupling constant of this state.

Using the formula from problem 12.33: $A_{21} = 52.95 \text{ cm}^{-1}$, $A_{10} = 52.10 \text{ cm}^{-1}$. Then $A = \left(\dfrac{A_{10} + A_{21}}{2}\right) = 52.5 \text{ cm}^{-1}$.

12.35 (a) What is the ground-state term symbol for the f^9 configuration?
(b) What J values are possible, and which is lowest in energy?
(c) What is the term symbol including J of the ground state and what is its degeneracy?

a) For the f^9 configuration:

	↑↓	↑↓	↑	↑	↑	↑	↑
m =	3	2	1	0	-1	-2	-3

$M_L(\text{max}) = 5 = L$ (ground state) and $S = \frac{5}{2}$, so that the ground state term is ^6H .

b) $J = L + S,\ L + S - 1 \ldots |L - S|$, thus:

$J = \frac{15}{2}, \frac{13}{2}, \frac{11}{2}, \frac{9}{2}, \frac{7}{2}, \frac{5}{2}$. By Hund's third rule, the state lowest in energy has $J = \frac{15}{2}$.

c) Ground state term is $^6H_{15/2}$. $g = 2J + 1 = 16$.

12.36 What are the permitted J values for the following terms?
(a) ^6S (b) ^1F (c) ^2H (d) ^4P (e) ^3D

a) $S = \frac{5}{2}$, $L = 0$.

$J = (L + S), (L + S - 1), \ldots, |L - S| = \frac{5}{2}$.

b) $S = 0$, $L = 3$. $J = 3$.

c) $S = \frac{1}{2}$, $L = 5$. $J = \frac{11}{2}, \frac{9}{2}$.

d) $S = \frac{3}{2}$, $L = 1$. $J = \frac{5}{2}, \frac{3}{2}, \frac{1}{2}$.

e) $S = 1$, $L = 2$. $J = 3, 2, 1$.

12.37 In the Na spectrum, the following wavelengths are absorbed:

$4^2P - 3^2S$: $\lambda = 330.26$ nm

$3^2P - 3^2S$: $\lambda = 589.593$ nm, 588.996 nm

$5^2S - 3^2P$: $\lambda = 616.073$ nm, 615.421 nm

Calculate the energies of the 4^2P and 5^2S states with respect to the ground (3^2S) state.

The energy of the 4^2P state is

$$E(4^2P) = \frac{1}{\lambda_1} = \frac{1}{(330.26 \times 10^{-7} \text{ cm})} = 30,279 \text{ cm}^{-1}.$$ The energy of

the 5^2S state is

$$E(5^2S) = \left(\frac{1}{\lambda_3}\right) + \left(\frac{1}{\lambda_2}\right)$$

$$E(5^2S) = \frac{1}{2}\left[\frac{1}{589.593} + \frac{1}{588.996} + \frac{1}{616.073} + \frac{1}{615.421}\right](10^7 \text{ cm}^{-1})$$

$$E(5^2S) = 33,210 \text{ cm}^{-1}.$$

12.38 The principal line of the potassium atomic spectrum ($4^2S \leftrightarrow 4^2P$) is a doublet with wavelengths 3933.66 Å and 3968.47 Å. Calculate the spin-orbit coupling constant.

The fine structure is due to the splitting of the 4^2P level into $4^2P_{3/2}$ and $4^2P_{1/2}$ levels. Using the equation derived in problem 12.33:

$$A = \left(\frac{E_J}{hc} - \frac{E_{J-1}}{hc}\right)\frac{1}{J} = (25421.6 \text{ cm}^{-1} - 25198.6 \text{ cm}^{-1})\frac{1}{3/2} = 149 \text{ cm}^{-1}.$$

12.39 The transition

$$Al[Ne](3s)^2(3p)^1 \leftrightarrow Al[Ne](3s)^2(4s)^1$$

has two lines, $\tilde{\nu}_1 = 25{,}354.8\ cm^{-1}$, $\tilde{\nu}_2 = 25{,}242.7\ cm^{-1}$. The transition

$$(ground) \leftrightarrow Al[Ne](3s)^2(3d)^1$$

has three lines, $\tilde{\nu}_3 = 32{,}444.8\ cm^{-1}$, $\tilde{\nu}_4 = 32{,}334.0\ cm^{-1}$, $\tilde{\nu}_5 = 32{,}332.7\ cm^{-1}$. Sketch an energy-level diagram of the states involved and explain the source of all lines. Calculate spin-orbit coupling constants when possible.

State	Terms
$Al[Ne](3s)^2(3p)^1$	$^2P_{3/2}$, $^2P_{1/2}$
$Al[Ne](3s)^2(4s)^1$	$^2S_{1/2}$
$Al[Ne](3s)^2(3d)^1$	$^2D_{5/2}$, $^2D_{3/2}$

Since $\Delta J = 0, \pm 1$, we can draw the following diagram of allowed transitions:

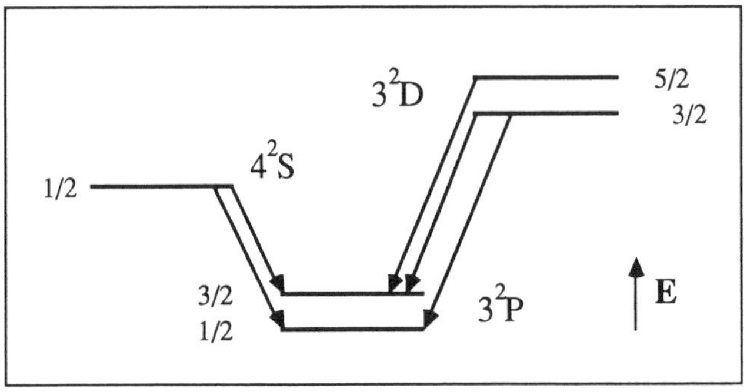

The ^2P ground state has $\Delta E = 112.1\ cm^{-1}$. Observed frequencies are due to the following transitions:

$\tilde{\nu}_1 = 25354.8\ cm^{-1}$ $\quad 4^2S_{1/2} \leftrightarrow 3^2P_{1/2}$

$\tilde{\nu}_2 = 25242.7\ cm^{-1}$ $\quad 4^2S_{1/2} \leftrightarrow 3^2P_{3/2}$

$\tilde{\nu}_3 = 32444.8\ cm^{-1}$ $\quad 3^2P_{1/2} \leftrightarrow 3^2D_{3/2}$

$\tilde{\nu}_4 = 32334.0\ cm^{-1}$ $\quad 3^2P_{3/2} \leftrightarrow 3^2D_{5/2}$

$\tilde{\nu}_5 = 32332.7\ cm^{-1}$ $\quad 3^2P_{3/2} \leftrightarrow 3^2D_{3/2}$

These assignments are made on the basis of the fact

$$\tilde{\nu}_1 - \tilde{\nu}_2 = \tilde{\nu}_3 - \tilde{\nu}_4 = 112.1 \text{ cm}^{-1} .$$

12.40 (a) Calculate the transition integrals for an electric dipole transition from 1*s* to 2*s* and show that it is forbidden.
(b) Calculate the transition integrals for an electric dipole transition from 1*s* to $2p_z$ and show that it is allowed.

The transition integrals are: $I_x \equiv \int \psi_i^* x \psi_j \, d\tau$ and similarly for I_y and I_z .

a) For the 1s and 2s functions, ψ is radially symmetric, but $x = r \sin\theta \cos\phi$, $y = r \sin\theta \sin\phi$, $z = r\cos\theta$ and $d\tau = r^2 \, dr \sin\theta \, d\theta \, d\phi$. The angular component of I_x is:

$I_x \propto \int_0^{2\pi}\int_0^{\pi} \sin^2\theta \cos\phi \, d\theta \, d\phi$. Because $\int_0^{2\pi} \cos\phi \, d\phi = 0$, $I_x = 0$.

Similarly, $I_y \propto \int_0^{2\pi} \sin\phi \, d\phi = 0$. Also,

$$I_z \propto \int_0^{\pi} \cos\theta \sin\theta \, d\theta = \sin^2\theta \Big|_0^{\pi} = 0 .$$

b) The $2p_z$ wavefunction has an angular component $\cos\theta$. Although the I_x and I_y components are still zero (integral over $d\phi$ is zero), now:

$I_z \propto \int_0^{\pi} \cos^2\theta \sin\theta \, d\theta = - \frac{\cos^3\theta}{3}\Big|_0^{\pi} \neq 0$. The radial component of I_z is: $I_z \propto \int_0^{\infty}\left(1 - \frac{\sigma}{2}\right)e^{-3\sigma/2}\sigma^3 d\sigma \neq 0$. With nonzero angular and radial components, I_z is nonzero and the transition is allowed.

12.41 The $^2S_{1/2}$ to $^2P_{1/2}$ transition of potassium has a wavelength of 3968.47 Å. If this spectrum were observed in a superconducting magnet with field 100,000 gauss, in a direction parallel to the field (along the axis of the solenoid), how many lines would be observed and what would be their wavelengths?

With B_0 = 100,000 gauss, $\frac{\mu_B B_0}{hc} = 4.67\ cm^{-1}$. The selection rule is $\Delta M_J = \pm 1$, $g_L = 2$ for $^2S_{1/2}$ and $g_L = \frac{2}{3}$ for $^2P_{1/2}$. M_J has possible values $\frac{1}{2}$ and $-\frac{1}{2}$, so that:

$$E_z = -M_J g_L\left(\frac{\mu_B B_0}{hc}\right).$$

$^2S_{1/2}$: $\frac{E_z}{hc} = \left(-\frac{1}{2}\right)(2)(4.67) = -4.67\ cm^{-1}$

$\frac{E_z}{hc} = \left(\frac{1}{2}\right)(2)(4.67) = 4.67\ cm^{-1}$

$^2P_{1/2}$: $\frac{E_z}{hc} = -1.56\ cm^{-1}$, $\frac{E_z}{hc} = 1.56\ cm^{-1}$

With $\lambda_0 = 3968.470$ and $\frac{E_0}{hc} = 25,198.63\ cm^{-1}$,

Transition	$\frac{\Delta E}{hc}$ (cm^{-1})	λ (Å)
$^2S_{1/2}\left(M_J = \frac{1}{2}\right) \rightarrow {}^2P_{1/2}\left(M_J = -\frac{1}{2}\right)$	25,192.40	3969.45
$^2S_{1/2}\left(M_J = -\frac{1}{2}\right) \rightarrow {}^2P_{1/2}\left(M_J = \frac{1}{2}\right)$	25,204.86	3967.49

Two lines will be observed.

12.42 A $^3P_2$ to $^3S_1$ transition is observed in a magnetic field. How many lines will be seen if the light transmitted perpendicular to the field is observed? How many lines if the light transmitted parallel to the field is observed?

For light polarized perpendicular to the magnetic field, $\Delta M_J = \pm 1$, whereas for light parallel to the field, $\Delta M_J = 0$.

State	Values of M_J
$^3P_2$	$M_J = 2, 1, 0, -1, -2$
$^3S_1$	$M_J = 1, 0, -1$

$$\Delta M_J = \pm 1 \qquad \left.\begin{bmatrix} 2 & \rightarrow & 1 \\ 1 & \rightarrow & 0 \\ 0 & \rightarrow & 1 \\ 0 & \rightarrow & -1 \\ -1 & \rightarrow & 0 \\ -2 & \rightarrow & -1 \end{bmatrix}\right\} 6$$

$$\Delta M_J = 0 \qquad \left.\begin{bmatrix} 1 & \rightarrow & 1 \\ 0 & \rightarrow & 0 \\ -1 & \rightarrow & -1 \end{bmatrix}\right\} 3$$

Light transmitted perpendicular to the field may be polarized either perpendicular or parallel, so that all 9 transitions are observed. Light transmitted parallel to the field can only be polarized perpendicular to the field, so that 6 transitions are observed.

12.43 Calculate the Landé g-factors for the states: $^4S_{3/2}$, $^4P_{5/2}$, $^4P_{3/2}$, $^4P_{1/2}$.

The Lande g-factor is: $g_L = 1 + \dfrac{J(J+1) + S(S+1) - L(L+1)}{2J(J+1)}$.

Draw up the following table:

State	S	L	J	g_L
$^4S_{3/2}$	3/2	0	3/2	2.0
$^4P_{5/2}$	3/2	1	5/2	1.600
$^4P_{3/2}$	3/2	1	3/2	1.733
$^4P_{1/2}$	3/2	1	1/2	2.667

12.44 A $^2P_{1/2}$ to $^2D_{3/2}$ transition is observed in a magnetic field; the light is coming out of the side of the magnet and, therefore, is propagating in a direction perpendicular to the direction of the magnetic field. How many lines will be observed and what will be the polarizations of these lines with respect to the direction of the field?

State	Values of M_J
$^2P_{1/2}$	M_J = 1/2, -1/2
$^2D_{3/2}$	M_J = 3/2, 1/2, -1/2, -3/2

$$\Delta M_J = \pm 1 \qquad \left.\begin{bmatrix} 1/2 & \rightarrow & 3/2 \\ 1/2 & \rightarrow & -1/2 \\ -1/2 & \rightarrow & 1/2 \\ -1/2 & \rightarrow & -3/2 \end{bmatrix}\right\} 4$$

There are 4 transitions with $\Delta M_J = \pm 1$ and hence with light polarized perpendicular to the magnetic field.

$$\Delta M_J = 0 \qquad \left.\begin{matrix} 1/2 & \rightarrow & 1/2 \\ -1/2 & \rightarrow & -1/2 \end{matrix}\right\} 2$$

There are 2 transitions with $\Delta M_J = 0$ and hence with light polarized parallel to the magnetic field.

12.45 Ce^{2+} has a $^3H_4$ ground state. What would be the g-factor for this state? What would be its magnetic moment (in multiples of the Bohr magneton)? If this ion were in solution, in what range would you expect its magnetic moment to fall?

$$g_L = 1 + \frac{J(J+1) + S(S+1) - L(L+1)}{2J(J+1)}$$. For $^3H_4$, $J = 4$, $S = 1$ and $L = 5$, so that $g_L = 0.8$. The upper bound of the magnetic moment is: $|\mu_J| = g_L\sqrt{J(J+1)}\,\mu_B = 3.6\,\mu_B$. The lower bound is the "spin only" magnetic moment:

$$|\mu_S| = 2\sqrt{S(S+1)}\,\mu_B = 2.8\,\mu_B .$$

12.46 Although the Landé formula is strictly valid only for gaseous atoms or ions, it is often used to interpret the magnetic moments of ions in solution. Calculate the magnetic moment (in Bohr magnetons) of $Co^{2+}(3d)^7$ (4.1 to $5.2\mu_B$ observed) and $Er^{3+}(4f)^{11}$ ($9.4\mu_B$ observed). What would the "spin-only" magnetic moments be for these ions?

For $Co^{2+}(3d)^7$, $S = \frac{3}{2}$, $L = 3$ and $J = \frac{9}{2}$. With

$$g_L = 1 + \frac{J(J+1) + S(S+1) - L(L+1)}{2J(J+1)}$$ we find $g_L = \frac{4}{3}$

$|\mu_J| = g_L\mu_B\sqrt{J(J+1)} = 6.63\,\mu_b$. Similarly, for $Er^{3+}(4f)^{11}$, $S = \frac{3}{2}$, $L = 6$ and $J = \frac{15}{2}$, so that $g_L = \frac{6}{5}$ and $|\mu_J| = 9.58\,\mu_B$.

The spin-only magnetic moment is $|\mu_S| = 2\mu_B\sqrt{S(S+1}$. For both Co^{2+} and Er^{3+}, with $S = \frac{3}{2}$, $|\mu_S| = 3.87\,\mu_B$.

12.47 What would be the ESR absorption frequency of sodium vapor in a magnetic field of 14,000 gauss? (This is a typical field for a large iron-core electromagnet.)

$\nu = g_L \mu_\beta \frac{B_0}{h}$. The ground state term for sodium is $^2S_{1/2}$, so that $J = \frac{1}{2}$, $S = \frac{1}{2}$, $L = 0$ and $g_L = 2.0$. Using $\mu_\beta = 9.274 \times 10^{-21}$ erg gauss^{-1} and $B_0 = 14{,}000$ gauss we find

$$\nu = 3.92 \times 10^{10}\ s^{-1} = 39.2\ GHz\ .$$

12.48 The application of an electric field ($\mathscr{E}$) to the H atom adds a potential:

$$V_S = e\mathscr{E}z = e\mathscr{E}r \cos\theta$$

to the Hamiltonian. This added potential could alter both the wave functions and the energy levels of the H atom. Show that the first-order Stark effect (that is, $\langle V_s \rangle$ as calculated with the unperturbed wave functions) is zero. Do the integrals for the 1s and 2p functions as an example.

$$\langle V_s \rangle = \frac{\int_{\text{all space}} \psi^* V_s \psi \, d\tau}{\int_{\text{all space}} \psi^* \psi \, d\tau} \ .$$

$$\int_{\text{all space}} \Psi_{100} V_s \Psi_{100} \, d\tau = \int_0^{2\pi}\int_0^{\pi}\int_0^{\infty} r^3 e^{-2Zr/a_0} dr \sin\theta \cos\theta \, d\theta \, d\phi \ .$$

The integral over θ is zero: $\int_0^{\pi} \sin\theta \cos\theta \, d\theta = \frac{\sin^2\theta}{2}\Big|_0^{\pi} = 0$.

Then $\langle V_s \rangle = 0$. For ψ_{210} , we have

$$\int_{\text{all space}} \psi_{210} V_s \psi_{210} \, d\tau = \int_0^{\pi}\int_0^{\infty} r^5 e^{-2Zr/a_0} \cos^3\theta \sin\theta \, dr \, d\theta \ .$$

The integral over θ is zero: $\int_0^{\pi} \cos^3\theta \sin\theta \, d\theta = \frac{\cos^4\theta}{4}\Big|_0^{\pi} = 0$.

Then $\int \psi_{210} V_s \psi_{210} \, d\tau = 0$ and $\langle V_s \rangle = 0$.

12.49 The second-order Stark effect in atoms gives energy-level perturbation that depends on the *square* of M_J; $E_s = KM^2$, where K is a collection of constant factors. Diagram this effect on a spectrum line for a ${}^1S_0 \rightarrow {}^1P_1$ transition.

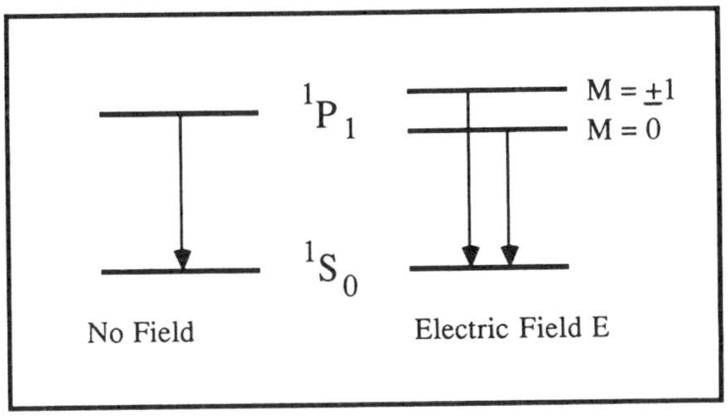

12.50 In the XPES spectrum of Au (Figure 12.18), what is the theoretical intensity ratio of the $p_{3/2}$ to the $p_{1/2}$ line? Show that the effect will be less pronounced for the $4d$ and $4f$ lines. Assign the lines of the $4d$ transition. (In this context, "intensity" refers to height above background.)

The theoretical intensity ratio is

$$\frac{I(P_{3/2})}{I(P_{1/2})} = \frac{g_{3/2}}{g_{1/2}} \left(\frac{\exp\left(-\frac{E_{3/2}}{kT}\right)}{\exp\left(-\frac{E_{1/2}}{kT}\right)} \right)$$

where $g = 2J + 1$. If $E_{3/2} \cong E_{1/2}$, then $\frac{I(P_{3/2})}{I(P_{1/2})} = \frac{g_{3/2}}{g_{1/2}}$. From Figure 12.18, the 4d and 4f lines are closer in energy, ΔE is less and hence $e^{\Delta E/kT}$ is closer to 1. The ratio of the degeneracies is also closer to 1, making the intensity ratio closer to 1. The high energy peak is due to $4d_{3/2}$ and the low energy peak to $4d_{5/2}$.

12.51 Calculate the spin-orbit coupling constant of a 4*d* electron in Au from its XPES spectrum (Figure 12.18).

For a transition between states J and J - 1 , $A = \frac{1}{J}\left(\frac{E_J}{hc} - \frac{E_{J-1}}{hc}\right)$ (problem 12.33). From Fig. 12.18,

$E_J - E_{J-1} = E_{5/2} - E_{3/2} = -19$ eV . Then

$$A = \frac{2}{5}[(-19 \text{ eV})(8065.3 \text{ cm}^{-1} \text{ eV}^{-1})] = -61{,}300 \text{ cm}^{-1} .$$

12.52 The magnetic moment of a nucleus is given by $|\mu| = g_N \mu_N \sqrt{I(I+1)}$, where $\mu_N = e\hbar/2Mc$ is the nuclear magneton. The mass of a proton is 1836 times the mass of an electron, and $g_N = 5.585$. Calculate the ratio of the electron/proton magnetic moments.

$\frac{|\mu_e|}{|\mu_p|} = \frac{g_e \mu_\beta \sqrt{S(S+1)}}{g_N \mu_N \sqrt{I(I+1)}}$. For a free electron, $S = \frac{1}{2}$. Similarly, for a free proton, $I = \frac{1}{2}$. Then

$$\frac{|\mu_e|}{|\mu_p|} = \frac{g_e \mu_\beta}{g_N \mu_N} = \frac{g_e M_N}{g_N M_e} = \frac{2.0(1836)}{5.585} = 657 .$$

12.53 If the particle on a ring, discussed in Section 11.7, had a charge (q), its Hamiltonian in a magnetic field (B) would be:

$$\hat{H} = \hat{L}_z^2/2\mu a^2 - (qB/2\mu c)\hat{L}_z/\hbar$$

(μ is the mass, a is the diameter of the ring.) Determine the eigenfunctions for this operator and derive a formula for the energies. Sketch the energy-level diagram.

The eigenvalue of $\hat{L}_z$ is $m\hbar$, and of $\hat{L}_z^2$ is $m^2\hbar^2$, so that the eigenvalues of $\hat{H}$ are:

$$E = \frac{m^2\hbar^2}{2\mu a^2} - \frac{mBq}{2\mu c} \qquad m = 0, \pm 1, \pm 2, \ldots$$

$$\frac{2Bq}{\mu c} \left\{ \begin{array}{l} \underline{\hspace{3cm}} \quad m = -2 \\ \underline{\hspace{3cm}} \quad m = +2 \end{array} \right.$$

$$\frac{Bq}{\mu c} \left\{ \begin{array}{l} \underline{\hspace{3cm}} \quad m = -1 \\ \underline{\hspace{3cm}} \quad m = +1 \end{array} \right. \qquad \uparrow E$$

$$\underline{\hspace{3cm}} \quad m = 0$$

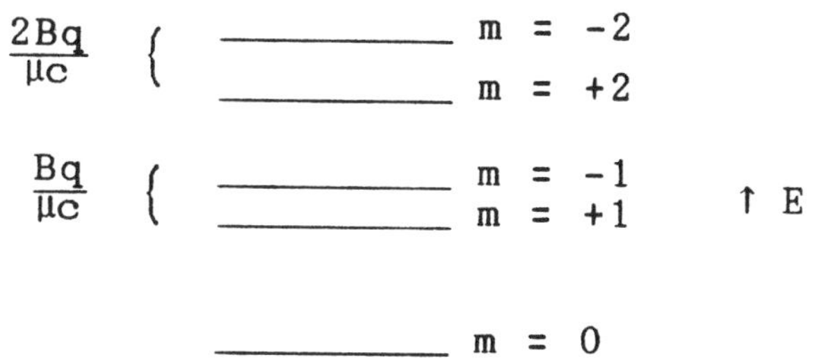

12.54 The ^{23}Na nucleus has spin $I = \frac{3}{2}$. What are the total nuclear spin quantum numbers (T) for Na(^{2}S) atoms?

For the ^{2}S state, S = $\frac{1}{2}$.   With I = $\frac{3}{2}$,

$$T = (I + S), \ldots, (I - S) = 2, 1 .$$

12.55 The selection rule for hyperfine transitions is $\Delta T = \pm 1$. Derive a formula relating the transition frequency to the coupling constant and the spin I (assuming $S = \frac{1}{2}$). Calculate the hyperfine coupling constant of cesium from its frequency (given in text).

a)   Starting with $E_{hf} = \frac{1}{2}$ Ah[T(T + 1) - I(I + 1) - S(S + 1)] and

with $\Delta E = E_{hf}(T) - E_{hf}(T - 1)$, we find $\Delta E = hAT = hA(I + S)$.

Also, $\Delta E = h\nu$, so with S = $\frac{1}{2}$, $\nu = A\left(I + \frac{1}{2}\right)$.

b)   For cesium atoms, $\nu = 9,192,631,770$ s^{-1} and I = $\frac{7}{2}$.

Then A = 2,298,157,943 s^{-1} .

12.56 (a) The Hamiltonian of an electron including the Zeeman effect and the hyperfine coupling is, in high magnetic field:

$$\hbar^2\hat{H} = -g\mu_B B_0 \hat{S}_z \hbar + Ah\hat{I}_z\hat{S}_z$$

[The meaning of "high magnetic field" is that the first term is much larger than the second, so the x- and y-terms of the **I** · **S** vector product of Eq. (12.56) can be neglected.] The eigenfunctions of this Hamiltonian are products of the nuclear and electron spin functions; for example, $\alpha_e\alpha_N$. Derive formulas for the energies of all of the eigenstates of this Hamiltonian for $I = \frac{1}{2}$.

(b) As a result of hyperfine coupling, the ESR transition will be split into two lines. Derive formulas for these transitions ($\Delta M_S = 1$, $\Delta M_I = 0$) and sketch the ESR spectrum. How is the hyperfine coupling constant related to the splitting?

a) With $I = \pm\frac{1}{2}$ and $S = \pm\frac{1}{2}$: $E_1 = -\frac{1}{2}g\mu_\beta B_0 + \frac{1}{4}hA$,

$E_2 = -\frac{1}{2}g\mu_\beta B_0 - \frac{1}{4}hA$, $E_3 = \frac{1}{2}g\mu_\beta B_0 - \frac{1}{4}hA$, $E_4 = \frac{1}{2}g\mu_\beta B_0 + \frac{1}{4}hA$.

b) For $\Delta M_S = 1$ and $\Delta M_I = 0$: $\nu_1 = \dfrac{E_4 - E_2}{h} = \dfrac{g\mu_\beta B_0}{h} + \frac{1}{2}A$ and

$$\nu_2 = \frac{E_3 - E_1}{h} = \frac{g\mu_\beta B_0}{h} - \frac{1}{2}A .$$

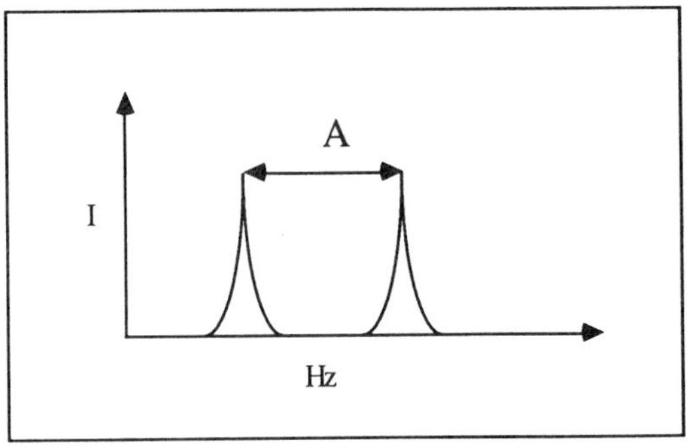

12.57 The theory of angular momentum shows that the integral of a triple product of Legendre polynomials:

$$\iint P_{l_1}^{m_1} P_{l_2}^{m_2} P_{l_3}^{m_3}\, d\Omega$$

is zero unless $m_1 + m_2 + m_3 = 0$ and the numbers l_1, l_2, and l_3 can form a triangle. Show that this requires a selection rule $\Delta L = \pm 1$ for atomic spectra.

A transition between ψ_1 and ψ_2 will be allowed if $\int \psi_1^* \begin{pmatrix} x \\ y \\ z \end{pmatrix} \psi_2 \, d\tau \neq 0$. Since in polar coordinates $z = r\cos\theta$, $x = r\sin\theta\cos\phi = \frac{r}{2}\sin\theta(e^{i\phi} + e^{-i\phi})$ and $y = r\sin\theta\sin\phi = \frac{r}{2i}(e^{i\phi} - e^{-i\phi})$, then $z \propto P_1^{|0|}$, $x \propto P_1^{|1|}$, and $y \propto P_1^{|1|}$. Factoring out the radial part of ψ, the integral above is proportional to $\int Y_{l_1}^{|m_1|} \begin{pmatrix} x \\ y \\ z \end{pmatrix} Y_{l_2}^{|m_2|}\, d\Omega$. This is proportional to $\int P_{l_1}^{|m_1|} P_{l_2}^{|m_2|} (P_1^{|m|})_{x,y \text{ or } z}\, d\Omega$. The z integral is $\int P_{l_1}^{|m_1|} P_{l_2}^{|m_2|} P_1^{|0|}\, d\Omega$. Since $m_1 + m_2 + m_3 = 0$, then $|m_1| + |m_2| = 0$ or $m_1 = m_2 = 0$. For l_1, l_2 and l_3 to form a triangle (sides have length proportional to l_1, l_2 or l_3), we must have $l_2 - l_1 = 1$ (two angles = zero). For the x or y case, $\int P_{l_1}^{|m_1|} P_{l_2}^{|m_2|} P_1^{|1|}\, d\Omega$. Since $m_1 + m_2 + m_3$ can't be zero, the integral is zero. Thus only the z transitions are allowed, with $\Delta L = \pm 1$.

13

Diatomic Molecules

13.1 The anharmonic potential can be written $V_{anh} = a(R - R_e)^3 + b(R - R_e)^4$.
(a) Identify a and b as they are related to $E_e(R)$.
(b) Calculate the first-order correction to the harmonic oscillator energy for the ground ($v = 0$) state.

a) By comparison with Eq. (13.20), $a = \frac{1}{6}\left(\frac{\partial^3 E_e}{\partial R^3}\right)_{R_e}$ and

$$b = \frac{1}{24}\left(\frac{\partial^4 E_e}{\partial R^4}\right)_{R_e} .$$

b) We use perturbation theory with

$\hat{H}' = a(R - R_e)^3 + b(R - R_e)^4$. Then

$\Delta E = \int \psi_0 [a(R - R_e)^3 + b(R - R_e)^4] \psi_0 \, d\tau$. The integral

$\int \psi_0 a(R - R_e)^3 \psi_0 \, d\tau$ is zero since it is an odd function

integrated over a symmetric interval. For

$\int \psi_0 b(R - R_e)^4 \psi_0 \, d\tau$, we use $\psi_0 = A_0 e^{-x^2/2\alpha^2}$ where $A_0 = \frac{1}{\sqrt{\alpha}(\pi)^{1/4}}$,

$\alpha = \left(\frac{\hbar^2}{k\mu}\right)^{1/4}$ and $x = (R - R_e)$. Then defining $y = \frac{x}{\alpha}$,

$\Delta E = \frac{1}{\alpha\sqrt{\pi}} \int_{-\infty}^{\infty} e^{-x^2/2\alpha^2} [bx^4] e^{-x^2/2\alpha^2} dx = \frac{b\alpha^4}{\sqrt{\pi}} \int_{-\infty}^{\infty} y^4 e^{-y^2} dy$. Using

Table 11.3,

$$\Delta E = \frac{b\alpha^4}{\sqrt{\pi}} \left(\frac{3\sqrt{\pi}}{4}\right) = \frac{b3\alpha^4}{4} = \frac{3b\hbar^2}{4k\mu} = \left(v + \frac{1}{2}\right)^2 \omega_e x_e = \frac{1}{4}\omega_e x_e \; .$$

The correction factor ΔE is subtracted, so that the 1st order perturbation energy of the harmonic oscillator is

$$E_v = \left(v + \frac{1}{2}\right) hc\omega_e - \left(v + \frac{1}{2}\right)^2 hc\omega_e x_e \; .$$

13.2 Calculate the harmonic force constant (k) of CO from its vibrational constant (Table 13.1); your answer should be in ergs/cm^2. If you had a spring with this force constant, how much weight would be required to extend it one cm?

$k = \mu(2\pi c\omega_e)^2$. For CO:

$$\mu = \frac{m_C m_O}{m_C + m_O} = \frac{(12.00)(15.9949)}{L(12.00 + 15.9949)} = 1.1385 \times 10^{-23} \text{ g} \; .$$

With $\omega_e = 2170.21 \text{ cm}^{-1}$, we find: $k = 1.9052 \times 10^6 \text{ erg cm}^{-2}$.

With $mg = kx$ and $x = 1$ cm : $m = \frac{kx}{g} = 1.95$ kg .

13.3 When speaking of "bond strength," two meanings could be envisioned: the energy required to break the bond (D_0) or the stiffness of the bond as measured by its force constant or vibrational constant (ω_e). Use the data on Table 13.1 (for single-bonded molecules only) to regress the vibrational constant vs. D_0 and calculate the correlation coefficient.

Use only species with single bonds:

Species	ω_e/cm^{-1}	D_0/eV
$^1H^1H$	4395.2	4.4773
$^1H^{35}Cl$	2989.74	4.436
$^{35}Cl^{35}Cl$	564.9	2.475
$^1H^{79}Br$	2649.67	3.775
$^1H^{127}I$	2309.5	3.053
$^{127}I^{35}Cl$	384.18	2.152
$^{127}I^{79}Br$	268.4	1.817
$^1H^{19}F$	4138.52	5.86

The regression equation is: $\omega_e = 1115D_0 - 1695$. $r = 0.93$.

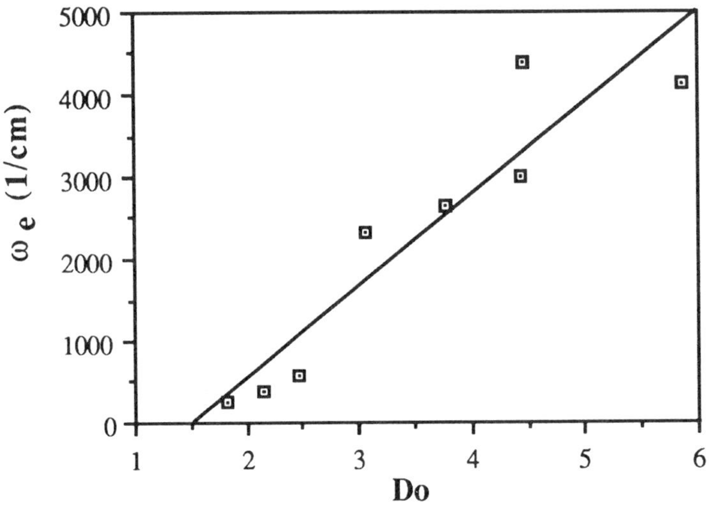

13.4 The standard enthalpy of formation for HCl at 0 K, $\Delta_f H_0^\circ$, is given by Table 6.4. Calculate this quantity from the spectroscopic energies of Table 13.1 and compare your result to that on Table 6.4.

$$\Delta_f H_0^\theta = \left[\tfrac{1}{2}D_0(Cl_2) + \tfrac{1}{2}D_0(H_2) - D_0(HCl)\right]$$

$$\Delta_f H_0^\theta = \left[\tfrac{1}{2}(2.475) + \tfrac{1}{2}(4.4773) - (4.436)\right]$$

$$\Delta_f H_0^\theta = (-0.9599\text{eV}) = -92.61 \text{ kJ mol}^{-1} .$$

13.5 The Morse potential is referred to as "semiempirical" because it uses experimental data to determine its parameters. What three experimentally measurable quantities can be used to determine the Morse potential of a particular molecule?

The Morse potential is: $E_e(R) = D_e(1 - e^{-\beta x})^2$ where $x = R - R_e$ and $\beta = \left(\frac{k}{2D_e}\right)^{1/2}$. The parameters are D_e (well depth), R_e (equilibrium distance), and k (harmonic force constant).

13.6 Calculate the vibration constants ω_e and $\omega_e x_e$ for $^2D^{35}Cl$ from those of $^1H^{35}Cl$ (Table 13.1).

$\omega_e = \frac{1}{2\pi c}\sqrt{\frac{k}{\mu}}$. If we assume that the force constant is unchanged with isotopic substitution: $\omega_e(^2H^{35}Cl) = \omega_e(^1H^{35}Cl)\sqrt{\frac{\mu(^1H^{35}Cl)}{\mu(^2H^{35}Cl)}}$.

With $\omega_e(^1H^{35}Cl) = 2989.74 \text{ cm}^{-1}$, $\mu(^2H^{35}Cl) = 1.9044$ amu, and $\mu(^1H^{35}Cl) = 0.9796$ amu we find $\omega_e(^2H^{35}Cl) = 2144.3 \text{ cm}^{-1}$. From Eq. (13.39): $\omega_e x_e(^2H^{35}Cl) = \omega_e x_e(^1H^{35}Cl)\,\frac{\mu(^1H^{35}Cl)}{\mu(^2H^{35}Cl)}$.

$\omega_e x_e(^1H^{35}Cl) = 52.05 \text{ cm}^{-1}$ so that $\omega_e x_e(^2H^{35}Cl) = 26.77 \text{ cm}^{-1}$.

13.7 Calculate the vibration constants ω_e and $\omega_e x_e$ of $^1H^{37}Cl$ from those of $^1H^{35}Cl$ (Table 13.1).

As in the previous problem: $\omega_e(^1H^{37}Cl) = \omega_e(^1H^{35}Cl)\sqrt{\frac{\mu(^1H^{35}Cl)}{\mu(^1H^{37}Cl)}}$,

$\omega_e(^1H^{35}Cl) = 2989.74\ cm^{-1}$, $\mu(^1H^{35}Cl) = 0.9796$ amu , and

$\mu(^1H^{37}Cl) = 0.9811$ amu . Thus: $\omega_e(^1H^{37}Cl) = 2987.52\ cm^{-1}$. Also,

$\omega_e x_e(^1H^{37}Cl) = \omega_e x_e(^1H^{35}Cl)\ \frac{\mu(^1H^{35}Cl)}{\mu(^1H^{37}Cl)}$. $\omega_e x_e(^1H^{35}Cl) = 52.05\ cm^{-1}$,

thus: $\omega_e x_e(^1H^{37}Cl) = 51.97\ cm^{-1}$.

13.8 Prove that the Morse potential approaches the harmonic potential ($\frac{1}{2}kx^2$) for small values of $x = R - R_e$.

From Eq. (13.32), $E_e(R) = D_e(1 - e^{-\beta x})^2$. At small values of x,

$e^{-\beta x}$ may be expanded as $1 + \beta x$:

$E_e(R) = D_e(1 - (1 + \beta x))^2 = D_e(-\beta x)^2$. Since $\beta = \left(\frac{k}{2D_e}\right)^{1/2}$,

then $E_e(R) = D_e x^2 \beta^2 = D_e\left(\frac{k}{2D_e}\right)x^2 = \frac{1}{2}\ kx^2$.

13.9 Calculate the Morse constant β for carbon monoxide. Calculate the Morse potential (in eV) for this molecule and R = 0.5, 1, 1.5, 2 and 4 Å. (If you have a computer or programmable calculator available, calculate many values from R = 0.5 to 4 and sketch the curve.)

$D_e \sim D_0 + \frac{1}{2}\ \omega_e$, $D_0(CO) = 11.108\ eV = 89{,}587.9\ cm^{-1}$,

$\omega_e(CO) = 2170.21\ cm^{-1}$, thus: $D_e \sim 90{,}673\ cm^{-1} = 11.243\ eV$.

$\beta = \left(\frac{k}{2D_e}\right)^{1/2}$. With $k(CO) = 1.908 \times 10^6\ erg\ cm^{-2}$ and

$D_e = 1.8012 \times 10^{-11}$ erg, $\beta = 2.301 \times 10^8\ cm^{-1} = 2.3\ Å^{-1}$.

$E_e(R) = D_e(1 - e^{-\beta x})^2$ and $x = R - R_e$, thus, with $R_e = 1.1282$ Å :

$E_e(0.5\ \text{Å}) = 118\ \text{eV}$, $E_e(1\ \text{Å}) = 1.32\ \text{eV}$, $E_e(1.5\ \text{Å}) = 3.71\ \text{eV}$,

$E_e(2.0\ \text{Å}) = 8.42\ \text{eV}$, and $E_e(\text{Å}) = 11.21\ \text{eV}$.

13.10 Use the constants from Table 13.1 to calculate the frequencies of the vibrational fundamental, first overtone and hot bands of CO. What would be the relative intensities of the fundamental and hot band if T = 1000 K?

For CO: $\omega_e = 2170.21\ \text{cm}^{-1}$ and $\omega_e x_e = 13.461\ \text{cm}^{-1}$. The vibration fundamental is: $\tilde{\nu}_0 = \omega_e - 2\omega_e x_e = 2143.29\ \text{cm}^{-1}$. The first overtone is: $\tilde{\nu}_1 = 2\omega_e - 6\omega_e x_e = 4295.65\ \text{cm}^{-1}$. The hot band is: $\tilde{\nu}_h = \omega_e - 4\omega_e x_e = 2116.37\ \text{cm}^{-1}$. The relative intensity of the fundamental and hot band is approximately: $\frac{N_h}{N_0} = \exp -\left(\frac{\omega_e}{k_b T}\right)$.

With T = 1000 K and $\frac{hc}{k_b} = 1.4388$ cm K , we find

$$\frac{N_h}{N_0}(1000\ \text{K}) = 0.044 .$$

13.11 Derive a formula for the vibrational frequency (band origin) of the second overtone.

The vibrational energy is given by

$$E_v = hc\left\{\left(v + \frac{1}{2}\right)\omega_e - \left(v + \frac{1}{2}\right)^2 \omega_e x_e + \left(v + \frac{1}{2}\right)^3 \omega_e y_e + \ldots\right\} .$$

The second overtone is given by the transition v = 0 to v = 3 .

Since $E_3 = hc\left\{\frac{7}{2}\ \omega_e - \left(\frac{7}{2}\right)^2 \omega_e x_e + \ldots\right\}$ and

$E_0 = hc\left\{\frac{1}{2}\ \omega_e - \left(\frac{1}{2}\right)^2 \omega_e x_e + \ldots\right\}$, then $\Delta E = hc\{3\omega_e - 12\omega_e x_e\}$.

The frequency is given by $\tilde{\nu} = \frac{\Delta E}{hc} = \{3\omega_e - 12\omega_e x_e\}$.

13.12 Analyze the vibrational frequencies (band origins) for $^1H^{35}Cl$ (below) to determine ω_e and $\omega_e x_e$.

Fundamental:	2885.9 cm^{-1}
1st overtone:	5668.0
2nd overtone:	8346.9

$$E_v = hc\left\{\left(v + \tfrac{1}{2}\right)\omega_e - \left(v + \tfrac{1}{2}\right)^2 \omega_e x_e + \ldots\right\} .$$

$$\Delta E = E_1 - E_0 = hc\{\omega_e - 2\omega_e x_e\} \text{ or } \tilde{\nu}_0 = \omega_e - 2\omega_e x_e = 2885.9 \text{ cm}^{-1} .$$

$$\Delta E = E_2 - E_0 = hc\{2\omega_e - 6\omega_e x_e\} \text{ or}$$

$$\tilde{\nu}_1 = \frac{\Delta E}{hc} = 2\omega_e - 6\omega_e x_e = 5668.0 \text{ cm}^{-1} .$$ For the 2nd overtone,

$$\Delta E = E_3 - E_0 = hc\{3\omega_e - 12\omega_e x_e\} \text{ or}$$

$$\tilde{\nu}_2 = 3\omega_e - 12\omega_e x_e = 8346.9 \text{ cm}^{-1} . \quad \omega_e = 2\tilde{\nu}_1 - \tilde{\nu}_2 = 2989.1 \text{ cm}^{-1}$$

and $$\omega_e x_e = -\frac{(\tilde{\nu}_0 - \omega_e)}{2} = 51.6 \text{ cm}^{-1} .$$

13.13 Estimate the bond energies for HD and D_2 from that of H_2. Since these molecules differ only by isotopic substitution you can assume that the potential curve $E_e(R)$ is unchanged, hence, D_e and k are unchanged. The observed values for these molecules are 4.513 and 4.555 eV.

$$\frac{\omega_e(D_2)}{\omega_e(H_2)} = \sqrt{\frac{\mu(H_2)}{\mu(D_2)}} = 0.7074 .$$ With $\omega_e(H_2) = 4395.2 \text{ cm}^{-1}$, we find

$\omega_e(D_2) = 3109.2 \text{ cm}^{-1}$. $D_e = D_0 + \frac{1}{2}\omega_e$. With

$D_0(H_2) = 36{,}111.8 \text{ cm}^{-1}$, we find $D_e = 38{,}309.4 \text{ cm}^{-1}$ so that

$$D_0(D_2) = D_e - \tfrac{1}{2}\omega_e(D_2) = 36{,}755 \text{ cm}^{-1} = 4.557 \text{ eV} .$$

$$\frac{\omega_e(HD)}{\omega_e(H_2)} = \sqrt{\frac{0.5039}{0.6717}} = 0.86613 .$$ $\omega_e(HD) = 3806.8 \text{ cm}^{-1}$ and

$$D_0(HD) = 36{,}406 \text{ cm}^{-1} = 4.514 \text{ eV} .$$

13.14 Calculate the classical rotation frequency, the number of rotations performed in one second, for a CO molecule in the $J = 10$ state. Do this by equating the classical kinetic energy, $\frac{1}{2}I\omega^2$, to the quantum mechanical energy.

From Eq. (13.41), $E_J = \dfrac{J(J + 1)h^2}{8\pi^2 I}$, where for CO,

$$I = \mu R_e^2 = (1.139 \times 10^{-23}\ g)(1.1282 \times 10^{-8}\ cm)^2$$

$$I = 1.450 \times 10^{-39}\ cm^2\ g\ .$$

Then $E_{10} = \dfrac{10(11)(6.626 \times 10^{-27}\ erg\ s)^2}{8\pi^2(1.450 \times 10^{-39}\ cm^2\ g)} = 4.218 \times 10^{-14}\ erg$.

The classical rotational energy is $E = \frac{1}{2}I\omega^2$. Then

$$\omega = \left(\frac{2E_{10}}{I}\right)^{1/2} = \left(\frac{2(4.218 \times 10^{-14}\ erg)}{1.45 \times 10^{-39}\ cm^2\ g}\right)^{1/2} = 7.627 \times 10^{12}\ s^{-1}$$

or $\nu = \dfrac{\omega}{2\pi} = 1.214 \times 10^{12}\ s^{-1}$.

13.15 The following frequencies were measured by microwave spectroscopy of $^{23}Na^{35}Cl$:

$$J = 1 \longrightarrow 2 \quad (v = 0) \quad \nu = 26.0511\ \text{GHz}$$
$$J = 1 \longrightarrow 2 \quad (v = 1) \quad \nu = 25.8576\ \text{GHz}$$

From these numbers, calculate the rotation-vibration constant (α_e) and bond length (R_e) for this molecule (neglect centrifugal stretching).

Neglecting centrifugal distortion: $\dfrac{E_J}{h} = J(J + 1)B_v$,

$B_0 = B_e - \frac{1}{2}\alpha_e$, $B_1 = B_e - \frac{3}{2}\alpha_e$. Thus, $\alpha_e = B_0 - B_1$. Also,

$\nu = \dfrac{\Delta E}{h}$, so that for $J = 1 \rightarrow 2$, $\nu_0 = 6B_0 - 2B_0 = 4B_0$.

Similarly, $\nu_1 = 4B_1$. Thus, $B_0 = \dfrac{\nu_0}{4} = 6.5128$ GHz ,

$B_1 = 6.4644$ GHz , and $\alpha_e = B_1 - B_0 = 48.4$ MHz ,

$B_e = B_0 + \frac{1}{2}\alpha_e = 6.5128$ GHz . Finally:

$$R_e = \left(\frac{h}{8\pi^2\mu B_e}\right)^{1/2} = 2.3609\ \text{Å}\ .$$

13.16 The rotational constant of $^{133}Cs^{35}Cl$ measured by microwave spectroscopy is 2163.8 MHz. Calculate R_e.

From Eq. (13.42), $B_e = \frac{h}{8\pi^2 I}$. With $I = \mu R_e^2$,

$$R_e = \left(\frac{h}{8\pi^2 B_e \mu}\right)^{1/2} = \left(\frac{6.626 \times 10^{-27} \text{ erg s}}{8\pi^2(2163.8 \times 10^6 \text{ s}^{-1})(4.601 \times 10^{-23} \text{ g})}\right)^{1/2}$$

$R_e = 2.903 \times 10^{-8}$ cm .

13.17 Calculate the bond lengths R_e from the rotational constants of HF and DF as listed on Table 13.1.

From Eq. (13.42), $R_e = \left(\frac{h}{8\pi^2 \tilde{B}_e \mu c}\right)^{1/2}$. For $^1H^{19}F$,

$$R_e = \left(\frac{6.626 \times 10^{-27} \text{ erg s}}{8\pi^2(20.939 \text{ cm}^{-1})(1.578 \times 10^{-24} \text{ g})(2.998 \times 10^{10} \text{ cm s}^{-1})}\right)^{1/2}$$

$R_e = 9.205 \times 10^{-9}$ cm .

For $^2D^{19}F$,

$$R_e = \left(\frac{6.626 \times 10^{-27} \text{ erg s}}{8\pi^2(11.007 \text{ cm}^{-1})(3.005 \times 10^{-24} \text{ g})(2.998 \times 10^{10} \text{ cm s}^{-1})}\right)^{1/2}$$

$R_e = 9.199 \times 10^{-9}$ cm .

13.18 Calculate the populations of the $J = 1$ through 5 rotational state of HBr at 300 K (relative to the $J = 0$ state population).

The relative population of two states is given by

$\frac{N'}{N} = \frac{(2J' + 1)}{(2J + 1)} \exp\left(-\frac{(E_{J'} - E_J)}{kT}\right)$. The rotational energy is

given by $E_J = \frac{J(J + 1)h^2}{8\pi^2 I}$. For HBr,

$$\frac{h^2}{8\pi^2 I} = \frac{(6.626 \times 10^{-27}\ \text{erg s})^2}{8\pi^2(1.656 \times 10^{-24}\ \text{g})(1.414 \times 10^{-8}\ \text{cm})^2} = 1.679 \times 10^{-15}\ \text{erg}.$$

For J' = 1 , J = 0 ,

$$\frac{N_1}{N_0} = 3\exp\left(\frac{-2(1.679 \times 10^{-15}\ \text{erg})}{(1.38 \times 10^{-16}\ \text{erg K}^{-1})(300\ \text{K})}\right) = 2.766 .$$

For J' = 2 , J = 0 , $\frac{N_2}{N_0} = 3.920$. For J' = 3 , J = 0 , $\frac{N_3}{N_0} = 4.303$. For J' = 4 , J = 0 , $\frac{N_4}{N_0} = 4.000$. For J' = 5 , J = 0 , $\frac{N_5}{N_0} = 3.259$.

13.19 Derive a formula for the J quantum number of the rotational state having the maximum population at some temperature T. For HCl, CO and ICl, calculate the J-value with the maximum population at 300 K.

$$\frac{N_J}{N_0} = (2J + 1)\exp\left[\frac{-J(J + 1)hc\tilde{B}_e}{k_bT}\right] .$$ Find $\frac{\partial\left(\frac{N_J}{N_0}\right)}{\partial J} = 0$:

$$\frac{\partial\left(\frac{N_J}{N_0}\right)}{\partial J} = \left[2 - (2J + 1)^2\frac{hc\tilde{B}_e}{k_bT}\right]\exp\left[-J(J + 1)\frac{hc\tilde{B}_e}{k_bT}\right] .$$ Thus

$$2 - (2J + 1)^2\frac{hc\tilde{B}_e}{k_bT} = 0 \text{ and } J_{max} = \frac{1}{2}\left[\left(\frac{2k_bT}{h\tilde{B}_e c}\right)^{1/2} - 1\right] .$$ With

$\tilde{B}_e\,(HCl) = 10.5909\ \text{cm}^{-1}$, $\tilde{B}_e(CO) = 1.9314\ \text{cm}^{-1}$, $\tilde{B}_e(ICl) = 0.11416\ \text{cm}^{-1}$, $\frac{hc}{k_b} = 1.4388$ cm K and T = 300 K , we find: $J_{max}(HCl) = 2.6 \sim 3$, $J_{max}(CO) = 6.8 \sim 7$, and $J_{max}(ICl) = 29.7 \sim 30$.

13.20 The $J = 0 \rightarrow 1$ microwave frequency for $^{2}D^{35}Cl$ was measured [Cowan and Gordy, *Phys. Rev.*, **111**, 209 (1958)] as 323 295.8 MHz. Estimate the centrifugal distortion constant from data and equations in this chapter and calculate B_0 from this number (keep six significant figures). From the IR of the same compound it was determined that $B_0 = 5.39226\ \text{cm}^{-1}$. Calculate the velocity of light from these data to six significant figures.

$$\tilde{B}_e(\text{DCl}) = \tilde{B}_e(\text{HCl})\,\frac{\mu(\text{HCl})}{\mu(\text{DCl})} = (10.5909\ \text{cm}^{-1})(0.5139) = 5.4425\ \text{cm}^{-1}\ .$$

Since $\omega_e(\text{HCl}) = 2989.74\ \text{cm}^{-1}$, $\omega_e(\text{DCl}) = (0.5139)^2(2989.72\ \text{cm}^{-1})$

or $\omega_e(\text{DCl}) = 2143.25\ \text{cm}^{-1}$.

$$D_c = \frac{4\tilde{B}_e^{\,3}}{\omega_e^{\,2}} = \frac{4(5.4425\ \text{cm}^{-1})^3}{(2143.25\ \text{cm}^{-1})^2} = 1.40381 \times 10^{-4}\ \text{cm}^{-1}\ .$$

From Eq. (13.46), $\frac{E_J}{h} = J(J + 1)B_0 - J^2(J + 1)^2 D_c$. For $J = 1$,

$$323{,}295.8 \times 10^6\ \text{s}^{-1} = 2B_0 - 4(1.40381 \times 10^{-4}\ \text{cm}^{-1}) \times (2.998 \times 10^{10}\ \text{cm s}^{-1})$$

or $B_0 = 1.61656 \times 10^{11}\ \text{s}^{-1}$. Then

$$c = \frac{B_0}{\tilde{B}_0} = \frac{1.61656 \times 10^{11}\ \text{s}^{-1}}{(5.39226\ \text{cm}^{-1})} = 2.99793 \times 10^{10}\ \text{cm s}^{-1}\ .$$

13.21 Microwave rotational frequencies have been measured for $^{12}C^{16}O$ ($v = 0$) as:

$$\nu(1 \rightarrow 2) = 230.53797\ \text{GHz}$$

$$\nu(3 \rightarrow 4) = 461.0468\ \text{GHz}$$

Use these data to calculate B_0 and D_c.

For a $J \rightarrow J + 1$ transition: $\nu = 2B_0(J + 1) - 4D_c(J + 1)^3$.

Thus, with $\nu(1 \rightarrow 2) = 230.53797$ GHz and $\nu(3 \rightarrow 4) = 461.0468$ GHz,

230.53797 GHz = $4B_0 - 32D_c$ and 461.0468 GHz = $8B_0 - 256D_c$.

Thus: 29.14 MHz = $192D_c$. D_c = 152 kHz and B_0 = 57.63571 GHz .

13.22 Derive the formulas for the *P* and *R* branches of the first-overtone vibrational band.

Using Eq. (13.49) for the first overtone, R branch:

$$\frac{E(2, J+1) - E(0, J)}{hc} = \frac{5}{2}\omega_e - \frac{25}{4}\omega_e x_e + (J+1)(J+2)\tilde{B}_e - (J+1)(J+2)\frac{5}{2}\alpha_e - \left[\frac{1}{2}\omega_e - \frac{1}{4}\omega_e x_e + J(J+1)\tilde{B}_e - J(J+1)\frac{1}{2}\alpha_e\right]$$

$$\frac{E(2, J+1) - E(0, J)}{hc} = 2\omega_e - 6\omega_e x_e + (2J+2)\tilde{B}_e - (2J+5)(2J+1)\alpha_e$$

$$\frac{E(2, J+1) - E(0, J)}{hc} = \tilde{\nu}_1 + 2(J+1)\tilde{B}_e - (2J+5)(J+1)\alpha_e \; .$$

For the P branch:

$$\frac{E(2, J-1) - E(0, J)}{hc} = \frac{5}{2}\omega_e - \frac{25}{4}\omega_e x_e + (J-1)J\tilde{B}_e - (J-1)J\frac{5}{2}\alpha_e - \left[\frac{1}{2}\omega_e - \frac{1}{4}\omega_e x_e + J(J+1)\tilde{B}_e - J(J+1)\frac{1}{2}\alpha_e\right]$$

$$\frac{E(2, J+1) - E(0, J)}{hc} = 2\omega_e - 6\omega_e x_e - 2J\tilde{B}_e - J(2J-3)\alpha_e$$

$$\frac{E(2, J+1) - E(0, J)}{hc} = \tilde{\nu}_1 - 2J\tilde{B}_e - J(2J-3)\alpha_e \; .$$

13.23 Analyze the vibrational frequencies (below) for the fundamental IR band of $^{12}C^{16}O$ to find the band origin, $\tilde{B}_e$ and α_e. (units: cm^{-1}):

J''	R	P
0	2147.084	—
1	2150.858	2139.427
2	2154.599	2135.548
3	2158.301	2131.633
4	2161.971	2127.684
5	2165.602	2123.700
6	2169.200	2119.681
7	2172.759	2115.632

First, note that the spacing between rotational bands is $\sim 4\ cm^{-1}$. We then label the bands with the integer m, where for the R branch $m = J'' + 1$ and for the P branch, $m = -J''$. Then the given table may be labelled as follows:

J"	m (R branch)	m (P branch)
0	1	-
1	2	-1
2	3	-2
3	4	-3
4	5	-4
5	6	-5
6	7	-6
7	8	-7

From Eqs. (13.50) and (13.51),

R: $\tilde{\nu}_R = \tilde{\nu}_0 + 2(J'' + 1)\tilde{B}_e - (J'' + 1)(J'' + 3)\alpha_e$ and

P: $\tilde{\nu}_P = \tilde{\nu}_0 - 2J''\tilde{B}_e - J''(J'' - 2)\alpha_e$. Substituting m into the appropriate eq., either of the above becomes:

$\tilde{\nu}_R = \tilde{\nu}_0 + 2m\tilde{B}_e - m(m + 2)\alpha_e = \tilde{\nu}_0 + m(2\tilde{B}_e - 2\alpha_e) - m^2\alpha_e$. The difference in frequency between m and m + 1 is then

$$\Delta\tilde{\nu} = ((m + 1) - m)(2\tilde{B}_e - 2\alpha_e) - [(m + 1)^2 - m^2]\alpha_e$$

$$\Delta\tilde{\nu} = 2\tilde{B}_e - 3\alpha_e - 2m\alpha_e .$$

A plot of $\Delta\tilde{\nu}$ vs. m should have slope = $-2\alpha_e$ and intercept = $2\tilde{B}_e - 3\alpha_e$. Linear regression gives intercept = 3.8054 with σ = 0.0052 and slope = -0.0432 with σ = 0.0014. Then α_e = 0.0216 cm^{-1}, $\tilde{B}_e$ = 1.935 cm^{-1} and

$$\tilde{\nu}_0 = 2143.28 \text{ cm}^{-1} .$$

13.24 In an IR spectrum of CO, the maximum-intensity line is associated with $J'' = 8$. What is the temperature of the sample? For CO, $\tilde{B}_0 = 1.9227 \text{ cm}^{-1}$.

From problem 13.19, $J_{max} = \frac{1}{2}\left\{\left(\frac{2k_bT}{\tilde{B}_e ch}\right)^{1/2} - 1\right\}$. For $J_{max} = 8$ and $\tilde{B}_e \cong \tilde{B}_0 = 1.9227 \text{ cm}^{-1}$, $(2J_{max} + 1)^2 = \frac{2kT}{\tilde{B}_e ch}$ or

$$T = (16 + 1)^2(1.9227 \text{ cm}^{-1}) \times \frac{(2.998 \times 10^{10} \text{ cm s}^{-1})(6.626 \times 10^{-27} \text{ erg s}^{-1})}{2(1.38 \times 10^{-16} \text{ erg K}^{-1})}$$

$$T \cong 400 \text{ K} .$$

13.25 If the rotational structure of an IR band can be resolved, the temperature of the sample can be calculated from Boltzmann's law, applied to the populations of the rotational states. Often, the bands cannot be resolved well enough to determine the J-values. However, in such cases, the temperature can be estimated from the frequency difference, $\Delta\tilde{\nu}$, between the maxima of the P- and R-branches. Show that this difference is related to the temperature as:

$$\Delta\tilde{\nu} = (8kT\tilde{B}_e/hc)^{1/2}$$

From Eqs. (13.50) and (13.51), if we neglect $\alpha_e \ll B_e$:

$\tilde{\nu}_R - \tilde{\nu}_P = \Delta\tilde{\nu} \sim 4J''\tilde{B}_e$ so that: $\Delta\tilde{\nu}_{max} \sim 4\tilde{B}_e J_{max}$. From problem 13.19: $J_{max} \sim \left[\frac{kT}{2hc\tilde{B}_e}\right]^{1/2}$ so that $\Delta\tilde{\nu}_{max} \sim \left[\frac{8kT\tilde{B}_e}{hc}\right]^{1/2}$.

13.26 We generally assume that the rotational energy is a small addition to the vibrational energy, but that clearly depends on the J quantum number. For CO, at what value of J would the energy of the $v = 0$ state exceed the energy of the $v = 1, J = 0$ state? Will there by many molecules rotating this fast at room temperature?

The combined rotational and vibrational energy is

$$\frac{E_{v,J}}{hc} = \left(v + \frac{1}{2}\right)\omega_e - \left(v + \frac{1}{2}\right)^2 \omega_e x_e + J(J + 1)\tilde{B}_e - J(J + 1)\left(v + \frac{1}{2}\right)\alpha_e .$$

$E_{1,0} = \frac{3}{2}\omega_e - \frac{9}{4}\omega_e x_e$ and

$E_{0,J} = \frac{1}{2}\omega_e - \frac{1}{4}\omega_e x_e + J(J + 1)\tilde{B}_e - \frac{1}{2} J(J + 1)\alpha_e$. Setting

$E_{1,0} = E_{0,J}$ we find: $J(J + 1) = \dfrac{\omega_e - 2\omega_e x_e}{\tilde{B}_e - \frac{1}{2}\alpha_e}$. For CO:

$\omega_e = 2170.21\ \text{cm}^{-1}$, $\omega_e x_e = 13.461\ \text{cm}^{-1}$, $\tilde{B}_e = 1.9314\ \text{cm}^{-1}$ and

$\alpha_e = 0.01748\ \text{cm}^{-1}$ so that $J(J + 1) = 1114.75$ and $J = 33$.

$\left(E_{1,0} = 3225\ \text{cm}^{-1}\right.$ with $\frac{k_bT}{hc} \sim 200\ \text{cm}^{-1}$. $\left.\right)$

13.27 The formula for the vibrational energy with one anharmonic term, Eq. (13.31), clearly implies that the vibrational quantum number cannot increase without limit, because the negative quadratic term implies that the energy at some point would *decrease*. It is usually assumed that the maximum quantum number v is the number at which this decrease begins, or, more conveniently, the value of v for which $E_{v+1} - E_v = 0$, and this energy is taken to be the dissociation energy. (a) Derive a formula relating v_{max} to the vibrational constant and anharmonicity. (b) Calculate this quantity for HF. (c) With this value, estimate the bond energy of HF. (Note: this formula is not usually considered to be a reliable way to estimate bond energies.)

$\frac{E_v}{hc} = \left(v + \frac{1}{2}\right)\omega_e - \left(v + \frac{1}{2}\right)^2 \omega_e x_e$. Set

$\dfrac{\partial\left(\frac{E_v}{hc}\right)}{\partial v} = \omega_e - 2\left(v + \frac{1}{2}\right)\omega_e x_e = 0$. $v_{max} = \dfrac{\omega_e}{2\omega_e x_e} - 1$. For HF:

ω_e = 4138.52 cm^{-1} , $\omega_e x_e$ = 90.069 cm^{-1} so that: v_{max} = 22 .

With v = 22: $\frac{E_v}{hc}$ = 47,519.3 cm^{-1} = 5.89 eV .

13.28 A diatomic molecule has a series of absorption bands in the far IR with frequencies 83.03, 104.1, 124.30, 145.03, 165.51, 185.86, 206.38, and 226.50 cm^{-1}. Identify the source of these lines and analyze their frequencies for the appropriate molecular constants.

Using Eq. (13.47) with v = 0 and m = J + 1 ,

$\tilde{\nu} = 2\tilde{B}_0 m - 4\tilde{D}_c m^3$. $\Delta\tilde{\nu} = 2\tilde{B}_0 - 4\tilde{D}_c[(m + 1)^3 - m^3]$. Since $4\tilde{D}_c$ is small compared to $2\tilde{B}_0$, then $\tilde{\nu} \cong 2\tilde{B}_0 m$ and $\Delta\tilde{\nu} \cong 2\tilde{B}_0$. For the first line given, m = 4 , so that:

$\tilde{\nu}$	m	$\frac{\tilde{\nu}}{m}$
83.03	4	20.75
104.1	5	20.82
124.30	6	20.72
145.03	7	20.72
165.51	8	20.69
185.86	9	20.65
206.38	10	20.64
226.50	11	20.59

Since $\frac{\tilde{\nu}}{m} = 2\tilde{B}_0 - 4\tilde{D}_c m^2$, plotting $\frac{\tilde{\nu}}{m}$ vs. m^2 will give us $\tilde{B}_0$ and $\tilde{D}_c$. From linear regression $\tilde{B}_0$ = 10.41 cm^{-1} and

$$\tilde{D}_c = 4.5 \times 10^{-4}\ cm^{-1} .$$

13.29 What are the degeneracies of the following diatomic states? (Neglect spin-orbit coupling.) (a) ${}^1\Sigma^+$ (b) ${}^1\Sigma_u^-$ (c) ${}^2\Pi$ (d) ${}^3\Delta_g$ (e) ${}^3\Sigma_g^-$

a) one

b) one

c) From $\Lambda = \pm 1$, $g = 2$. Also $g_S = 2$, so that

degeneracy = 2 x 2 = 4 .

d) From $\Lambda = \pm 2$, $g = 2$. $g_S = 3$, so degeneracy = 2 x 3 = 6 .

e) three

13.30 What types of MO will result from the following LCAO combinations?

$$p_{zA} + p_{zB};\quad p_{xA} + p_{xB};\quad d_{xzA} + d_{xzB};\quad d_{xyA} + d_{xyB}$$

$p_{zA} + p_{zB}$: 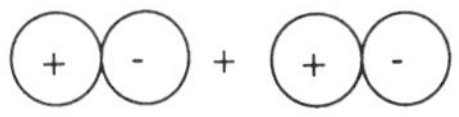 $\rightarrow \sigma^*$

$p_{xA} + p_{xB}$: 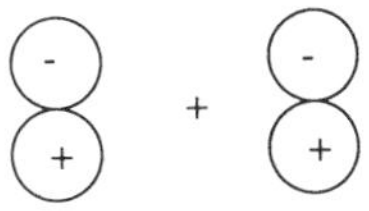 $\rightarrow \pi$

$d_{xzA} + d_{xzB}$: 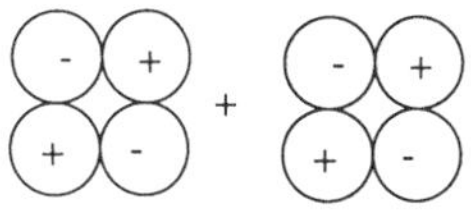 $\rightarrow \pi^*$

(in plane of paper)

$d_{xyA} + d_{xyB}$: 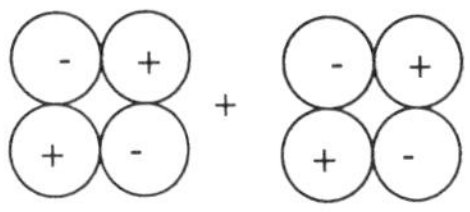 $\rightarrow \delta$

(perpendicular to plane of paper)

13.31 Determine all possible terms that will result from the following configurations:

$(2s\sigma_g)^1(2s\sigma_u^*)^1 \qquad (2p\sigma_g)^2(2p\pi_u)^2$

$(2p\sigma_g)^1(2p\pi_u)^3 \qquad (2p\sigma_g)^2(2p\pi_u)^1(2p\pi_g^*)^1$

$(2s\sigma_g)^1(2s\sigma_u^*)^1$: $(\Lambda = 0;\ S = 0, 1)$. Thus the terms are: $^1\Sigma_u^+$ and $^3\Sigma_u^+$.

$(2p\sigma_g)^1(2p\pi_u)^3$: $(\Lambda = \pm1;\ S = 0, 1)$. Thus the terms are: $^1\Pi_u$ and $^3\Pi_u$.

$(2p\sigma_g)^2(2p\pi_u)^2$: $(\Lambda = 0;\ S = 0, 1)$ or $(\Lambda = \pm2;\ S = 0)$. Thus the terms are: $^1\Sigma_g^+$, $^1\Delta_g$, and $^3\Sigma_g^-$.

$(2p\sigma_g)^2(2p\pi_u)^1(2p\pi_g^*)^1$: $(\Lambda = 0;\ S = 0, 1)$ or $(\Lambda = \pm2;\ S = 0, 1)$. Thus the terms are: $^1\Sigma_u^+$, $^1\Sigma_u^-$, $^3\Sigma_u^+$, $^3\Sigma_u^-$, $^1\Delta_u$, and $^3\Delta_u$.

13.32 Determine the configuration and state symbol and bond order for the ground states of B_2^+, B_2, B_2^-, C_2.

For B_2^+, $(\sigma_g 1s)^2(\sigma_u^* 1s)^2(\sigma_g 2s)^2(\sigma_u^* 2s)^2(\pi_u 2p)^1$. Then the state symbol is $^2\Pi_u$ and bond order $= \frac{1}{2}(5 - 4) = \frac{1}{2}$. For B_2, $(\sigma_g 1s)^2(\sigma_u^* 1s)^2(\sigma_g 2s)^2(\sigma_u^* 2s)^2(\pi_u 2p)^2$. Then we have the state symbol $^3\Sigma_g^-$ and bond order $= \frac{1}{2}(6 - 4) = 1$. For B_2^-,

$(\sigma_g 1s)^2(\sigma_u^* 1s)^2(\sigma_g 2s)^2(\sigma_u^* 2s)^2(\pi_u 2p)^3$. There are two possible configurations: $(\pi_+)^2(\pi_-)^1$ and $(\pi_-)^2(\pi_+)^1$, thus the state symbol is $^2\Pi_u$ and bond order = $\frac{1}{2}(7 - 4) = \frac{3}{2}$. For C_2 , we have $(\sigma_g 1s)^2(\sigma_u^* 1s)^2(\sigma_g 2s)^2(\sigma_u^* 2s)^2(\pi_u 2p)^4$. Since this is a filled shell, the state symbol is $^1\Sigma_g$. Bond order = $\frac{1}{2}(8 - 4) = 2$.

13.33 Use MO theory to explain the trends in bond lengths observed in the O_2 ions below:

	R_e/Å
O_2^+	1.1227
O_2	1.20741
O_2^-	1.26

O_2^+ $(\sigma_g 1s)^2(\sigma_u^* 1s)^2(\sigma_g 2s)^2(\sigma_u^* 2s)^2(\pi_u 2p)^4(\sigma_g 2p)^2(\pi_g^* 2p)^1$

O_2 $(\sigma_g 1s)^2(\sigma_u^* 1s)^2(\sigma_g 2s)^2(\sigma_u^* 2s)^2(\pi_u 2p)^4(\sigma_g 2p)^2(\pi_g^* 2p)^2$

O_2^- $(\sigma_g 1s)^2(\sigma_u^* 1s)^2(\sigma_g 2s)^2(\sigma_u^* 2s)^2(\pi_u 2p)^4(\sigma_g 2p)^2(\pi_g^* 2p)^3$

The bond orders are: O_2^+ b.o. = $\frac{1}{2}(10 - 5) = \frac{5}{2}$, O_2 b.o. = $\frac{1}{2}(10 - 6) = 2$, O_2^- b.o. = $\frac{1}{2}(10 - 7) = \frac{3}{2}$. In this series, the bond order decreases, implying weakening bonding. For weaker bonds, the bond length should be longer as shown by the given data.

13.34 Determine the state symbol and bond order for F_2, F_2^+, and F_2^-. Which molecule should be the most stable?

For F_2, $[N_2](\pi_g^*2p)^4$. Since this is a closed shell, the state symbol is $^1\Sigma_g$. Bond order $= \frac{1}{2}(10 - 8) = 1$. For F_2^+, $[N_2](\pi_g^*2p)^3$. The state symbol is $^2\Pi_g$ and b.o. $= \frac{1}{2}(10 - 7) = \frac{3}{2}$. For F_2^-, $[N_2](\pi_g^*2p)^4(\sigma_u^*2p)^1$. The state symbol is $^2\Sigma_u^+$ with b.o. $= \frac{1}{2}(10 - 9) = \frac{1}{2}$. F_2^+ should be the most stable.

13.35 There is some inconsistency in the literature as to the ground state of C_2, involving the order of the $\pi_u 2p$ and $\sigma_g 2p$ orbitals. According to JANAF tables, the order is:

$$X\,^1\Sigma_g^+,\quad ^3\Pi_u(610\ \text{cm}^{-1}),\quad ^3\Sigma_g^-(6243.5\ \text{cm}^{-1})$$

(Some sources give $^3\Pi_u$ as the ground state). What are the likely configurations for these states?

State	Configuration
$X\,^1\Sigma_g^+$	$(\sigma_g1s)^2(\sigma_u^*1s)^2(\sigma_g2s)^2(\sigma_u^*2s)^2(\pi_u2p)^4$
$^3\Pi_u$	$(\sigma_g1s)^2(\sigma_u^*1s)^2(\sigma_g2s)^2(\sigma_u^*2s)^2(\pi_u2p)^3(\sigma_g2p)^1$
$^3\Sigma_g^-$	$(\sigma_g1s)^2(\sigma_u^*1s)^2(\sigma_g2s)^2(\sigma_u^*2s)^2(\pi_u2p)^2(\sigma_g2p)^2$

13.36 Calculate the relative equilibrium populations of the $X^3\Sigma_g^-$ and the $a^1\Delta_g$ states of O_2 at 1000 K.

From Table 13.6, $X^3\Sigma_g^-$ has $T_e = 0\ cm^{-1}$ and a $^1\Delta_g$ has $T_e = 7918.1\ cm^{-1}$. The relative population is given by

$$\frac{N(a^1\Delta_g)}{N(X^3\Sigma_g^-)} = \frac{g(a^1\Delta_g)}{g(X^3\Sigma_g^-)} \exp\left(-\frac{(T_e(a^1\Delta_g) - T_e(X^3\Sigma_g^-))hc}{k_BT}\right).$$

Using data from Table 13.6,

$$\frac{N(a)}{N(X)} = \frac{2}{3} \exp\left(-\frac{7918.1(2.9979 \times 10^{10})(6.626 \times 10^{-27})}{(1.38 \times 10^{-16})(1000)}\right)$$

$$\frac{N(a)}{N(X)} = 7.4 \times 10^{-6}.$$

13.37 Determine the probable configuration and ground-state symbol of the diatomic molecule BO. What is the bond order?

$(\sigma 1s)^2(\sigma^*1s)^2(\sigma 2s)^2(\sigma^*2s)^2(\pi 2p)^4(\sigma 2p)^1$, $^2\Sigma^+$.

bond order $= \frac{1}{2}(9 - 4) = \frac{5}{2}$.

13.38 (a) Figure 13.19 shows the ground and two excited states for CN. What are the most probable electron configurations for these states?
(b) From the same figure, when NO dissociates into N + O from its ground state, what are the states of the atoms? Are these ground state atoms?

a) For CN:

Ground State $X^2\Sigma^+$: $(\sigma 1s)^2(\sigma^*1s)^2(\sigma 2s)^2(\sigma^*2s)^2(\pi 2p)^4(\sigma 2p)^1$

$A^2\Pi$: $(\sigma 1s)^2(\sigma^*1s)^2(\sigma 2s)^2(\sigma^*2s)^2(\pi 2p)^3(\sigma 2p)^2$

$B^2\Sigma^+$: $(\sigma 1s)^2(\sigma^*1s)^2(\sigma 2s)^2(\sigma^*2s)^2(\pi 2p)^4(\sigma 2p)^1$

b) Ground states of N and O atoms are ^4S and ^3P, respectively.

13.39 The following molecules have the ground states indicated: CH, $^2\Pi$; NH, $^3\Sigma$; OH, $^1\Pi$; HF, $^1\Sigma$. From this, deduce the MO configuration for these molecules.

Species	Term Symbol	S	Λ	Valence Electrons
CH	$^2\Pi$	1/2	±1	5
NH	$^3\Sigma$	1	0	6
OH	$^1\Pi$	0	±1	7
HF	$^1\Sigma$	0	0	8

Ground state MO configurations are:

CH	$(1\sigma)^2(2\sigma)^2(3\sigma)^2(1\pi)^1$
NH	$(1\sigma)^2(2\sigma)^2(3\sigma)^2(1\pi)^2$
OH	$(1\sigma)^2(2\sigma)^2(3\sigma)^2(1\pi)^3$
HF	$(1\sigma)^2(2\sigma)^2(3\sigma)^2(1\pi)^4$

13.40 Some observed states of NH are: $X\,^3\Sigma^-$, $a\,^1\Delta$, $b\,^1\Sigma^+$, $A\,^3\Pi$, $c\,^1\Sigma^+$. List all electric-dipole allowed transitions among these states.

The relevant selection rules are $\Delta\Lambda = 0, \pm 1$ and $\Sigma^+ \not\leftrightarrow \Sigma^-$ and $\Delta S = 0$. The following transitions are then allowed:

$$X^3\Sigma^- \leftrightarrow A^3\Pi \;,\; b^1\Sigma^+ \leftrightarrow c^1\Sigma^+ \;.$$

13.41 Of the three states shown for CN on Figure 13.19, which of the three possible transitions are fully allowed?

State	Λ	S
$X^2\Sigma^+$	0	1
$A^2\Pi$	±1	1
$B^2\Sigma^+$	0	1

Selection rules are: $\Delta\Lambda = 0, \pm 1$, $\Delta S = 0$ and $\Sigma^+ \not\leftrightarrow \Sigma^-$.

Examination of the table above shows that all transitions are allowed.

13.42 A transition between the O_2 states $^3\Sigma_g$ and $^1\Delta_g$ violates three selection rules. Name them. Since "forbidden" in spectroscopy merely means "weak" or "improbable," the violation of multiple selection rules is significant.

State	Λ	S
$^3\Sigma_g$	0	2
$^1\Delta_g$	±2	0

Selection rules which would be violated by this transition in O_2 are:

(1) $\Delta\Lambda = 0, \pm 1$

(2) $\Delta S = 0$

(3) $g \leftrightarrow u$ in homonuclear diatomics

13.43 For CH, the ground state is $^2\Pi$ and the first excited state is $^2\Sigma$. Give the configurations for these states. Is this an allowed transition?

Species	Term	Configuration
CH	$^2\Pi$	$(1\sigma)^2(2\sigma)^2(3\sigma)^2(1\pi)^1$
	$^2\Sigma$	$(1\sigma)^2(2\sigma)^2(3\sigma)^2(4\sigma)^1$

For this transition, $\Delta\Lambda = \pm 1$, $\Delta S = 0$ so that it is allowed.

13.44 What transitions from the ground state of N_2 (Fig. 13.16) are fully allowed? At what wavelength would these transitions begin? What about O_2 (Figure 13.17)? What implications does this have for doing uv spectroscopy in air?

The ground state of N_2 is $^1\Sigma_g^+$. Imposing the selection rules $\Delta\Lambda = \pm 1$, $\Sigma^+ \not\leftrightarrow \Sigma^-$, $\Delta S = 0$, and $g \leftrightarrow u$, allowed transitions are: $^1\Sigma_g^+ \rightarrow {}^1\Sigma_u^+$ and $^1\Sigma_g^+ \rightarrow {}^1\Pi_u$. The ground state of O_2 is $^3\Sigma_g^-$, so that allowed transitions are: $^3\Sigma_g^- \rightarrow {}^3\Sigma_u^-$ and $^3\Sigma_g^- \rightarrow {}^3\Pi_u$. N_2 transitions begin around 10^5 cm^{-1} , O_2 transitions around 4×10^4 cm^{-1} .

13.45 (a) Use data in Table 13.5 to calculate the wavelength of the 0-0 band of the H_2 $X \rightarrow b$ transition. Is this an allowed transition?
(b) From this, calculate the wavelengths of the 1-0 and 2-0 absorption bands. [The first number is the vibrational quantum number (v') for the excited state.]

a) From Eq. (13.75a),

$$T_{00} = \tilde{\nu}_{00} = 91{,}689\ \text{cm}^{-1} + \tfrac{1}{2}(1356.90 - 4395.2)\text{cm}^{-1} - \tfrac{1}{4}(19.932 - 117.9)\text{cm}^{-1}$$

$$T_{00} = 90{,}194.3\ \text{cm}^{-1}\ .$$

$\lambda = \frac{1}{\tilde{\nu}}\left(\frac{10^7\ \text{nm}}{1\ \text{cm}}\right) = 110.87\ \text{nm}$. The transition is allowed since $\Sigma^+ \rightarrow \Sigma^+$, $\Delta S = 0$ and $\Delta\Lambda = 0$.

b) Using Eq. (13.75b) for the 1 - 0 band,

$$\tilde{\nu}_{1\text{-}0} = 90{,}194.3\ \text{cm}^{-1} + (1)(1356.90 - 19.932)\text{cm}^{-1} - (1)^2(19.932\ \text{cm}^{-1})$$

$$\tilde{\nu}_{1\text{-}0} = 91{,}511.3\ \text{cm}^{-1}\ .$$

$\lambda = \frac{1}{\tilde{\nu}}\left(\frac{10^7\ \text{nm}}{1\ \text{cm}}\right) = 109.28\ \text{nm}$. For the 2 - 0 band,

$$\tilde{\nu}_{2\text{-}0} = 90{,}194.3\ \text{cm}^{-1} + (2)(1356.90 - 19.932)\text{cm}^{-1} - (2)^2(19.932\ \text{cm}^{-1})$$

$$\tilde{\nu}_{2\text{-}0} = 92{,}788.21\ \text{cm}^{-1}\ .$$

$$\lambda = \frac{1}{\tilde{\nu}_{2\text{-}0}}\left(\frac{10^7\ \text{nm}}{1\ \text{cm}}\right) = 107.77\ \text{nm}\ .$$

13.46 The uv spectrum shows the following frequencies for the $v'' = 0 \to v'$ bands of PN:

v'	$\tilde{\nu}/\text{cm}^{-1}$
0	39 699.1
1	40 786.8
2	41 858.9
3	42 919.0
4	43 962.0
5	44 991.3

Calculate the vibrational constants ω_e and $\omega_e x_e$ for the excited state.

Dividing Eq. (13.75b) by v' and rearranging,

$$\frac{\tilde{\nu}_{v'-0}}{v'} - \frac{\tilde{\nu}_{00}}{v'} = (\omega_e' - \omega_e' x_e') - v'(\omega_e' x_e') .$$

Thus a plot of $\frac{\Delta\tilde{\nu}}{v'}$ vs. v' has slope = $-\omega_e' x_e'$ and intercept = $(\omega_e' - \omega_e' x_e')$.

Rearranging the data:

v'	$\Delta\tilde{\nu}$	$\frac{\Delta\tilde{\nu}}{v'}$
0	-	-
1	1087.7	1087.7
2	2159.8	1079.9
3	3219.9	1073.3
4	4262.9	1065.7
5	5292.2	1058.4

From linear regression, intercept = 1094.84 with σ = 0.31 and slope = -7.280 with σ = 0.092 . Thus $\omega_e' x_e'$ = 7.28 cm^{-1} and

$$\omega_e' = 1102.12 \text{ cm}^{-1} .$$

13.47 Use the wavelengths of the C_2 Swan bands (Figure 13.20) to calculate the vibrational constants of this molecule.

From Figure 13.20,

v' - v"	λ	$\tilde{\nu}_{v'-v''}$
0 - 2	6191 Å	16152 cm^{-1}
0 - 1	5636 Å	17743 cm^{-1}
0 - 0	5165 Å	19361 cm^{-1}
1 - 0	4737 Å	21110 cm^{-1}
2 - 0	4383 Å	22815 cm^{-1}

Eq. (13.75b) gives us $\dfrac{\tilde{\nu}_{v'-0} - \tilde{\nu}_{00}}{v'} = (\omega_e' - \omega_e'x_e') - v'(\omega_e'x_e')$.

Rearranging the data:

v' - v"	$\dfrac{\tilde{\nu}_{0-v''} - \tilde{\nu}_{00}}{v''}$	$\dfrac{\tilde{\nu}_{v'-0} - \tilde{\nu}_{00}}{v'}$
0 - 2	-1604.5	
0 - 1	-1618.0	
1 - 0		1749.0
2 - 0		1727.0

Using the first two points above, we find that for the ground state, $\omega_e'x_e' = 13.5\ cm^{-1}$ and $\omega_e' = 1645.0\ cm^{-1}$. Similarly, for the next two points (excited states), $\omega_e'x_e' = 22.0\ cm^{-1}$ and $\omega_e' = 1793.0\ cm^{-1}$.

13.48 The absorption frequencies for the Schumann-Runge bands of O_2 include (near the dissociation limit):

v	$\tilde{\nu}/\mathrm{cm}^{-1}$	v	$\tilde{\nu}/\mathrm{cm}^{-1}$
16	56 719.50	19	57 030.18
17	56 852.41	20	57 082.83
18	56 954.54	21	57 114.77

(a) Plot the differences $\delta = \tilde{\nu}_{i+1} - \tilde{\nu}_i$ vs. $\tilde{\nu}$ and determine the dissociation energy by extrapolating to $\delta \to 0$.
(b) From this and the atomic oxygen energies, $O(^1D) - O(^3P) = 15{,}867.862\ \mathrm{cm}^{-1}$, calculate D_0 for ground-state O_2.

a) A plot of $\tilde{\nu}$ vs. δ is shown below:

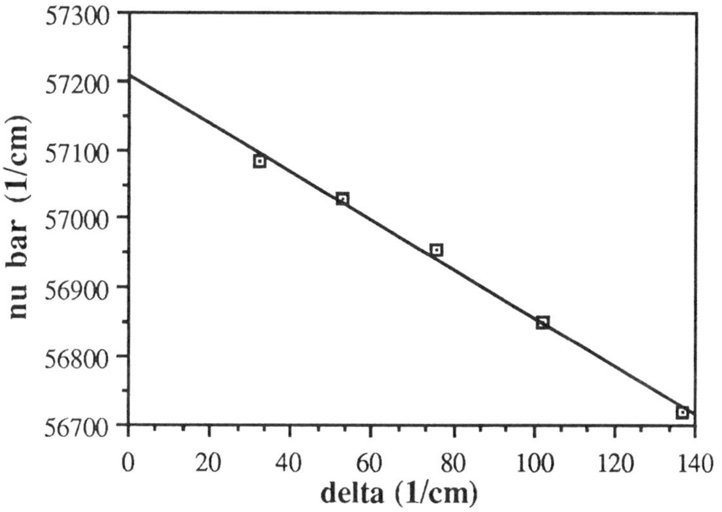

From the graph, intercept = 57,214 cm^{-1} .

b) The dissociation energy minus the atomic oxygen energies gives us D_0. Then $D_0 = 57{,}214 - 15{,}868 = 41{,}346\ \mathrm{cm}^{-1} = 5.13\ \mathrm{eV}$.

13.49 Calculate the percent ionic character of LiF from its dipole moment (Table 13.6).

From Eq. (13.82),

$$\%\ \text{ionic character} = \frac{100(\mu_0)}{eR_e}$$

$$\%\ \text{ionic character} = \frac{100(6.32 \times 10^{-18}\ \text{esu-cm})}{(4.803 \times 10^{-10}\ \text{esu})(1.5639 \times 10^{-8}\ \text{cm})}$$

$$\%\ \text{ionic character} = 84.14\%\ .$$

13.50 Calculate the energy of the gas-phase ionization at $R = \infty$:

$$Na + Cl \longrightarrow Na^+ + Cl^-$$

from the data in Table 13.8.

Since the ionization reaction is

$$Na \rightarrow Na^+ + e^- \qquad IP = 5.138\ \text{eV}$$
$$Cl + e^- \rightarrow Cl^- \qquad EA = 3.613\ \text{eV}$$

then the ionization energy is

$$IP - EA = 5.138 - 3.613 = 1.525\ \text{eV}\ .$$

13.51 Use the potential function of Eq. (13.77) and data for NaCl to calculate the constants (A, B) and bond energy of this diatomic molecule.

The derivative of Eq. (13.77) with respect to R will be zero when $R = R_e$. Then $\frac{\partial E_e(R)}{\partial R} = -\frac{AB}{R_e} e^{-BR/R_e} + \frac{300e}{R^2} = 0$ or

$\frac{300e}{R_e} = ABe^{-B} = \frac{300(4.803 \times 10^{-10})}{(2.3609 \times 10^{-8})} = 6.1032\ \text{eV}$. The second derivative of Eq. (13.77) is

$$k' = \frac{300k}{e} = \frac{300}{e}[\mu(2\pi c\omega_e)^2]$$

$$k' = \frac{300}{4.803 \times 10^{-10}}\left[\frac{35 \times 23}{58(6.022 \times 10^{23})}((2\pi c)^2(364.6)^2)\right]$$

$$k' = 6.790 \times 10^{16} \text{ eV cm}^{-2} .$$

Since $\frac{\partial^2 E}{\partial R^2} = \frac{AB^2}{R_e^{\,2}} e^{-BR/R_e} - \frac{2(300e)}{R^3} = 0$ or $k' = \frac{AB^2}{R_e^{\,2}} e^{-B} - \frac{600e}{R_e^{\,3}}$ and

$ABe^{-B} = 6.1032$ eV , then we have

$$6.790 \times 10^{16} \text{ eV cm}^{-2} = \frac{B(6.1032 \text{ eV})}{(2.3609 \times 10^{-8} \text{ cm})}{}^{2} - \frac{(6.1032 \text{ eV})2}{(2.3609 \times 10^{-8} \text{ cm})^2}$$

or $B = 8.20$. Then $A = \frac{6.1032 \text{ eV}}{Be^{-B}} = 2710$ eV . From Eq. (13.77)

at $R = R_e$,

$$E_e(R_e) = -D_e = (2710)e^{-8.2} - 6.1032 + 1.525 = -3.83 \text{ eV} .$$

13.52 The potential energy between two ions such as $K^+ + Cl^-$ is:

$$V = F(R) - 300e/R + \Delta E_\infty ,$$

where $F(R)$ is the repulsive potential and $\Delta E_\infty = \text{IP} - \text{EA}$ is the ionization energy at $R = \infty$.
(a) Prove that if $F(R) = a/R^{12}$, then $a = 300eR_e^{11}/12$ and $D_e = 11(300e)/12R_e - \Delta E_\infty$ (units: eV).
(b) Use $\Delta E_\infty = 0.726$ eV and $R_e = 2.67 \times 10^{-8}$ cm to estimate D_e for KCl using this model.

a) $V = \frac{a}{R^{12}} - \frac{300e}{R} + \Delta E_\infty$ where V and ΔE_∞ are now in units of eV's. $\frac{\partial V}{\partial R} = -\frac{12a}{R^{13}} + \frac{300e}{R^2}$. At $R = R_e$, $\frac{\partial V}{\partial r} = 0$ and $a = \frac{300eR_e^{\,11}}{12}$,

so that $V = -\frac{300e}{R}\left(1 - \frac{R_e^{\,11}}{12R^{11}}\right) + \Delta E_\infty$.

$$V(R_e) = -D_e = -300\left(\frac{11}{12}\right)\left(\frac{e}{R_e}\right) + \Delta E_\infty .$$

b) With $\Delta E_\infty = 0.726$ eV , $e = 4.803 \times 10^{-10}$ esu and $R_e = 2.67 \times 10^{-8}$ cm we find $D_e = 4.22$ eV .

13.53 If a microwave $J = 2 \rightarrow 3$ transition is observed in an electric field, how many lines will appear? Assume the electric field is perpendicular to the electric vector of the microwaves.

In an electric field, J = 2 splits into 3 lines and J = 3 splits into 4 lines. Since the selection rule is $\Delta m = 1$,

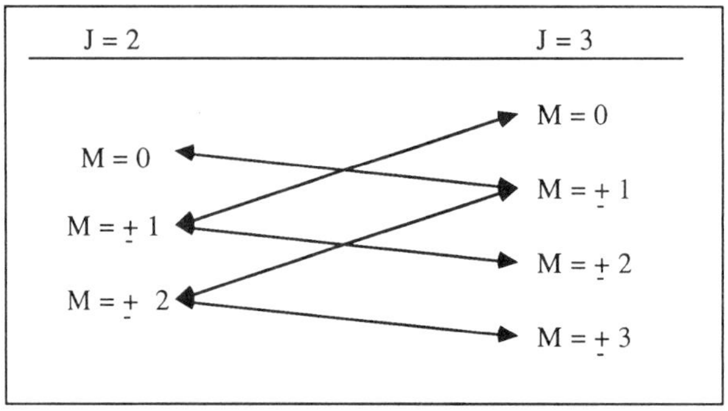

five transitions are allowed.

13.54 Calculate the Stark splitting (in Hz) of the $J = 1$ state of KCl in an electric field of 3000 volts/cm. (The cgs unit of voltage is 1 esu = 300 volts, so, in cgs units, $\mathscr{E} = 10$.)

For KCl,

$$I = \mu R_e^2 = \frac{39.10(35.45\ g)}{74.55(6.022 \times 10^{23})} (2.6668 \times 10^{-8}\ cm)^2$$

$$I = 2.212 \times 10^{-38}\ erg\ s^{-2} .$$

Using Eq. (13.86),

$$E_{Stark} = -\frac{(2.212 \times 10^{-38}\ erg\ s^{-2})(10.48 \times 10^{-18}\ esu\ cm^{-1})^2}{\left(\frac{6.626 \times 10^{-27}\ erg\ s}{2\pi}\right)} \times$$

$$(10\ esu\ cm^{-1})^2 \left[\frac{2 - 3M^2}{10}\right]$$

$$E_{Stark} = -2.185 \times 10^{-16}\ erg \left[\frac{2 - 3M^2}{10}\right]$$

The splitting of M = 0 → M = 1 is then $\Delta E = 6.555 \times 10^{-17}$ erg .

Converting to Hz (s^{-1}), $\frac{\Delta E}{h} = \frac{6.555 \times 10^{-17} \text{ erg}}{6.626 \times 10^{-27} \text{ erg s}} = 9.89$ GHz .

13.55 If a linear rotating molecule interacts with radiation polarized with its electric vector along the z axis, the transition dipole is:

$$I = \iint \psi_{JM} \mu_z \psi^*_{J'M'} \, d\Omega$$

where z is a direction in space, not the molecular axis.
(a) Prove $I = 0$ unless $M = M'$.
(b) Do the integral for $\psi_{0,0} = 1/\sqrt{4\pi}$, $\psi_{1,0} = \sqrt{3/4\pi} \cos\theta$.

a) The integral may be written

$$I = \int_0^{2\pi} e^{i(M-M')\Phi} d\Phi \int_0^{\pi} P_J^{M} P_{J'}^{M'} \mu_0 \cos\theta \sin\theta \, d\theta \;.$$ The Φ integral is

$$I = \left. \frac{e^{i(M-M')\Phi}}{i(M - M')} \right|_0^{2\pi} = \frac{e^{i2\pi(M-M')} - 1}{i(M - M')}$$ which is zero unless M = M'

(using l'Hôpital's rule).

b) $$I = \iint \frac{1}{(4\pi)^{1/2}} \mu_z \sqrt{\frac{3}{4\pi}} \cos\theta \, d\Omega = \int_0^{2\pi}\int_0^{\pi} \frac{\sqrt{3}}{4\pi} \mu_0 \cos^2\theta \sin\theta \, d\theta \, d\Phi$$

$$I = \frac{\sqrt{3}\mu_0}{4\pi} \int_0^{2\pi} d\Phi \int_0^{\pi} \cos^2\theta \sin\theta \, d\theta = \frac{\sqrt{3}\mu_0 (2\pi)}{4\pi} \left[- \frac{\cos^3\theta}{3} \right]_0^{\pi} = \frac{\mu_0}{\sqrt{3}} \;.$$

13.56 The molar polarization:

$$P = \frac{\varepsilon - 1}{\varepsilon + 2}\frac{M}{\rho}$$

has been measured for $CHCl_3$ (below). Use these data to calculate the polarizability (α) and dipole moment (μ_0) of this molecule. (These values are for solutions in hexane.)

T/K	P/cm^3	T/K	P/cm^3
193	62.1	273	51.1
213	58.9	293	49.7
233	56.0	313	48.3
253	53.1	323	47.5

From Eq. (13.84), $P = \frac{4\pi L}{3}\left(\alpha + \frac{\mu_0^{\,2}}{3k_BT}\right)$. Thus a plot of P vs. $\frac{1}{T}$ has slope $= \frac{4\pi L}{3}\left(\frac{\mu_0^{\,3}}{3k_B}\right)$ and intercept $= \frac{4\pi L}{3}\alpha$. Regressing the data, we find slope = 7060.6 cm^3 K and intercept = 25.547 cm^3.

Then $\alpha = \frac{3(25.547\ \text{cm}^3)}{4\pi(6.022 \times 10^{23})} = 1.013 \times 10^{-23}\ \text{cm}^3$ and

$$\mu_0 = \left(\frac{9(1.38 \times 10^{-16}\ \text{erg K}^{-1})(7060.6\ \text{cm}^3\ \text{K})}{4\pi(6.022 \times 10^{23})}\right)^{1/2}$$

$$\mu_0 = 1.08 \times 10^{-18}\ \text{esu} = 1.08\ \text{D} .$$

13.57 In Figure 13.25, what is the "meaning of" (what words describe) the numbers 4.48, 13.60, 2.65 (all eV)?

4.48 eV is the bond energy of H_2. 13.60 eV is the ionization potential of H_2. 2.65 eV is the bond energy of H_2^+.

14
Polyatomic Molecules

14.1 Give the point-group symmetries of:

$H{-}C{\equiv}C{-}H$, $H{-}C{\equiv}C{-}Cl$, $H{-}C{\equiv}N$, CCl_4

$H - C \equiv C - H$, $D_{\infty h}$ $\qquad$ $H - C \equiv C - Cl$, $C_{\infty v}$

$H - C \equiv N$, $C_{\infty v}$ $\qquad$ CCl_4 , T_d

14.2 What are the point groups of CH_4, CH_3Cl, CH_2Cl_2, CCl_3H, PCl_3 (pyramidal), BF_3 (planar), CH_2FCl?

CH_4 , T_d $\qquad$ CH_3Cl , C_{3v}

CH_2Cl_2 , C_{2v} $\qquad$ CCl_3H , C_{3v}

PCl_3 , C_{3v} $\qquad$ BF_3 , D_{3h}

CH_2FCl , C_s

14.3 Give the point groups of (a) the isomers of dichloroethylene:

cis 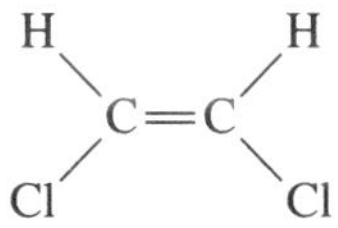 *trans* 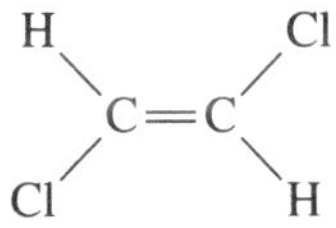 (1, 1) 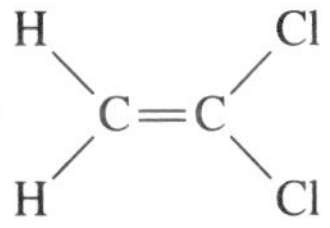

and (b) the isomers of dichlorobenzene:

ortho-

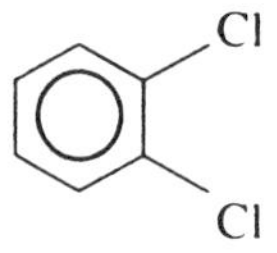

meta-

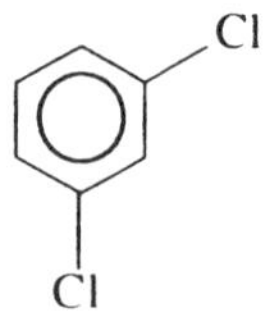

para-

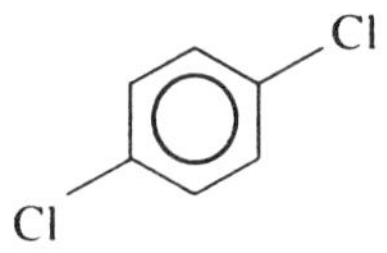

and (c) the pyridines:

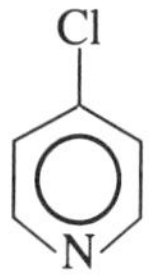

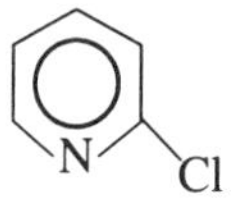

a) *cis* 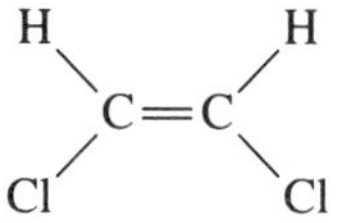 , C_{2v} *trans* 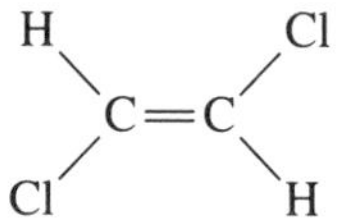 , C_{2h}

(1, 1) 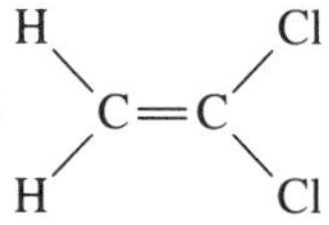 , C_{2v}

b) *ortho-*

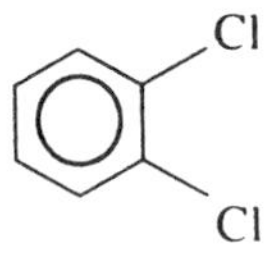 , C_{2v}

meta-

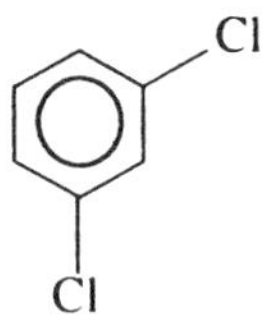 , C_{2v}

para-

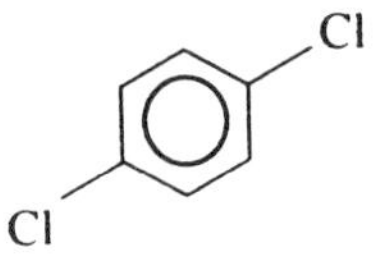 , D_{2h}

c)  , C_{2v} 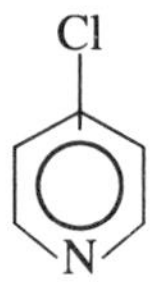 , C_{2v}

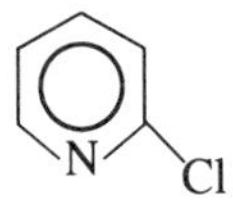 , C_s

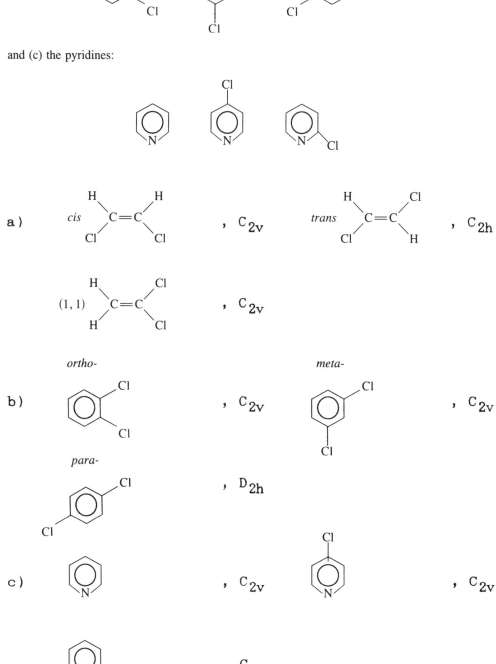

14.4 What is the point group of (a) diborane:

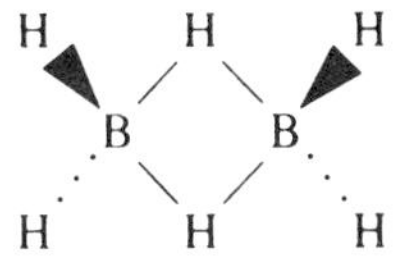

(b) diborane substituted in a terminal position,
(c) diborane substituted in a bridge position,
(d) diborane substituted in both bridge positions? [In parts (b), (c), and (d) assume that the substituent has the symmetry of a point.]

a) D_{2h} b) C_s c) C_{2v}

d) Assuming the two substituents are the same, D_{2h} .

14.5 Sulfur often will occur as cyclic S_8 molecules. The structure is that of a puckered octagon:

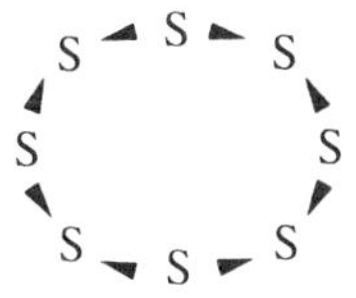

(alternate atoms up and down). What is the point group?

The S_8 molecule may be depicted as having alternating "up" and "down" sites. Symmetry elements are: a C_4 principal axis; 4 C_2 perpendicular to C_4; no σ_h; 4 σ_d and S_8 parallel to C_4. The molecule thus has D_{4d} symmetry.

14.6 The dihedral angle in hydrogen peroxide:

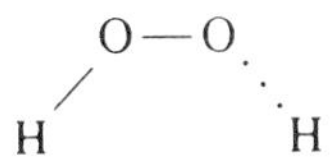

is defined as the angle between the HO bonds, looking down the OO axis:

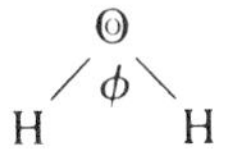

What is the point group if $\phi = 0$, $\phi = 180°$, or $\phi =$ any other angle?

$\Phi = 0°$, C_{2v} $\Phi = 180°$, C_{2h} $\Phi =$ any other, C_2

14.7 What is the point group of ethane (CH_3—CH_3) in the (a) eclipsed, (b) staggered conformation? What is the point group of 1,2-dichloroethane in the (c) *gauche:*

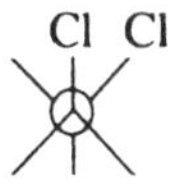

or (d) *trans:*

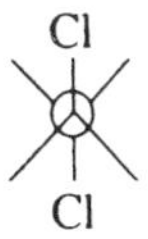

conformation?

a) D_{3h} b) D_{3d} c) C_2 d) C_{2h}

14.8 Draw the structures for all isomers of trichloroethane ($C_2H_3Cl_3$) and give the point group for each. Include all distinct rotamers, but only those that are perfectly staggered (that is, the CX bond from one carbon exactly bisects the CX bonds from the other carbon, for X equal Cl or H).

Cl_3C - CH_3 :

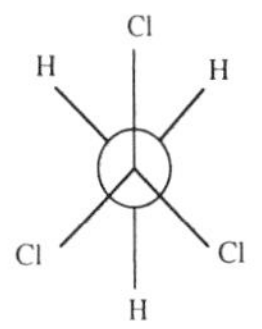

C_3 axis with $3\sigma_v$ → C_{3v} .

Cl_2HC - CH_2Cl :

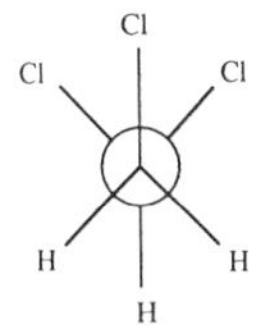

Contains a single mirror plane σ → C_s .

or

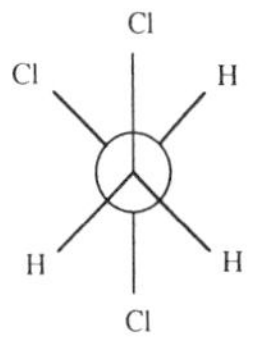

No symmetry elements → C_1 .

14.9 In hexamethylbenzene, the most stable structure is probably one in which one of the methyl CH bonds point straight up on alternating carbons and straight down on the intervening carbons — see the extended side view of this structure below. What would be the point group of hexamethylbenzene in this structure?

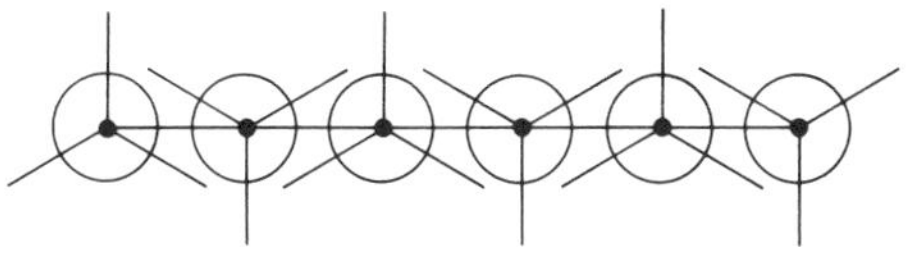

The structure may be represented as: 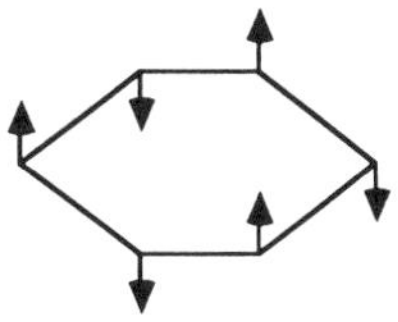

Symmetry elements are: a C_3 axis; 3 C_2 perpendicular; 3 σ_d and S_6 parallel to C_3. Thus the point group is D_{3d}.

14.10 What is the point group of boric acid:

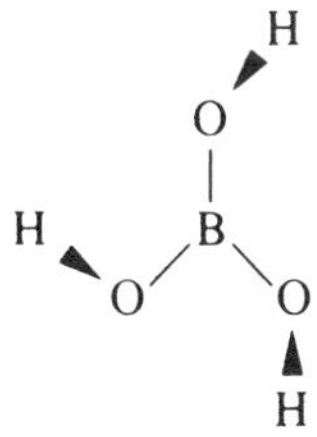

if (a) the H's lie in the BO_3 plane, (b) the H's are above the plane in a propeller fashion?

a) C_{3h}

b) C_3

14.11 (a) What are the point groups of a regular hexagon with arrows pointing up or down as follows:

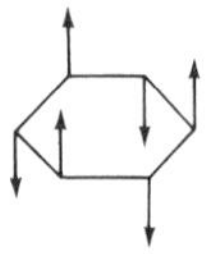

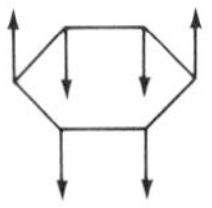

(b) Use a molecular model kit to build a model of cyclohexane (C_6H_{12}) in the "chair" and "boat" conformations. What are the point groups for these conformations?

a) 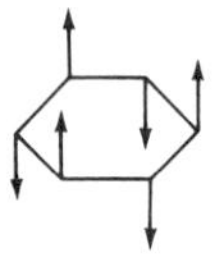

D_{3d} . (See problem 14.9.)

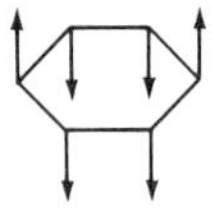

C_2 axis, $2\sigma_v \rightarrow C_{2v}$.

b) The structures in part a) represent cyclohexane chair and boat forms, D_{3d} and C_{2v} , respectively.

14.12 In D_{2h} symmetry, what are the products $B_{2g} \otimes B_{3g}$, $B_{1u} \otimes B_{1g}$, $A_u \otimes B_{2u}$?

From the D_{2h} character table,

B_{2g}	1	-1	1	-1	1	-1	1	-1
B_{3g}	1	-1	-1	1	1	-1	-1	1
	1	1	-1	-1	1	1	-1	-1

This product may be identified as B_{1g} from the character table.

For $B_{1u} \otimes B_{1g}$,

B_{1u}	1	1	-1	-1	-1	-1	1	1
B_{1g}	1	1	-1	-1	1	1	-1	-1
	1	1	1	1	-1	-1	-1	-1

The product is A_u . For $A_u \otimes B_{2u}$,

A_u	1	1	1	1	-1	-1	-1	-1
B_{2u}	1	-1	1	-1	-1	1	-1	1
	1	-1	1	-1	1	-1	1	-1

The product is B_{2g} .

14.13 Find the following direct products:
(a) $A_2 \otimes E$ in C_{3v}.
(b) $A_1'' \otimes A_2''$ in D_{3h}.
(c) $A_2 \otimes T_1$ in T_d.

a)

A_2	1	1	-1
E	2	-1	0
	2	-1	0

The direct product is E.

b)

A_1''	1	1	1	-1	-1	-1
A_2''	1	1	-1	-1	-1	1
	1	1	-1	1	1	-1

The direct product is A_2' .

c)

A_2	1	1	1	-1	-1
T_1	3	0	-1	1	-1
	3	0	-1	-1	1

The direct product is T_2 .

14.14 Find the result of operating with all of the symmetry operations of C_{2h} on the following functions, and classify them (if possible) according to the representations of that group:

$$x, y, z, xy, xz, yz, x^2 - y^2, xe^{-x}, xe^{-x^2}, r^2, xyz$$

The symmetry operations of C_{2h} are $\hat{C}_2$, $\hat{i}$, and $\hat{\sigma}_h$, and have the following effect on the coordinates (x, y, z):

$$\hat{i}\begin{pmatrix} x \\ y \\ z \end{pmatrix} = \begin{pmatrix} -x \\ -y \\ -z \end{pmatrix}, \quad \hat{C}_2\begin{pmatrix} x \\ y \\ z \end{pmatrix} = \begin{pmatrix} -x \\ -y \\ z \end{pmatrix}, \quad \hat{\sigma}_h\begin{pmatrix} x \\ y \\ z \end{pmatrix} = \begin{pmatrix} x \\ y \\ -z \end{pmatrix}$$

Draw up the following table, based upon Table 14.1:

Function	Symmetry			Representation
	$C_2(z)$	i	σ_h	
x	-1	-1	1	B_u
y	-1	-1	1	B_u
z	1	-1	-1	A_u
xy		$B_u \otimes B_u$		A_g
xz		$B_u \otimes A_u$		B_g
yz		$B_u \otimes A_u$		B_g
$x^2 - y^2$				A_g
xe^{-x}		No Symmetry		
xe^{-x^2}	-1	-1	1	B_u
r^2				A_g
xyz		$B_u \otimes B_u \otimes A_u$		A_u

14.15 The permanent dipole moment of a molecule is calculated with the average value theorem as:

$$\langle \boldsymbol{\mu} \rangle = \int \psi^* \boldsymbol{\mu} \psi \, d\tau$$

What are the symmetry requirements for these integrals to be nonzero? For which of the following groups can one or more of these integrals be nonzero?

$$C_s, C_i, C_{nv}, C_{nh}, D_{nd}, D_{nh}, T_d, O_h$$

The symmetry requirement is that $\psi^*\psi$ be symmetrical, that is:

$\Gamma_\psi \otimes \begin{pmatrix} x \\ y \\ z \end{pmatrix} \otimes \Gamma_{\psi^*} = \Gamma_s$ in at least one dimension. Point groups for which x, y or z are in Γ_s are: C_s and C_{nv} .

14.16 Optical activity is possible for molecules belonging to which of the following groups?

$$C_s, C_i, C_{nv}, C_{nh}, D_{nd}, D_{nh}, T_d, O_h$$

A molecule which exhibits optical activity will not be superimposable on its mirror image. The symmetry requirement is that the molecule have no improper axis of rotation (S_n). Recalling that the $\hat{S}_1 = \hat{\sigma}$ and $\hat{S}_2 = \hat{i}$, we draw up the following table:

Point Group	Symmetry Elements
C_s	$\hat{\sigma}$
C_i	$\hat{i}$
C_{nv}	$\hat{C}_n$, $n\hat{\sigma}_v$
C_{nh}	$\hat{C}_n$, $n\hat{\sigma}_h$
D_{nd}	$\hat{C}_n$, $n\hat{C}_2$, $n\hat{\sigma}_d$
D_{nh}	$\hat{C}_n$, $n\hat{C}_2$, $\hat{\sigma}_h$
T_d	
O_h	

None of the groups may be optically active.

14.17 Enthalpies of formation as used in Chapter 6 refer to carbon (graphite) as the standard state, whereas the bond energies of Table 14.4 refer to C(gas). The heat of vaporization of graphite is needed; at 298 K this is:

$$C(\text{graphite}) \longrightarrow C(\text{gas}), \qquad \Delta H = 717 \text{ kJ}$$

Use this together with the average bond energies of Table 14.4 to estimate the ΔH of formation of the following molecules (compare Table 6.1): (a) CH_3OH, (b) $COCl_2$, (c) C_2H_4.

a) From Table 14.4,

bonds made:	3 C - H	3(415 kJ)
	1 C - O	350 kJ
	1 O - H	464 kJ
		2059 kJ

The formation reaction is

$$C(gr) + 2\ H_2 + \frac{1}{2}\ O_2 = CH_3OH$$

bonds broken:	C(gr) → C(g)	717 kJ
	2 H - H	2(435 kJ)
	1/2 O = O	(1/2)(492 kJ)
		1833 kJ

Then ΔH = 1833 kJ - 2059 kJ = -226 kJ mol^{-1}. (Table 6.1: ΔH = -201 kJ mol^{-1}.)

b) From Table 14.4,

bonds made:	2 C - Cl	3(326 kJ)
	1 C = O	724 kJ
		1376 kJ

The formation reaction is

$$C(gr) + Cl_2 + \frac{1}{2}\ O_2 = COCl_2$$

bonds broken:	C(gr) → C(g)	717 kJ
	1 Cl - Cl	239 kJ
	1/2 O = O	(1/2)(492 kJ)
		1202 kJ

Then ΔH = 1202 kJ - 1376 kJ = -174 kJ mol^{-1} . (Table 6.1: ΔH = -219 kJ mol^{-1}.)

c) From Table 14.4,

bonds made:	1 C = C	615 kJ
	4 C - H	4(415 kJ)
		2275 kJ

The formation reaction is

$$2\ C(gr) + 2\ H_2 = C_2H_4$$

bonds broken:	2 C(gr) → 2 C(g)	2(717 kJ)
	2 H - H	2(435 kJ)
		2304 kJ

Then ΔH = 2304 kJ - 2275 kJ = 29 kJ mol^{-1} . (Table 6.1: ΔH = 52.26 kJ mol^{-1}.)

14.18 (a) Show that the sp^2 hybrids:

$$\chi_1 = \frac{\sqrt{5}\,(s) + 2(p_x) + 3(p_y)}{\sqrt{18}}$$

$$\chi_2 = \frac{\sqrt{5}\,(s) + 2(p_x) - 3(p_y)}{\sqrt{18}}$$

are normalized and orthogonal to each other. (b) What is the angle between the maxima of these hybrids? [*Hint:* The orbitals p_x and p_y have the properties of unit vectors along the x and y axes, respectively.] (c) There is, of course, a third orbital (χ_3), which must be normalized and orthogonal to these two. Derive the form and direction of this orbital.

a) $\int \chi_1\chi_1\,d\tau = \int \frac{1}{18}[\sqrt{5}(s) + 2(p_x) + 3(p_y)]^2 d\tau$

$$\int \chi_1\chi_1\,d\tau = \frac{1}{18}\int [5(s)^2 + 4(p_x)^2 + 9(p_y)^2 + 4\sqrt{5}(s)(p_x) + 6\sqrt{5}(s)(p_y) + 12(p_x)(p_y)]d\tau$$

Since (s), (p_x), and (p_y) are orthonormal,

$\int \chi_1\chi_1\, d\tau = \frac{1}{18}[5 + 4 + 9] = 1$. Also,

$$\int \chi_2\chi_2\, d\tau = \int \frac{1}{18}[\sqrt{5}(s) + 2(p_x) - 3(p_y)]^2 d\tau$$

$$\int \chi_2\chi_2\, d\tau = \frac{1}{18}\int [5(s)^2 + 4(p_x)^2 + 9(p_y)^2] d\tau = 1 .$$

$$\int \chi_1\chi_2\, d\tau = \frac{1}{18}\int [5(s)^2 + 4(p_x)^2 - 9(p_y)^2] d\tau = \frac{1}{18}(5 + 4 - 9) = 0 .$$

b) χ_1 has the form $\sqrt{5} + 2\sqrt{\frac{3}{2}} \sin\theta \cos\Phi + 3\sqrt{\frac{3}{2}} \sin\theta \sin\Phi$.

χ_2 has the form $\sqrt{5} + 2\sqrt{\frac{3}{2}} \sin\theta \cos\Phi - 3\sqrt{\frac{3}{2}} \sin\theta \sin\Phi$. Since p_x and p_y have maxima in the xy plane, we take $\theta = 90^\circ$. Then $\frac{\partial\chi_1}{\partial\Phi} = 0 = -2\sqrt{\frac{3}{2}} \sin\Phi + 3\sqrt{\frac{3}{2}} \cos\Phi$ or $\Phi = 56.3^\circ$. For χ_2 , $\Phi = 56.3^\circ$ also. The angle between the maxima is then

$$56.3^\circ + 56.3^\circ = 112.6^\circ .$$

c) The normalization constants of χ_1 and χ_2 are:

	(s)	(p_x)	(p_y)
χ_1	$\sqrt{\frac{5}{18}}$	$\sqrt{\frac{4}{18}}$	$\sqrt{\frac{9}{18}}$
χ_2	$\sqrt{\frac{5}{18}}$	$\sqrt{\frac{4}{18}}$	$-\sqrt{\frac{9}{18}}$

For χ_3 to be normalized and orthonormal we choose

χ_3	$\sqrt{\frac{8}{18}}$	$-\sqrt{\frac{10}{18}}$	0

Then $\chi_3 = \frac{1}{\sqrt{18}}(\sqrt{8}(s) - \sqrt{10}(p_x)) = \frac{1}{3}(2(s) - \sqrt{5}(p_x))$.

14.19 Consider a hypothetical H_2X_2 molecule with structure:

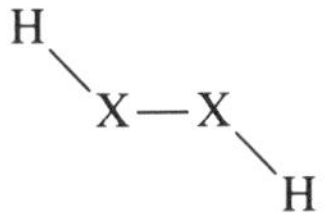

(z axis perpendicular to paper)

What are the proper symmetry designations of the following SALC's?

$$\chi_1 = (H_A 1s) + (H_B 1s), \qquad \chi_2 = (H_A 1s) - (H_B 1s)$$
$$\chi_3 = (X_A p_z) + (X_B p_z), \qquad \chi_4 = (X_A p_z) - (X_B p_z)$$

We find the symmetry designations of the orbitals by finding their representations.

		$\hat{E}$	$\hat{C}_2$	$\hat{i}$	$\hat{\sigma}_h$
$\chi_1 = (H_A 1s) + (H_B 1s)$	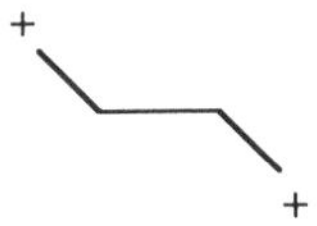	1	1	1	1
$\chi_2 = (H_A 1s) - (H_B 1s)$	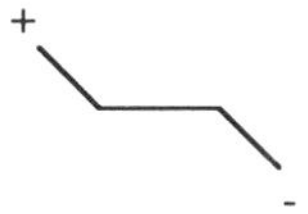	1	-1	-1	1
$\chi_3 = (X_A p_z) + (X_B p_z)$	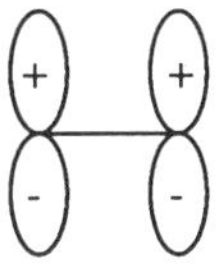	1	1	-1	-1
$\chi_4 = (X_A p_z) - (X_B p_z)$	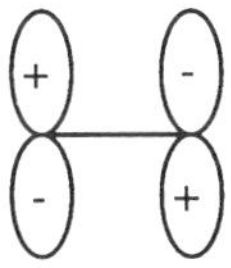	1	-1	1	-1

Then, χ_1: a_g; χ_2: b_u; χ_3: a_u; χ_4: b_g.

14.20 For the hydrogen 1*s* orbitals of ethylene, give all appropriate SALC's and their symmetry designations. (The *z* axis is the C=C bond, and the molecular plane is *yz*.)

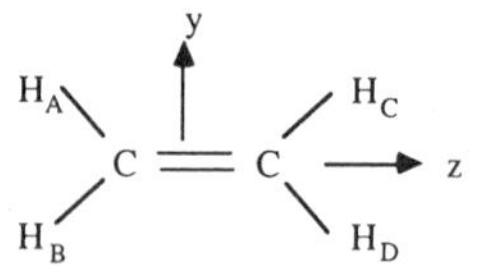

x axis perpendicular to plane of paper

Ethylene has D_{2h} symmetry.

Draw up the following table:

SALC				$\hat{C}_2(z)$	$\hat{C}_2(y)$	$\hat{C}_2(x)$	$\hat{i}$	Sym.
$(H_A 1s)$ +	$(H_B 1s)$ +	$(H_C 1s)$ +	$(H_D 1s)$	1	1	1	1	a_g
+	+	−	−	1	−1	−1	−1	b_{1u}
+	−	−	+	−1	−1	1	1	b_{3g}
+	−	+	−	−1	1	−1	−1	b_{2u}

Pictorial represesentations are:

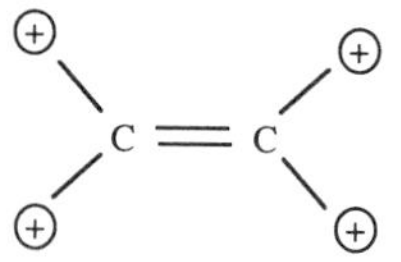

a_g

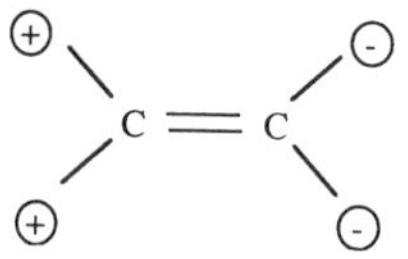

b_{1u}

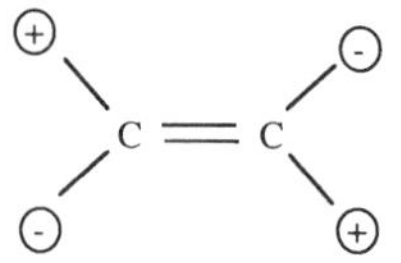

b_{3g}

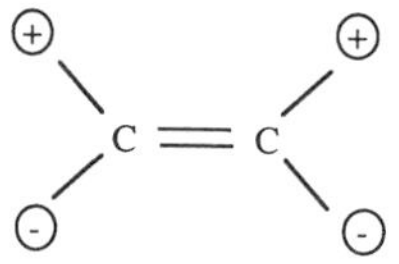

b_{2u}

14.21 The electronic spectrum of a conjugated molecule such as butadiene is largely due to the pi electrons; it can be explained by considering only the p_z orbitals of the carbons, ignoring the σ electrons and the protons. Consider the carbon framework in a *trans* planar configuration (C_{2h}). The p_z orbitals (perpendicular to the plane) will give the following linear combinations:

$$\Phi_1 = p_{z1} + p_{z2} + p_{z3} + p_{z4}$$

$$\Phi_2 = p_{z1} + p_{z2} - p_{z3} - p_{z4}$$

$$\Phi_3 = p_{z1} - p_{z2} - p_{z3} + p_{z4}$$

$$\Phi_4 = p_{z1} - p_{z2} + p_{z3} - p_{z4}$$

Give the symmetry designation for each of these MO's. Give the configuration for the ground and the first 4 excited states. Which are electric dipole-allowed transitions?

Draw up the following table:

	Symmetry	Nodes	Designation
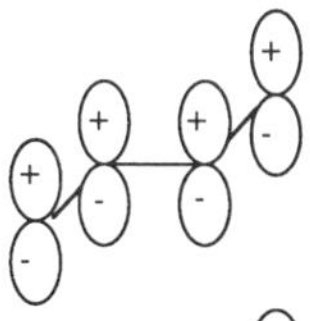	a_u	0	$1a_u$
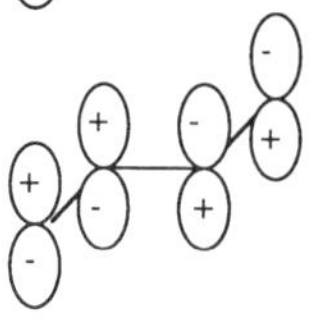	b_g	1	$1b_g$
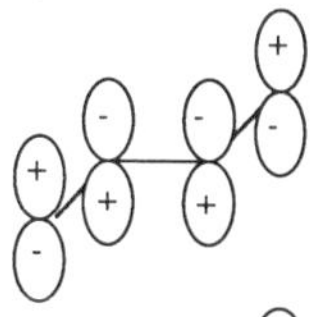	a_u	2	$2a_u$
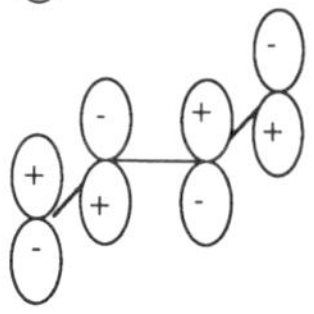	b_g	3	$2b_g$

E↑

	$(1a_u)$	$(1b_g)$	$(2a_u)$	$(2b_g)$	State
4	↑↓	↑		↓	^1A_g
3	↑↓	↑		↑	^3A_g
2	↑↓	↑	↓		^1B_u
1	↑↓	↑	↑		^3B_u
ground	↑↓	↑↓			^1A_g

Selection rules require $\Delta S = 0$ and $g \leftrightarrow u$, so that the only allowed transition is $^1A_g \rightarrow {}^1B_u$.

14.22 The symmetry orbitals for XH_3 with C_{3v} symmetry are (in order of energy):

$$(1a_1)(2a_1)(1e)(3a_1)(4a_1)(2e)$$

[Note that $(1a_1) \equiv (X1s)$, a nonbonding orbital.] What are the configurations and ground-state term symbols for (a) NH_3, (b) NH_3^+, (c) NH_3^-?

a) For NH_3, there are 10 electrons, thus we have $(1a_1)^2(2a_1)^2(1e)^4(3a_1)^2$. The term symbol is $^1A_1$.

b) For NH_3^+, $(1a_1)^2(2a_1)^2(1e)^4(3a_1)^1$. The term symbol is $^2A_1$.

c) For NH_3^-, $(1a_1)^2(2a_1)^2(1e)^4(3a_1)^2(4a_1)^1$. Then the term symbol is $^2A_1$.

14.23 The symmetry orbitals for XH_3 with D_{3h} symmetry are (in order of energy):

$$(1a_1')(2a_1')(1e')(1a_2'')(3a_1')(2e')$$

What are the configurations and ground-state term symbols for (a) BH_3, (b) BH_3^+, (c) BH_3^-?

a) For BH_3, $(1a_1')^2(2a_1')^2(1e')^4$. The term symbol is $^1A_1'$.

b) For BH_3^+, $(1a_1')^2(2a_1')^2(1e')^3$. We treat this as a hole configuration. Thus the term symbol is $^2E'$.

c) For BH_3^-, $(1a_1')^2(2a_1')^2(1e')^4(1a_2'')^1$. Thus $^2A_2''$ is the term symbol.

14.24 Water has a $^1A_1$ ground state (Table 14.8) and an excited state with a configuration . . . $(3a_1)^2(1b_1)^1(2b_2)^1$. What state(s) result from this configuration? Is it an allowed transition from the ground state to any of these states?

The excited configuration gives us

b_1	1	-1	1	-1
b_2	1	-1	-1	1
A_2	1	1	-1	-1

Thus the resulting states could be $^1A_2$ or $^3A_2$. Since $A_1 \otimes A_2 = A_2$ and A_2 does not have the symmetry of x, y or z, then a transition from A_1 to A_2 is forbidden.

14.25 What are the state symbols for the ground state of NH_2^+, NH_2^-, BH_2^-, CH_2^-? (Assume these are nonlinear.)

NH_2^+: $(1a_1)^2(2a_1)^2(1b_2)^2(3a_1)^2$. Thus the state symbol is $^1A_1$.

NH_2^-: $(1a_1)^2(2a_1)^2(1b_2)^2(3a_1)^2(1b_1)^2$. The state symbol is $^1A_1$.

BH_2^-: $(1a_1)^2(2a_1)^2(1b_2)^2(3a_1)^2$. The state symbol is $^1A_1$.

CH_2^-: $(1a_1)^2(2a_1)^2(1b_2)^2(3a_1)^2(1b_1)^1$. The state symbol is $^2B_1$.

14.26 The MO's of naphthalene (ref. 1, p. 164) give the following ground-state configuration: $(1b_{1u})^2(1b_{2g})^2(1b_{3g})^2(2b_{1u})^2(1a_u)^2$; the next (empty) orbital is $(2b_{2g})$.
(a) What are the symmetries of the ground and first excited states?
(b) Is this an allowed transition for absorption of a photon by electric dipole rules?

a) The symmetry of the ground state is a_{1g}. For the first excited state we have $(1b_{1u})^2(1b_{2g})^2(1b_{3g})^2(2b_{1u})^2(1a_u)^1(2b_g)^1$. Since the point group is D_{2h},

a_u	1	1	1	1	-1	-1	-1	-1
b_{2g}	1	-1	1	-1	1	-1	1	-1
b_{2u}	1	-1	1	-1	-1	1	-1	1

and the term symbols are $^1B_{2u}$ and $^3B_{2u}$.

b) The direct product is $A_{1g} \otimes B_{2u} = B_{2u}$. Since B_{2u} has the symmetry of y, the transition is allowed.

14.27 In benzene, what state(s) would result if an e_{1g} electron were excited to the b_{2g} orbital?

The ground state in benzene has the configuration $\ldots (a_{2u})^2(e_{1g})^4$. The excited state would be $\ldots (a_{2u})^2(e_{1g})^3(b_{2g})^1$. Since benzene is D_{6h},

e_{1g}	2	1	-1	-2	0	0	2	1	-1	-2	0	0
b_{2g}	1	-1	1	-1	-1	1	1	-1	1	-1	-1	1
e_{2g}	2	-1	-1	2	0	0	2	-1	-1	2	0	0

Thus the states are $^3E_{2g}$, $^1E_{2g}$.

14.28 The C_s point-group character table is:

C_s	$\hat{E}$	$\hat{\sigma}$
A'	1	1
A''	1	−1

Which types of transitions are electric-dipole allowed?

$$A' \leftrightarrow A'', \qquad A' \leftrightarrow A', \qquad A'' \leftrightarrow A''$$

Since $A' \otimes A'' = A''$, the transition $A' \leftrightarrow A''$ is allowed. For $A' \leftrightarrow A'$, $A' \otimes A' = A'$, thus the transition is allowed. For $A'' \leftrightarrow A''$, $A'' \otimes A'' = A'$ and this transition is also allowed.

14.29 How many vibrational normal modes will the following molecules have? H_2O_2, H—C≡C—H (acetylene), $CH_2{=}CH_2$ (ethylene), $CHCl{=}CH_2$ (ethylene chloride), C_6H_6 (benzene), C_6H_5Cl (chlorobenzene).

Nonlinear molecules: 3N - 6 normal modes. Linear molecules: 3N - 5 normal modes. H_2O_2: 3(4) - 6 = 6 ; H - C ≡ C - H: 3(4) - 5 = 7 ; $H_2C = CH_2$: 3(6) - 6 = 12 ; $HClC = CH_2$: 3(6) - 6 = 12 ; C_6H_5Cl: 3(12) - 6 = 30 .

14.30 Determine the symmetry of the following normal modes of *trans*-dichloroethylene (C_{2h}):

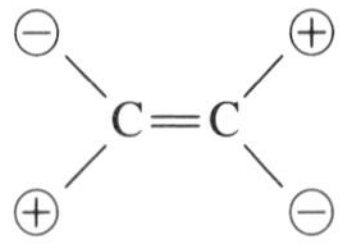

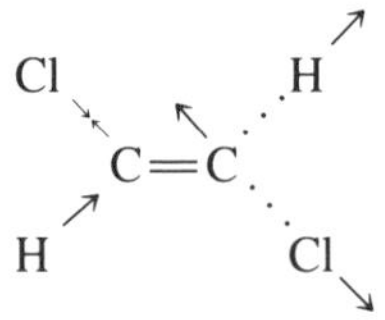

For the point group C_{2h},

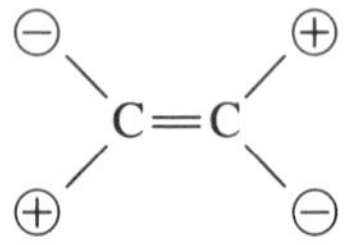

$\hat{E}$	$\hat{C}_2$	$\hat{i}$	$\hat{\sigma}_h$
1	1	-1	-1

This is the representation a_u. For

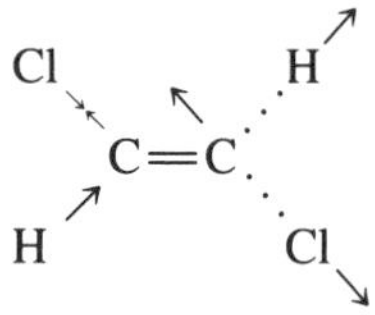

$\hat{E}$	$\hat{C}_2$	$\hat{i}$	$\hat{\sigma}_h$
1	-1	-1	1

This is the representation b_u.

14.31 Calculate the energies of the lowest nine vibrational states of F_2O. [*Hint:* All will have energies less than 3000 cm^{-1}.]

From Table 14.10, $\omega_{e1} = 830\ cm^{-1}$, $\omega_{e2} = 490\ cm^{-1}$ and $\omega_{e3} = 1110\ cm^{-1}$. From Eq. (14.46), $\tilde{\nu} = \dfrac{E_{vib}}{hc} = \sum_{i=1}^{3N-6}\left(v_i + \frac{1}{2}\right)\omega_{ei}$.

Then we have

(0, 0, 0)	$\tilde{\nu} = 1215\ cm^{-1}$
(0, 1, 0)	$\tilde{\nu} = 1705\ cm^{-1}$
(1, 0, 0)	$\tilde{\nu} = 2045\ cm^{-1}$
(0, 2, 0)	$\tilde{\nu} = 2195\ cm^{-1}$
(0, 0, 1)	$\tilde{\nu} = 2325\ cm^{-1}$
(1, 1, 0)	$\tilde{\nu} = 2535\ cm^{-1}$
(0, 3, 0)	$\tilde{\nu} = 2685\ cm^{-1}$
(0, 1, 1)	$\tilde{\nu} = 2815\ cm^{-1}$
(2, 0, 0)	$\tilde{\nu} = 2875\ cm^{-1}$

14.32 In D_{6h} symmetry, what types of vibrations are IR active? Which are Raman active?

From the D_{6h} character table, we find that the a_{2u} and e_{1u} vibrations are IR active since they have the symmetry of x, y or z. The Raman active vibrations are a_{1g} , e_{1g} and e_{2g} (these have x^2, y^2, z^2, xy, yz or zx symmetry).

14.33 For formaldehyde (Figure 14.12) what are the symmetries of the vibrational states:

$$(0,0,0,1,0,0), \quad (1,0,0,0,0,1), \quad (0,0,0,0,1,1)$$

Which of these will be dipole allowed for absorption from the ground state?

The vibrational state (0, 0, 0, 1, 0, 0) has the symmetry of Q_4 (the mode with ω_{e4}), which is b_1 . The state (1, 0, 0, 0, 0, 1) has the symmetry of the product of Q_1 and Q_6, $a_1 \otimes b_2 = b_2$. The state (0, 0, 0, 0, 1, 1) has the symmetry $b_1 \otimes b_2 = a_2$. For a transition from the ground state to be allowed, the direct product of a_1 and the excited state representation must be a_1, b_1 or b_2 . Then

(0, 0, 0, 1, 0, 0)	$a_1 \otimes b_1 = B_1$	allowed
(1, 0, 0, 0, 0, 1)	$a_1 \otimes b_2 = B_2$	allowed
(0, 0, 0, 0, 1, 1)	$a_1 \otimes a_2 = A_2$	not allowed

14.34 Estimate the frequency of the overtone band (0, 0, 0) → (2, 1, 1) in the IR spectrum of H_2O.

Using Eq. (14.46) and data from Table 14.10,

$$\frac{E(0,0,0)}{hc} = \frac{1}{2}(3652) + \frac{1}{2}(1595) + \frac{1}{2}(3756) = 4501.5 \text{ cm}^{-1} \quad \text{and}$$

$$\frac{E(2,1,1)}{hc} = \frac{5}{2}(3652) + \frac{3}{2}(1595) + \frac{3}{2}(3756) = 17{,}156.5 \text{ cm}^{-1} .$$ The

transition frequency is then

$$\frac{\Delta E}{hc} = 17{,}156.5 - 4501.5 = 12{,}655 \text{ cm}^{-1} .$$

14.35 Which normal modes of acetylene (Figure 14.11) will be IR active?

A mode will be IR active if there is a change in dipole moment. From Figure 14.12, Q_3 and Q_5 show a dipole moment change and are thus IR active.

14.36 In the IR spectrum of SO_2 the fundamental (0, 0, 0) → (0, 1, 0) is at 1290 cm^{-1} and the overtone (0, 0, 0) → (0, 2, 0) is at 2422 cm^{-1}. Calculate the vibrational constant and anharmonicity of this normal mode.

The vibrational energy is given by

$E_v = \left(v + \frac{1}{2}\right)\omega_e + \left(v + \frac{1}{2}\right)^2 \omega_e x_e$. Then $E_0 = \frac{1}{2}\,\omega_e - \frac{1}{4}\,\omega_e x_e$, $E_1 = \frac{3}{2}\omega_e - \frac{9}{4}\omega_e x_e$ and $E_2 = \frac{5}{2}\omega_e - \frac{25}{4}\omega_e x_e$. The fundamental is then $E(0,1,0) - E(0,0,0) = \omega_e - 2\omega_e x_e = 1290 \text{ cm}^{-1}$ and for the overtone, $E(0,2,0) - E(0,0,0) = 2\omega_e - 6\omega_e x_e = 2422 \text{ cm}^{-1}$. We then find $\omega_e = 1448 \text{ cm}^{-1}$ and $\omega_e x_e = 79 \text{ cm}^{-1}$.

14.37 Ethylene (C_2H_4) has the following normal vibrations (Figure 14.12):

$$3a_g,\ a_u,\ 2b_{1g},\ b_{1u},\ b_{2g},\ 2b_{2u},\ 2b_{3u}$$

(a) Which are IR active?
(b) Which are Raman active?
(c) Are any inactive?
(d) Is the first overtone of a b_{1u} mode IR active?
(e) Is a combination band $a_u + b_{1g}$ IR active?

a) Ethylene is D_{2h} . From the character table, the IR active modes are b_{1u} , b_{2u} and b_{3u} . From Figure 14.13b, we then have 5 IR active modes: b_{1u} , $2b_{2u}$ and $2b_{3u}$.

b) There are 6 Raman active modes, $3a_g$, $2b_{1g}$ and $1b_{2g}$.

c) a_u is inactive in both IR and Raman.

d) Since $b_{1u} \otimes b_{1u} = a_g$, the overtone is not IR active.

e) $a_u \otimes b_{1g} = b_{1u}$, which is IR active.

14.38 In a Raman experiment, SO_2 is irradiated with 600-nm light. What will be the wavelengths of the strongest lines (fundamentals) in the scattered light?

$\tilde{\nu} = \frac{1}{\lambda} = \frac{1}{600 \times 10^{-7}\ \text{cm}} = 16{,}667\ \text{cm}^{-1}$. From Table 14.10, $\omega_{e1} = 1151\ \text{cm}^{-1}$, $\omega_{e2} = 524\ \text{cm}^{-1}$ and $\omega_{e3} = 1361\ \text{cm}^{-1}$. The frequency of the scattered light will be $16{,}667\ \text{cm}^{-1} - \omega_e = \tilde{\nu}_s$. Then $\tilde{\nu}_{s1} = 16{,}667 - 1151 = 15{,}516\ \text{cm}^{-1} = 645\ \text{nm}$, $\tilde{\nu}_{s2} = 620\ \text{nm}$ and $\tilde{\nu}_{s3} = 654\ \text{nm}$.

14.39 What are the directions of the principal inertial axes in dichloroethylene?

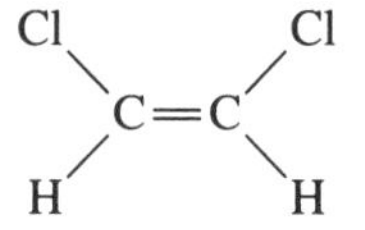

One principal axis will be perpendicular to the plane of the molecule. Another principal axis will be perpendicular to the C = C bond and in the plane of the molecule. The third principal axis will be parallel to the C = C bond and in the plane of the molecule.

14.40 (a) Classify the following molecules as (1) asymmetric top, (2) symmetric top, (3) spherical top: CH_4, CH_3Cl, CH_2Cl_2, $CH_2{=}CH_2$, benzene, SF_6.
(b) Which of these molecules will show a pure rotational (microwave) spectrum?

a)	CH_4	spherical top	CH_3Cl	symmetric top
	CH_2Cl_2	asymmetric top	$CH_2 = CH_2$	asymmetric top
	benzene	symmetric top	SF_6	spherical top

b) CH_3Cl and CH_2Cl_2 both have permanent dipole moments and will hence have a pure rotational spectrum.

14.41 Derive formulas for the moments of inertia of a planar trigonal molecule XY_3. Note that I_a is for rotation about the z axis (the C_3 axis) and I_b is for rotation about any axis in the plane of the molecule. Which of these is measurable by microwave spectroscopy?

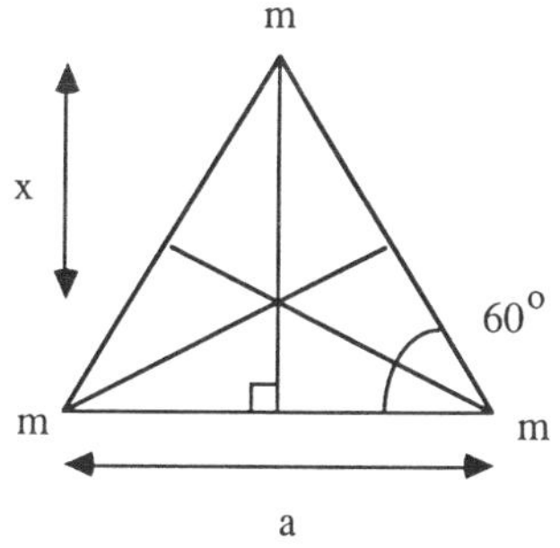

The distance from any m to the center of mass, x, is given by

$x = \dfrac{a}{2\cos 30^\circ} = \dfrac{a}{\sqrt{3}}$. Thus for the perpendicular axis,

$I_a = m(3x^2) = ma^2$. For the axis in the plane,

$$I_b = m\left(\frac{a^2}{4} + \frac{a^2}{4}\right) = \frac{ma^2}{2} .$$

14.42 The rotational constant (B) of BF_3 (a D_{3h} molecule) is 0.35 cm^{-1}. Calculate the BF bond length. (Use the results of Problem 14.41.)

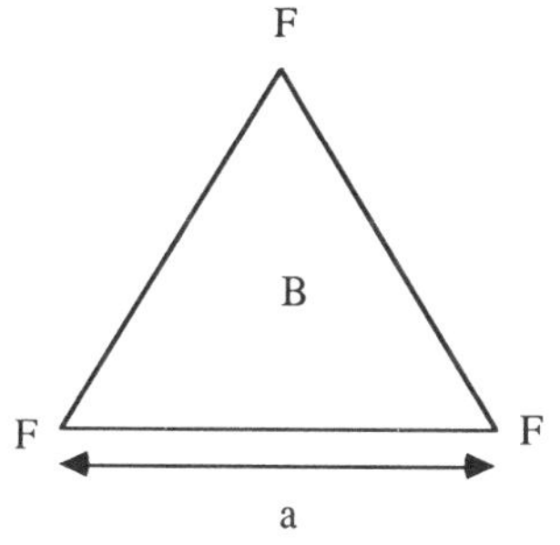

$$\tilde{B} = 0.35 cm^{-1} = \frac{2h}{8\pi^2 c m a^2}$$

$$\tilde{B} = \frac{2(6.626 \times 10^{-27} \text{ erg s})}{8\pi^2 c\left(\frac{18.998}{L}\right)a^2}$$

or $a = 2.25 \times 10^{-8}$ cm . From problem 14.41, we have

$x = \dfrac{a}{2\cos 30^\circ}$, where in this case x is the B - F bond distance.

Then $x = 1.30 \times 10^{-8}$ cm = 1.30 Å .

14.43 Show that the moment of inertia of a linear XYZ molecule is given by:

$$I = m_1 R_{12}^2 + m_3 R_{23}^2 - \frac{(m_1 R_{12} - m_3 R_{23})^2}{(m_1 + m_2 + m_3)}$$

Consider a molecule of the following geometry:

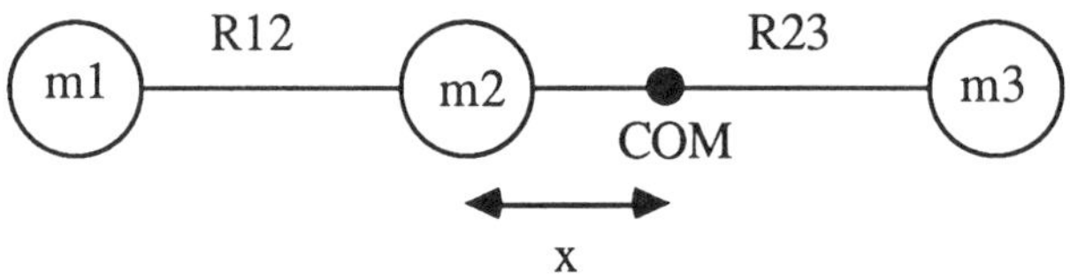

If the COM is located a distance x from m_2, then with

$\sum m_i r_i = 0$ we have: $m_3(R_{23} - x) - m_2 x - m_1(R_{12} + x) = 0$ so that

$x = \dfrac{m_1 R_{12} - m_3 R_{23}}{(m_1 + m_2 + m_3)}$. The moment of inertia is

$$I = \sum m_i r_i^2 = m_1(R_{12} + x)^2 + m_2 x^2 + m_3(R_{23} - x)^2$$

$$I = m_1(R_{12}^2 + 2R_{12}x + x^2) + m_2 x^2 + m_3(R_{23}^2 - 2R_{23}x + x^2)$$

$$I = m_1 R_{12}^2 + m_3 R_{23}^2 + (m_1 + m_2 + m_3)x^2 - 2x(m_3 R_{23} - m_1 R_{12})$$

But $-x(m_3 R_{23} - m_1 R_{12}) = (m_1 + m_2 + m_3)x^2$ so that

$$I = m_1 R_{12}^2 + m_3 R_{23}^2 - \frac{(m_1 R_{12} - m_3 R_{23})^2}{(m_1 + m_2 + m_3)} .$$

14.44 The bond lengths for Cl—C≡N (linear) are:

$$R_{C-Cl} = 1.629 \text{ Å}, \qquad R_{C-N} = 1.163 \text{ Å}$$

Calculate the moment of inertia of this molecule.

Denoting the distance of the COM from Cl as x,

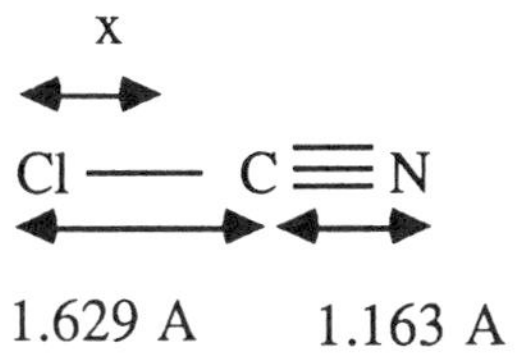

$$35x - 12(1.629 - x) - 14(1.629 - x + 1.163) = 0 \text{ or}$$

$x = 0.9612$ Å. Then

$$I = \sum_i m_i x_i^2$$

$$= \frac{35(0.9612)^2 + 12(1.629 - 0.9612)^2 + 14(2.782 - 0.9612)^2}{6.0227 \times 10^{23}}$$

$$I = 1.405 \times 10^{-22} \text{ g Å}^2 = 1.405 \times 10^{-38} \text{ g cm}^2 .$$

14.45 Using the formula for the moment of inertia of a linear XYZ molecule (Problem 14.43) to determine the bond distances requires measurements on two molecules differing in the mass of one of the atoms. Show that the formula of Problem 14.43 can be written as:

$$I(m_1 + m_2 + m_3) = m_1(m_2 + m_3)R_{12}^2 + m_3(m_1 + m_2)R_{23}^2 + 2m_1m_3R_{12}R_{23}$$

This is a particularly convenient form if the mass of a terminal atom (1 or 3) is changed. Table 14.12 gives rotation constants for $^{16}O^{12}C^{32}S$ and $^{16}O^{12}C^{34}S$. Use these to calculate the bond distances of this molecule (set up simultaneous equations for each molecule using the equation above, and solve for R_{12} and R_{23}). It is best to use the exact masses of Table 13.2, but the approximate masses — 16, 12 and 32 or 34 — will give pretty good answers.

If we let $M = m_1 + m_2 + m_3$, then:

$$IM = m_1MR_{12}^2 + m_3MR_{23}^2 - (m_1R_{12} - m_3R_{23})^2$$

$$IM = m_1MR_{12}^2 + m_3MR_{23}^2 - m_1^2R_{12}^2 + 2m_1m_3R_{12}R_{23} - m_3^2R_{23}^2$$

$$IM = m_1(m_2 + m_3)R_{12}^2 + m_3(m_1 + m_2)R_{23}^2 + 2m_1m_3R_{12}R_{23} .$$

Designating the isotopes as m_1 and m_1':

$\frac{IM}{m_1} = (m_2 + m_3)R_{12}^2 + \frac{m_3}{m_1}(m_1 + m_2)R_{23}^2 + 2m_3R_{12}R_{23}$ and similarly for m_1'. Thus: $\frac{IM}{m_1} - \frac{I'M'}{m_1'} = R_{23}^2\left\{\frac{m_3}{m_1}(m_1 + m_2) - \frac{m_3}{m_1'}(m_1' + m_2)\right\}$ and

$$R_{23}^2 = \frac{\left(\frac{IM}{m_1} - \frac{I'M'}{m_1'}\right)}{\left\{\frac{m_3}{m_1}(m_1 + m_2) - \frac{m_3}{m_1'}(m_1' + m_2)\right\}} = \frac{m_1'IM - m_1I'M'}{m_2m_3(m_1' - m_1)}$$

With $I = \frac{h}{8\pi^2B_e}$, $B_e(OCS) = 6.081494 \times 10^9\ s^{-1}$ and

$B_e(OC^{34}S) = 5.93284 \times 10^9\ s^{-1}$, we find:

$I(OCS) = 1.379928 \times 10^{-38}\ g\ cm^2$ and

$I(OC^{34}S) = 1.414503 \times 10^{-38}\ g\ cm^2$. Using the masses:

$m_1 = m(S) = 31.9720/L$, $m_1' = m(^{34}S) = 33.9679/L$,

$m_2 = m(C) = 12.00/L$ and $m_3 = m(O) = 15.9949/L$, we find

$M = 59.96698/L$ and $M' = 61.9628/L$ so that

$R_{23} = 1.16292 \times 10^{-8}\ cm = 1.16292$ Å. Use the quadratic formula to solve for R_{12}: $AR_{12}^2 + BR_{12} + C = 0$. $A = 895.0552$,

$B = 1189.4124$, $C = -4032.1533$ and $R_{12} = 1.5596$ Å.

14.46 In acetylene (C_2H_2) the C—C bond length is 1.205 Å, and the C—H bond length is 1.060 Å. Calculate the moment of inertia.

$I = \sum_i m_i(z_i - z_0)^2$. By symmetry, the COM is at the center of the C - C bond, so that $|z_C - z_0| = \frac{1}{2}(1.205\ \text{Å}) = 0.6025\ \text{Å}$ and $|z_H - z_0| = \frac{1}{2}(1.205\ \text{Å}) + 1.060\ \text{Å} = 1.6625\ \text{Å}$. With $m_H = 1.6736 \times 10^{-24}$ g and $m_C = 1.9927 \times 10^{-23}$ g we calculate

$$I = 2.372 \times 10^{-39}\ \text{g cm}^2 .$$

14.47 Ethylene has rotational constants:

$\tilde{A} = 4.828\ \text{cm}^{-1}$, $\tilde{B} = 1.0012\ \text{cm}^{-1}$, $\tilde{C} = 0.8282\ \text{cm}^{-1}$

What are the principal axes? Which is the "*A*" axis?

Ethylene is an asymmetric top, thus $I_A \neq I_B \neq I_C$. The principal axes are

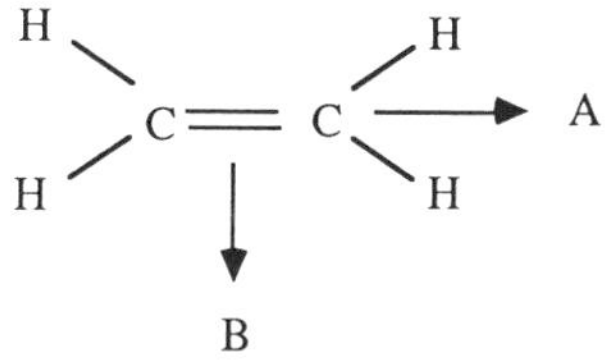

where the C axis is perpendicular to the plane of the molecule (not shown).

14.48 The rotational constant of CO_2 was measured from the rotational Raman spectrum and found to be $\tilde{B}_e = 0.3937\ \text{cm}^{-1}$. Calculate the CO bond length.

$I = \dfrac{h}{8\pi^2\tilde{B}_e c} = 7.105 \times 10^{-39}\ \text{g cm}^2$. For CO_2,

$I = \sum m_i r_i^2 = 2m_O r_{CO}^2$. With $m_O = 2.656 \times 10^{-23}$ g , we find:

$$r_{CO} = 1.157 \times 10^{-8}\ \text{cm} = 1.157\ \text{Å} .$$

14.49 Derive a formula for the moment of inertia of a tetrahedral molecule, A_4X. Begin by considering a cube, with X at the body center and the A atoms on alternate corners. Then derive relationships between the lengths of the cube's sides, its face diagonal, and its body diagonal (which is twice the bond length). It is probably easiest to calculate the moment of inertia about an axis perpendicular to the center of a face, but calculate it also about a body diagonal; you should get the same answers, since all moments of inertia of a T_d molecule are the same.

$$I = \sum_i m_i r_i^2 .$$

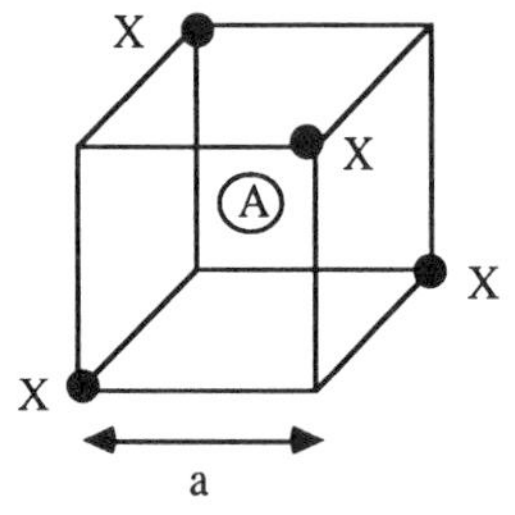

The AX_4 molecule is presumed to be centered in a cube of edge length a.

Any face diagonal has length squared: $r_{xx}^2 = a^2 + a^2 = 2a^2$ and any body diagonal has length squared: $(2r_{xa})^2 = a^2 + 2a^2 = 3a^2$ so that the distance from any X to A is: $r_{xa} = \frac{\sqrt{3}}{2}\, a$ (this is the bond length). The moment of inertia about an axis perpendicular to a face is: $I = 4m_x\left(\frac{\sqrt{2}a}{2}\right)^2 = 2m_x a^2$ or

$$I = \frac{8}{3}\, m_x r_{xa}^2 .$$

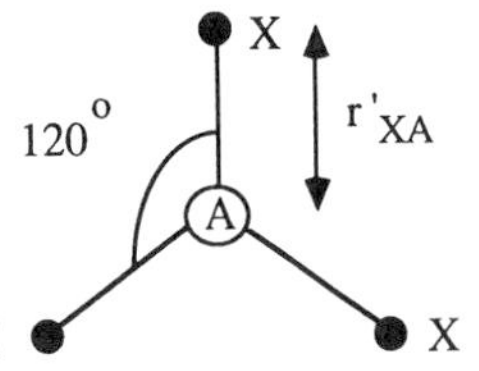

From the geometry of the problem, the in-plane x to A distance is $r_{xa}' = \frac{\sqrt{2}}{2}\, a\left(\frac{1}{\cos 30°}\right) = \sqrt{\frac{2}{3}}\, a$.

$$I = 3m_x(r_{xa}')^2 = 2m_x a^2 = \frac{8}{3}\, m_x r_{xa}^2 .$$

14.50 The moment of inertia of an A_4X tetrahedral molecule is:

$$I = \frac{8}{3} m_A r^2$$

where r is the AX bond length. Estimate the CH bond length in methane from its IR spectrum (Figure 14.16).

From Figure 14.16 the splitting is approximately $2\tilde{B} = 10 \text{ cm}^{-1}$ or

$\tilde{B} = 5 \text{ cm}^{-1}$. Then $I = \dfrac{h}{3\pi^2 \tilde{B} c} = 5.602 \times 10^{-40} \text{ g cm}^2$. Since

$I = \frac{8}{3} m_A r^2$ where $m_A = m_H = 1.66 \times 10^{-24}$ g , then

$5.602 \times 10^{-40} \text{ g cm}^2 = \frac{8}{3}(1.66 \times 10^{-24} \text{ g}) r^2$ or

$$r = 1.1 \times 10^{-8} \text{ cm} = 1.1 \text{ Å} .$$

14.51 The formula for the rotation-vibration energy of polyatomic linear molecules and spherical tops is the same as that given for diatomics, Eq. (13.49); of course, the moment of inertia is different and α_e is different for each vibration. Another important difference is that, for some vibrations of polyatomic molecules, a Q branch ($\Delta J = 0$) is allowed. Derive a formula for the frequencies of the Q branch of the first overtone band for such cases, in terms of the rotational quantum number for the lower state, J''.

For the first overtone, $v = 0 \rightarrow 2$. For $v = 0$, Eq. (13.49)

becomes: $\dfrac{E_{0,J''}}{hc} = \frac{1}{2}\omega_e - \frac{1}{4}\omega_e x_e + J''(J'' + 1)\tilde{B}_e - \frac{1}{2} J''(J'' + 1)\alpha_e$.

For $v = 2$, Eq. (13.49) becomes:

$$\frac{E_{2,J''}}{hc} = \frac{5}{2}\omega_e - \frac{25}{4}\omega_e x_e + J''(J'' + 1)\tilde{B}_e - \frac{5}{2}J''(J'' + 1)\alpha_e .$$

$$\tilde{\nu} = \frac{E_{2,J''}}{hc} - \frac{E_{0,J''}}{hc} = 2\omega_e - 6\omega_e x_e - 2J''(J'' + 1)\alpha_e .$$

14.52 Table 14.12 gives the rotational constants for formaldehyde (CH_2O). From these, assuming typical bond distances r_{CH} = 1.07 Å and r_{CO} = 1.22 Å, estimate the HCH angle.

From Table 14.12: $A = \frac{h}{8\pi^2 I_{zz}} = 282.106 \times 10^9\ s^{-1}$. This corresponds to rotation about the C - O axis:

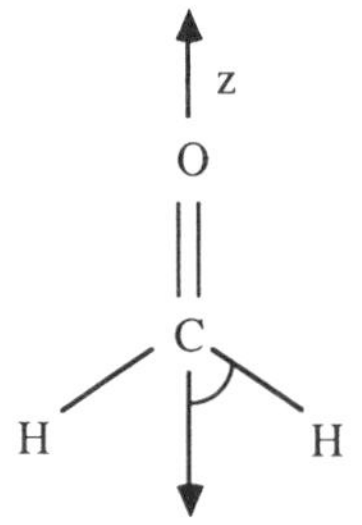

Using $h = 6.626 \times 10^{-27}$ erg s^{-1} , we find

$I_{zz} = 2.975 \times 10^{-40}$ g cm^2 . Also,

$I_{zz} = \sum_i m_i r_i^2 = 2m_H(r_{CH}\sin\Phi)^2$. With $m_H = 1.674 \times 10^{-24}$ g and $r_{CH} = 1.07 \times 10^{-8}$ cm we find $\sin\Phi = 0.8811$. The HCH angle is $2\Phi = 123.5°$.

15

Statistical Mechanics

15.1 The average translational energy of a particle can be defined with the state density function, $g(\varepsilon)$:

$$\langle \varepsilon \rangle = \frac{\int_0^\infty \varepsilon g(\varepsilon) e^{-\varepsilon/kT}\, d\varepsilon}{\int_0^\infty g(\varepsilon) e^{-\varepsilon/kT}\, d\varepsilon}$$

Use this to show that $\langle \varepsilon \rangle = \frac{3}{2}kT$, the equipartition value.

From Eq. (15.26), $\langle \epsilon \rangle = \dfrac{\int_0^\infty \epsilon^{3/2} e^{-\epsilon/kT} d\epsilon}{\int_0^\infty \epsilon^{1/2} e^{-\epsilon/kT} d\epsilon}$. Since

$\int_0^\infty x^n e^{-ax} dx = \dfrac{\Gamma(n+1)}{a^{n+1}}$, then we have

$$\langle \epsilon \rangle = \frac{\Gamma\left(\frac{5}{2}\right)/\left(\frac{1}{kT}\right)^{5/2}}{\Gamma\left(\frac{3}{2}\right)/\left(\frac{1}{kT}\right)^{3/2}} = \frac{kT\Gamma\left(\frac{5}{2}\right)}{\Gamma\left(\frac{3}{2}\right)} = \frac{kT\ \frac{3\sqrt{\pi}}{4}}{\frac{\sqrt{\pi}}{2}} = \frac{3}{2}\ kT\ .$$

15.2 Use Eq. (15.26) to derive the Maxwell-Boltzmann law [Eq. (1.36)] for the distribution of molecular velocities of particles with energy:

$$\varepsilon = \tfrac{1}{2}mv^2$$

For molecules with energies between ϵ and $\epsilon + d\epsilon$,

$g(\epsilon)d\epsilon = \frac{\pi}{4}\left(\frac{8ma^2}{h^2}\right)^{3/2} \epsilon^{1/2} d\epsilon$. With $\epsilon = \frac{1}{2}\ mv^2$, then $d\epsilon = mv\ dv$ and

$g(\epsilon)d\epsilon = \frac{\pi}{4}\left(\frac{8ma^2}{h^2}\right)^{3/2}\left(\frac{m^{3/2}}{\sqrt{2}}\right)v^2 dv$. The translational partition function is $z_{tr} = \left(\frac{\pi^{3/2}}{8}\right)\left(\frac{8ma^2kT}{h^2}\right)^{3/2}$ so that using Boltzmann's law, we have

$$P(\epsilon)d\epsilon = g(\epsilon(v))d\epsilon(v)\ \frac{e^{-\epsilon(v)/kT}}{z_{tr}} = \left(\frac{2}{\pi}\right)^{1/2}\left(\frac{1}{kT}\right)^{3/2} m^{3/2} v^2 e^{-mv^2/2kT} dv$$

and $P(\epsilon)d\epsilon = F(v)dv = 4\pi\left(\frac{m}{2\pi kT}\right)^{3/2} e^{-mv^2/2kT} v^2 dv$.

15.3 Calculate the contribution of nuclear spins to the molar entropy of $^{11}BF_3$.

S_m(nuclear spin) = R ln g_N where $g_N = 2I + 1$. From Table 15.1, $I_B = \frac{3}{2}$ and $I_F = \frac{1}{2}$ so $g_B = 4$ and $g_F = 2$. Then $g_{BF_3} = \Pi g_i = g_B g_F^{\,3} = 32$. For $^{11}BF_3$,

$$S_m = R \ln(32) = 28.815 \text{ J K}^{-1} .$$

15.4 Calculate the contribution of nuclear spins to the molar entropy of $^{31}PH_3$.

From Table 15.1, ^{31}P has $I = \frac{1}{2}$, $g = 2$ and ^1H has $I = \frac{1}{2}$, $g = 2$. Then $g_N = (2)(2)^3 = 16$ and $S_m = R \ln(16) = 23.05$ J K^{-1} .

15.5 Calculate the value of the partition function, z_{nsr}, for H_2 at 100 K; compare your answer to the approximate value

$$z_{nsr} = \frac{g_N T}{\sigma \theta_r}$$

(Use $\theta_r = 85.35$ K.) Repeat the calculation at 500 K.

For H_2,

$$z_{nsr} = \sum_{even}([2J + 1]\exp\{-J(J + 1)\theta_r/T\}) + 3\sum_{odd}([2J + 1]\exp\{-J(J + 1)\theta_r/T\}) .$$

With $\theta_r = 85.35$ K and T = 100 K , we find

$z_{nsr} = (1.0 + 1.6327 + 0.0299 + 0.0007 + \ldots) = 2.663$. The approximation $z_{nsr} = \frac{g_N T}{\sigma\theta_r}$ where $\sigma = 2$ and $g_N = 4$ gives $z_{nsr} = 2.343$. At 500 K,

$$z_{nsr} = 1.0 + 6.3970 + 1.7954 + 2.7078 + 0.2962 + 0.1970 + 0.0100 + 0.0032 + 0.0001$$

$$z_{nsr} = 12.4067 .$$

Using the approximation, $z_{nsr} = 11.7165$.

15.6 Calculate the percent *ortho* hydrogen in an equilibrium mixture at 200 K. (Use $\theta_r = 85.35$ K.)

The ratio of ortho to para is

$$\frac{\text{ortho}}{\text{para}} = \frac{3\sum_{odd}\{(2J + 1)\exp[-J(J + 1)\theta_r/T]\}}{\sum_{even}\{(2J + 1)\exp[-J(J + 1)\theta_r/T]\}}$$

$$\frac{\text{ortho}}{\text{para}} = \frac{3[1.2778 + 0.0418 + \ldots]}{[1.0 + 0.3863 + 0.0018 + \ldots]} = 2.8520$$

and % ortho = 74.04% .

15.7 Calculate the rotational internal energy per mole of *para* hydrogen at $T = 200$ K. Use $\theta_r = 85.35$ K and compare your answer to the equipartition value.

The average energy per particle is $\langle\epsilon\rangle = kT^2 \frac{\partial \ln z}{\partial T}$. On a per mole basis, $\langle E_{rot}\rangle = RT^2 \frac{\partial \ln z_{nsr}}{\partial T} = \frac{R\,T^2}{z_{nsr}} \frac{\partial z_{nsr}}{\partial T}$. Using Eq. (15.35b), for para H_2:

$$\frac{\partial z_{nsr}}{\partial T} = \sum_{even} \left\{ \frac{J(J + 1)(2J + 1)\theta_r}{T} \exp\left[\frac{-J(J + 1)\theta_r}{T}\right]\right\}$$

or $\frac{\partial z_{nsr}}{\partial T} = 5.021 \times 10^{-3}\ K^{-1}$ at $T = 200$ K . From problem 15.6, $z_{nsr}(200\ K,\ para) = 1.3881$, so $\langle E_{rot}\rangle = 1203$ J . From equipartition of energy, $\langle E_{rot}\rangle = RT = 1663$ J .

15.8 The deuterium nucleus has a spin $I = 1$. What is the nuclear spin-rotation partition function for D_2? What is the high-temperature limit?

From Eq. (15.38),

$$z_{nsr} = 6 \sum_{even} \left\{ (2J + 1) \exp\left[\frac{-J(J + 1)\theta_r}{T}\right]\right\} + 3 \sum_{odd} \left\{ (2J + 1) \exp\left[\frac{-J(J + 1)\theta_r}{T}\right]\right\} .$$

The high temperature limit (derived in the text for $^{14}N_2$) is

$$z_{nsr} = \frac{9}{2} \frac{T}{\theta_r} .$$

15.9 Derive a formula for the Stokes and antiStokes frequencies of a rotational Raman spectrum with exciting line $\tilde{\nu}_i$.

For the Stokes branch: J' = J" + 2 where J" = initial state and J' = final state. Using Eq. (15.41),

$$\tilde{\nu}_s(S) = \tilde{\nu}_i - \tilde{B}[(J'' + 2)(J'' + 3) - J''(J'' + 1)] = \tilde{\nu}_i - \tilde{B}(4J'' + 6)$$

where J" = 0, 1, 2, ... For the antiStokes branch: J' = J" − 2 , thus

$$\tilde{\nu}_s(aS) = \tilde{\nu}_i - \tilde{B}[(J'' - 2)(J'' - 1) - J''(J'' + 1)] = \tilde{\nu}_i + \tilde{B}(4J'' - 2)$$

where J" = 2, 3, ...

15.10 What would be the ratio of spin statistical weights (observable from alternation of Raman intensities) for a homonuclear diatomic molecule with $I = \frac{5}{2}$? (Assume ${}^1\Sigma_g^+$ electronic state.)

If $I = \frac{5}{2}$ for each atom, then $M = \frac{5}{2}, \frac{3}{2}, \frac{1}{2}, -\frac{1}{2}, -\frac{3}{2}, -\frac{5}{2}$ for each atom and there are a total of 36 possible spin combinations. Total spin quantum numbers are: T = 0 (g = 1), T = 1 (g = 3), T = 2 (g = 5), T = 3 (g = 7), T = 4 (g = 9) and T = 5 (g = 11). The T = 0, 2 and 4 states go with even J values and the T = 1, 3 and 5 states go with odd J values. Then

$$z_{nsr} = 15 \sum_{\text{even}} \left\{ (2J + 1) \exp\left[\frac{-J(J + 1)\theta_r}{T}\right] \right\} + 21 \sum_{\text{odd}} \left\{ (2J + 1) \exp\left[\frac{-J(J + 1)\theta_r}{T}\right] \right\} .$$

The spin statistical weights are thus: $\frac{\text{odd}}{\text{even}} = \frac{21}{15} = \frac{7}{5}$.

15.11 What will be the ratio of the statistical-nuclear spin weights for the odd J/even J levels of a homonuclear diatomic molecule with $I = \frac{3}{2}$? (Assume the electronic state is $^1\Sigma_g^+$.)

Since $I = \frac{3}{2}$, $M = \frac{3}{2}, \frac{1}{2}, -\frac{1}{2}, -\frac{3}{2}$ for each nucleus. For a homonuclear diatomic: T = 0 (g = 1), T = 1 (g = 3), T = 2 (g = 5) and T = 3 (g = 7). Odd J go with odd T so that, from Eq. (15.32),

$$z_{nsr} = 6\sum_{even}\left\{(2J+1)\exp\left[\frac{-J(J+1)\theta_r}{T}\right]\right\} +$$

$$10\sum_{odd}\left\{(2J+1)\exp\left[\frac{-J(J+1)\theta_r}{T}\right]\right\}.$$

Then the statistical weights are $\frac{\text{odd } J}{\text{even } J} = \frac{10}{6} = \frac{5}{3}$.

15.12 For a rotational Raman spectrum of a homonuclear diatomic molecule, what are the ratios of the differences ($|\tilde{\nu}_s - \tilde{\nu}_i|$) of the second side band to the first if (a) all J's are present; (b) only even J's are present; (c) only odd J's are present?

Using Figure 15.6a,

a) All peaks present; 1st peak: $|\tilde{\nu}_s - \tilde{\nu}_i| = 6B$, 2nd peak: $|\tilde{\nu}_s - \tilde{\nu}_i| = 10B$. $\frac{|\tilde{\nu}_s - \tilde{\nu}_i|_2}{|\tilde{\nu}_s - \tilde{\nu}_i|_1} = \frac{10}{6} = \frac{5}{3}$.

b) Only even peaks present; 1st peak: $|\tilde{\nu}_s - \tilde{\nu}_i| = 6B$, 2nd peak: $|\tilde{\nu}_s - \tilde{\nu}_i| = 14B$. $\frac{|\tilde{\nu}_s - \tilde{\nu}_i|_2}{|\tilde{\nu}_s - \tilde{\nu}_i|_1} = \frac{14}{6} = \frac{7}{3}$.

c) Only odd peaks present; 1st peak: $|\tilde{\nu}_s - \tilde{\nu}_i| = 10B$, 2nd peak: $|\tilde{\nu}_s - \tilde{\nu}_i| = 18B$. $\frac{|\tilde{\nu}_s - \tilde{\nu}_i|_2}{|\tilde{\nu}_s - \tilde{\nu}_i|_1} = \frac{18}{10} = \frac{9}{5}$.

15.13 The Raman spectrum of a homonuclear diatomic molecule is analyzed to give the rotational constant, $\theta_r = 3.00$ K. Analyze the relative intensity pattern below (for $T = 300$ K) to determine the nuclear spin.

J''	Rel. int.	J''	Rel. int.
0	1.00	4	7.37
1	4.90	5	13.6
2	4.71	6	8.54
3	10.4	7	14.2

From Eq. (15.34), $\frac{g_N}{z_{nsr}} = \frac{1}{(2J + 1)}\left(\frac{N_J}{N}\right) \exp\left\{\frac{J(J + 1)\theta_r}{T}\right\}$. Using $\theta_r = 3.0$ K and T = 300 K,

J"	rel. int. = $\frac{N_{J''}}{N}$	$\frac{g_N}{z_{nsr}}$
0	1.0	1.000
1	4.90	1.666
2	4.71	1.000
3	10.4	1.675
4	7.37	1.000
5	13.6	1.699
6	8.54	1.000
7	14.2	1.657

Comparison with problem 15.11 shows $\frac{\text{odd}}{\text{even}} = \frac{5}{3}$ and $I = \frac{3}{2}$.

15.14 Show that the Debye formula for the internal energy (per mole) of a crystal approaches $U_m = 3RT$ and that the heat capacity approaches $C_{vm} = 3R$ (the law of Dulong and Petit) as $T \to \infty$. [*Hint:* Use $e^u \cong 1 + u$ as $u \to 0$.]

According to the Debye theory, $U_m = 9RT\left(\frac{T^3}{\theta_D^3}\right)\int_0^{\theta_D/T} \frac{u^3 du}{e^u - 1}$. As $T \to \infty$, $u = \frac{\theta_D}{T} \to 0$. Using $\lim_{u\to 0} e^u = 1 + u$,

$U_m = 9RT\left(\frac{T^3}{\theta_D^3}\right)\int_0^{\theta_D/T} u^2 du = 3RT$. The molar heat capacity is given by $C_{vm} = 9R\left(\frac{T}{\theta_D}\right)^3 \int_0^{\theta_D/T} \frac{u^4 e^u du}{(e^u - 1)^2}$. Using $\lim_{T\to\infty} e^u = 1 + u$,

$$C_{vm} = 9R\left(\frac{T}{\theta_D}\right)^3 \int_0^{\theta_D/T} u^2(1 + u)du = \left[9R\left(\frac{T}{\theta_D}\right)^3\left[\frac{u^3}{3} + \frac{u^4}{4}\right]\right]_0^{\theta_D/T}$$

$$C_{vm} = 3R + \frac{9}{4}\left(\frac{\theta_D}{T}\right) .$$

But $u = \frac{\theta_D}{T} \to 0$ as $T \to \infty$, thus $C_{vm} = 3R$ as $T \to \infty$.

15.15 The heat capacity of aluminum oxide at 5 K is $C_{pm} = 0.0012$ J/K. Use this value to estimate the Debye temperature for this material. Use this value to estimate the heat capacity at 10 K (obs. 0.0094 J/K).

At low T, $\theta_D = \left(\frac{36\pi^4 R}{15C_{vm}}\right)^{1/3} T$. With $C_p \cong C_v$,

$$\theta_D = \left(\frac{36\pi^4(8.3145 \text{ J K}^{-1})}{15(0.0012 \text{ J K}^{-1})}\right)^{1/3} (5 \text{ K}) = 587 \text{ K} .$$ Using this value for θ_D at T = 10 K, we find $C_{vm}(10 \text{ K}) \cong C_{pm}(10 \text{ K}) = 0.0096 \text{ J K}^{-1}$.

15.16 Calculate the molar heat capacity (constant volume) of NaCl at 10 K, 100 K, and 300 K, using the Debye theory.

For $T \ll \theta_D$,

$$C_{vm} = \left\{\frac{36\pi^4 R}{15\theta_D^3}\right\}T^3 = \left\{\frac{36\pi^4(8.3145 \text{ J K}^{-1})}{15(281 \text{ K})^3}\right\}(10 \text{ K})^3 = 0.0876 \text{ J K}^{-1}.$$

At T = 100 K , we use Figure 15.10 to find

$D\left(\frac{\theta_D}{T}\right) = D(2.81) = 0.7$. Then $C_{vm} = 3RD\left(\frac{\theta_D}{T}\right) = 17 \text{ J K}^{-1}$. At

T = 300 K , $T > \theta_D$ and $C_{vm} = 3R\left(1 - \frac{\theta_D^2}{20T^2}\right) = 23.8 \text{ J K}^{-1}$.

15.17 The Einstein formula is considerably more convenient to use than Debye's, but its constants (θ_E) are not usually tabulated. Show that if the Einstein frequency (ν_E) is interpreted as the average of the Debye frequencies, then:

$$\theta_E = \tfrac{3}{4}\theta_D$$

Compare these theories by calculating the heat capacity for $\theta_D/T = 3$.

For the Einstein theory, $\theta_E = \dfrac{h\nu_E}{k}$, whereas for the Debye theory,

$\theta_D = \dfrac{h\nu_m}{k}$. If $\nu_E = \langle\nu_m\rangle$, then using Eq. (15.53),

$$\nu_E = \langle\nu_m\rangle = \frac{\int_0^{\nu_m} \nu g(\nu)\,d\nu}{\int_0^{\nu_m} g(\nu)\,d\nu} = \frac{\int_0^{\nu_m} \nu^3 d\nu}{\int_0^{\nu_m} \nu^2 d\nu} = \frac{3}{4}\nu_m . \quad \text{This gives } \theta_E = \frac{3}{4}\theta_D .$$

For the Einstein theory, $C_{vm} = \dfrac{3Ru^2e^u}{(e^u - 1)^2}$, so that

with $u = \dfrac{3}{4}\dfrac{\theta_D}{T} = \dfrac{9}{4}$, then $\dfrac{C_{vm}}{3R} = 0.667$. For the Debye theory,

$\dfrac{C_{vm}}{3R} = D\left(\dfrac{\theta_D}{T}\right)$. Using Figure 15.10, for $\dfrac{\theta_D}{T} = 3$,

$$\frac{C_{vm}}{3R} = D\left(\frac{\theta_D}{T}\right) = 0.67 .$$

15.18 Calculate the Stefan-Boltzmann constant (σ) from Eq. (15.66).

Combining Eqs. (15.62) and (15.66),

$$\sigma = \frac{2\pi^5 k^4}{15h^3c^2} = \frac{2\pi^5(1.3805 \times 10^{-23}\ \mathrm{J\ K^{-1}})^4}{15(6.6256 \times 10^{-34}\ \mathrm{J\ s})^3c^2}$$

$$\sigma = 5.6698 \times 10^{-8}\ \mathrm{J\ s^{-1}\ m^{-2}\ K^{-4}} .$$

15.19 Show that the frequency at the maximum of the radiation density from a black body is:

$$\nu_{max} = \frac{2.8214kT}{h}$$

(This is one form of the Wien displacement law.)

From Eq. (15.64), $\rho(\nu)d\nu = \dfrac{8\pi k^4T^4u^3du}{h^3c^3(e^u - 1)}$. With $u = \dfrac{h\nu}{kT}$,

$du = \dfrac{h}{kT}\, d\nu$ and $\rho(u) = \dfrac{8\pi k^3T^3u^3}{h^2c^3(e^u - 1)}$,

$\dfrac{\partial\rho}{\partial u} = \dfrac{8\pi k^3T^3}{h^2c^3}\left(\dfrac{3u^2}{e^u - 1} - \dfrac{u^3e^u}{(e^u - 1)^2}\right)$. $\rho(u)$ is at a maximum when

$\dfrac{\partial\rho}{\partial u} = 0$ or $u = 3(1 - e^{-u})$. Solving by iteration, $u^{(0)} = 0$,

$u^{(1)} = 3$, . . . , $u^{(10)} = 2.821439$. Then with $\nu = \dfrac{ukT}{h}$,

$$\nu_{max} = 2.821439\,\frac{kT}{h} .$$

15.20 Derive the black-body radiation law for wavelength $\rho(\lambda)$. Then show that the wavelength for the maximum radiation density is:

$$\lambda_{max} = \frac{hc}{4.965kT}$$

(Compare to Problem 15.19.)

a) From Eq. (15.64): $\rho(\nu)d\nu = \dfrac{8\pi k^4T^4u^3du}{h^3c^3(e^u - 1)}$. Substituting

$u = \dfrac{hc}{\lambda kT}$, $du = -\dfrac{hc}{\lambda^2kT}\, d\lambda$ and $d\nu = -\dfrac{c}{\lambda^2}\, d\lambda$ we find after

substitution: $\rho(\lambda)d\lambda = \dfrac{8\pi hcd\lambda}{\lambda^5\left[\exp\left(\dfrac{hc}{\lambda kT}\right) - 1\right]}$.

b) At the maxima, $\frac{d\rho}{d\lambda} = 0$:

$$\frac{d\rho}{d\lambda} = -\frac{3}{\lambda}\rho(\lambda) + \frac{hc}{\lambda^2 kT}\frac{\exp\left(\frac{hc}{\lambda kT}\right)}{\left[\exp\left(\frac{hc}{\lambda kT}\right) - 1\right]}\rho(\lambda) \quad \text{or}$$

$\lambda = \frac{hc}{3kT}\frac{1}{\left[1 - \exp\left(-\frac{hc}{\lambda kT}\right)\right]}$. With $u = \frac{hc}{\lambda kT} = 3(1 - e^{-u})$ and

$\lambda = \lambda_{max}$, the solution is $u(\lambda_{max}) = 2.82144$.

16

Structure of Condensed Phases

16.1 Derive a formula for the volume of a hexagonal unit cell in terms of the lattice constants only.

For the general parallelepiped: $V = \underline{a} \cdot \underline{b} \times \underline{c}$. For the hexagonal unit cell: $\underline{a} = \underline{b}$, $\alpha = \beta = 90°$ and $\gamma = 120°$. Using the formula

$$V = abc[1 - \cos^2(\alpha) - \cos^2(\beta) - \cos^2(\gamma) + 2\cos(\alpha)\cos(\beta)\cos(\gamma)]^{1/2}$$

with $\cos \alpha = \cos \beta = 0$ and $\cos \gamma = -0.5$, we find

$$V = abc(0.75)^{1/2} = 0.866\ a^2c\ .$$

16.2 X-ray diffraction of lysozyme showed a unit cell with dimensions 71.2 Å × 71.2 Å × 31.4 Å, with all angles 90°. The density of the material was 1.305 g/cm^3, and it contained 9% water. The molecular weight by another method was estimated at 13900. Calculate the number of molecules per unit cell and the molecular weight by the X-ray method.

The volume of the unit cell is:

$$V = (71.2\ \text{Å})^2(31.4\ \text{Å})(10^{-8}\ \text{cm/Å})^3 = 1.592 \times 10^{-19}\ \text{cm}^3\ .$$

The weight of the molecules contained within the unit cell is:

$$m = \rho V = (1.592 \times 10^{-19}\ \text{cm}^3)(1.305\ \text{g cm}^{-3}) = 2.077 \times 10^{-19}\ \text{g}\ .$$

The weight of the lysozyme is:

$$m' = (0.91)(2.077 \times 10^{-19}\ \text{g}) = 1.89 \times 10^{-19}\ \text{g}\ .$$

The number of molecules per unit cell is:

$$n = \frac{m'N}{M.W.} = \frac{(1.89 \times 10^{-19} \text{ g})(6.022 \times 10^{23} \text{ mol}^{-1})}{(13900 \text{ g mol}^{-1})} = 8.19 \sim 8 .$$

Taking n = 8 , we calculate

$$M.W. = \frac{(1.89 \times 10^{-19} \text{ g})(6.022 \times 10^{23} \text{ mol}^{-1})}{8} = 14{,}200 \text{ g mol}^{-1} .$$

16.3 The salt [HO(C_6H_4)COO]KH, was found by X-ray diffraction to have a monoclinic cell with dimensions 16.4, 3.82, 11.3 Å, β = 92.5°. The density was 1.55 g/cm^3. Calculate the composition of the unit cell (which contains some water).

The M.W. of p-hydroxybenzoate, $(C_7H_5O_3)_2KH$, is 314.3 g mol^{-1} .

$$V = abc[1 - \cos^2 \alpha - \cos^2 \beta - \cos^2 \gamma + 2\cos \alpha \cos \beta \cos \gamma]^{1/2} .$$

For a monoclinic cell, $\alpha = \gamma = 90°$, $\cos \alpha = \cos \gamma = 0$,

$\beta = 92.5°$, $\cos \beta = -0.044$ and $\cos^2 \beta = 0.002$. Thus

$$V \sim abc = (3.82 \text{ Å})(16.4 \text{ Å})(11.3 \text{ Å}) = 7.079 \times 10^{-22} \text{ cm}^3 .$$

The weight of the unit cell is:

$$m = (1.55 \text{ g cm}^{-3})(7.079 \times 10^{-22} \text{ cm}^3) = 1.097 \times 10^{-21} \text{ g} .$$

If there are x units of H_2O per molecule of $(C_7H_5O_3)_2KH$, then the number of molecules per unit cell is:

$$n = \frac{(1.097 \times 10^{-21} \text{ g})(6.022 \times 10^{23} \text{ mol}^{-1})}{(314.3 + 18x)\text{g mol}^{-1}}$$

If x = 1 , n = 2.0 .

16.4 Match the following Schoenfliess and Herman-Mauguin point-group symbols:

$mmm \quad m3m \quad 422 \quad 2/m \quad 2mm \quad m \quad 6/mmm$

$O_h \quad C_{2h} \quad D_{6h} \quad D_{2h} \quad D_4 \quad C_{2v} \quad C_s$

Answer in Table 16.2.

16.5 What would be the Herman-Mauguin symbol for the C_{5v} point group?

C_{5v}(Schoenflies) = 5m(Hermann - Mauguin) . Logic: 5 - fold rotation axis → 5 , mirror plane → m .

16.6 What are the indices (*hkl*) for the "C-face" of a unit cell?

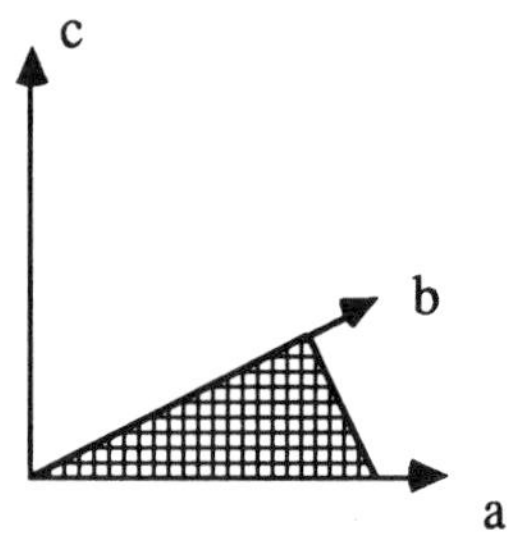

The "c - face" is defined by the ab plane, and is parallel to a and b. The Miller indices are 001.

16.7 Make drawings to show the following crystal planes: 002, 022, 120, 112.

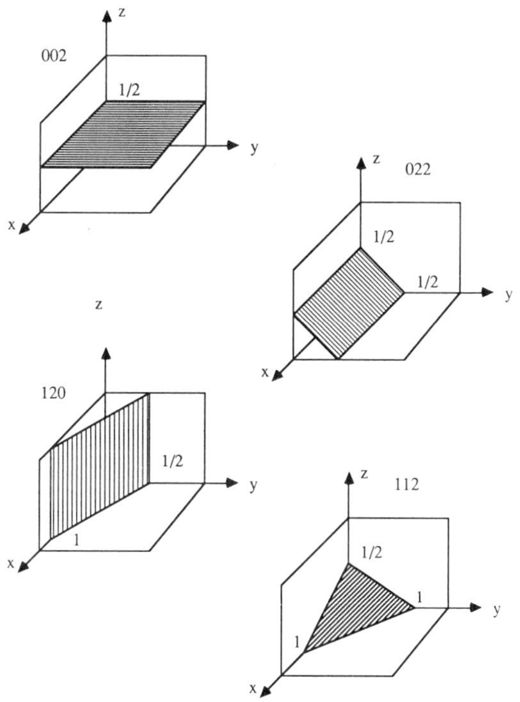

16.8 What would be the minimum interplanar spacing which would give reflections for X-ray radiation with wavelength 1.54 Å.

The Bragg Equation may be rearranged to: $d = \frac{n\lambda}{2\sin\theta}$. The minimum interplaner spacing d corresponds to $n = 1$, $\theta = 90^\circ$ and $\sin\theta = 1$ so that $d_{min} = \frac{\lambda}{2} = 0.77$ Å .

16.9 Often, with complicated patterns that have a great many reflections, it is useful to limit resolution by using only reflections with small angles. What would be the resolution using 1.54 Å X-rays if only reflections at angles less than $\pm 10^\circ$ were used?

Using $\lambda = 1.54$ Å and $\theta = 10^\circ$: $d = \frac{\lambda}{2\sin(10^\circ)} = 4.43$ Å . Because $\sin\theta$ approaches 0 as θ approaches 0, d increases at smaller angles.

16.10 With the von Laue method (Figure 16.13), and X-rays with wavelength 1.44 Å, incident parallel to the *a* axis, the rings were spaced 2.4 mm apart for a film radius of 66 mm. Calculate the lattice constant *a*.

Using Eq. (16.5): $a = \dfrac{h\lambda}{\left[\sin\left(\tan^{-1}\left(\frac{y}{r}\right)\right)\right]}$. With h = 1 ,

$\lambda = 1.44$ Å , y = 2.4 mm and r = 66 mm , we find: a = 39.6 Å .

16.11 The following is a list of reflections found for a primitive lattice; indicate which would be observed for: (a) a body-centered lattice; (b) a face-centered lattice. 100, 110, 111, 200, 210, 211, 220, 221, 300, 301, 311, 222, 302, 321, 400, 410, 322

For body-centered cells, Σhkl is even: 110, 200, 211, 220, 301, 222, 321, 400. For face-centered cells, hkl are all even or all odd: 111, 200, 220, 311, 222, 400.

16.12 Derive a specific formula for the interplanar spacings (as a function of *hkl* and the lattice constants) in a hexagonal lattice.

From Table 16.1, for a hexagonal lattice: $a = b \neq c$, $\alpha = \beta = 90°$ and $\gamma = 120°$. Thus: $\cos\alpha = \cos\beta = 0$, $\sin\alpha = \sin\beta = 1$, $\cos\gamma = -\frac{1}{2}$ and $\sin\gamma = \frac{\sqrt{3}}{2}$. Substituting these values into Eq. (16.8), we find

$$d^2_{hkl} = \frac{\frac{3}{4}}{\left(\frac{h^2}{a^2} + \frac{k^2}{a^2} + \frac{l^2}{c^2}\left(\frac{3}{4}\right) + \frac{hk}{a^2}\right)} .$$

Rearranging: $d^{-2}_{hkl} = \frac{4}{3}\left(\frac{h^2 + hk + k^2}{a^2}\right) + \frac{l^2}{c^2}$.

16.13 Calculate the angles for all allowed reflections from a body-centered cubic cell, a = 3.4 Å, from X-rays with wavelength 1.8 Å.

For a body-centered cubic cell, Σhkl assumes only even values.

Using $d_{hkl} = \dfrac{a}{(h^2 + k^2 + l^2)^{1/2}}$ and $\theta = \sin^{-1}\left(\dfrac{\lambda}{2d_{hkl}}\right)$, we may draw up the following table:

hkl	d_{hkl}(A°)	$\theta = \sin^{-1}\left(\dfrac{\lambda}{2d_{hkl}}\right)$
110	2.40	22
200	1.70	32
211	1.39	40
220	1.20	49
301	1.08	57
222	0.98	67
321	0.91	82
400	0.85	--

Must have $\lambda > 2d_{hkl}$.

16.14 A cubic cell shows Bragg reflections at the following angles: 20.27, 23.58, 34.45, 41.55, 43.85, 53.13°. What is the cell type? Calculate the lattice constant assuming the X-rays have a wavelength of 1.55 Å.

With $d_{hkl} = \dfrac{\lambda}{2\sin\theta} = \dfrac{a}{\sqrt{h^2 + k^2 + l^2}}$ we have

$a = \dfrac{\lambda}{2\sin\theta}(h^2 + k^2 + l^2)^{1/2}$. Draw up the following table:

θ	hkl(prim)	hkl(bcc)	hkl(fcc)
20.27	100	110	111
23.58	110	200	200
34.45	111	211	220
41.55	200	220	311
43.85	210	301	222
53.13	211	222	400

Now calculate a for each case with $\lambda = 1.55\ \text{Å}$:

θ	a(prim)	a(bcc)	a(fcc)
20.27	2.237	3.164	3.875
23.58	2.740	3.875	3.875
34.45	2.373	3.356	3.875
41.55	2.337	3.305	3.875
43.85	2.501	3.538	3.875
53.13	2.373	3.356	3.875

Clearly, the best fit is for the fcc cell with a lattice constant of 3.875 Å .

16.15 NaCl has a cell constant $a = 5.64$ Å. Calculate its density. What is the distance between Na and the nearest Cl? What is the distance between Na and the nearest Na?

The Na - Cl separation is: $\frac{1}{2}\ a = \frac{1}{2}(5.64\ \text{Å}) = 2.82\text{Å}$. The Na - Na separation is: $\frac{\sqrt{2}}{2}\ a = 3.99\ \text{Å}$. A cube 2.82 Å on a side contains $\frac{1}{2}\ Cl^-$ and $\frac{1}{2}\ Na^+$, so that the density is:

$$\rho = \frac{\frac{1}{2}(22.9\ \text{g mol}^{-1} + 35.45\ \text{g mol}^{-1})}{(2.82 \times 10^{-8}\ \text{cm})^3(6.022 \times 10^{23}\ \text{mol}^{-1})} = 2.164\ \text{g cm}^{-3}\ .$$

16.16 Based on the radius-ratio rules, what structure would you expect for crystals of LiF, NaF and KF? What would it mean if your predictions were incorrect?

Calculate the following radius ratios:

Species	RR	CN	Structure Type
LiF	0.441	6	NaCl
NaF	0.699	6	NaCl
CsCl	0.934	8	CsCl

Violations would indicate non-ionic bonding.

16.17 Calcium fluoride has a lattice constant $a = 5.462$ Å. Calculate its density.

With a cube of side length 5.462 Å, containing 8 F and 4 Ca, one may calculate:

$$\rho = \frac{4(40.08\ \text{g mol}^{-1}) + 8(18.99\ \text{g mol}^{-1})}{(5.462 \times 10^{-8}\ \text{cm})^3(6.022 \times 10^{23}\ \text{mol}^{-1})} = 3.182\ \text{g cm}^{-3}\ .$$

16.18 Derive the Madelung constant for a linear array of ions, alternating plus and minus, separated by a uniform distance.

For a linear array of alternating positive and negative charges separated by R: $M = 2(1 - \frac{1}{2} + \frac{1}{3} - \frac{1}{4} \ldots)$. The term in parentheses is the series expansion for $\ln(1 + x)$, with $x = 1$:

$\ln(1 + x) = x - \frac{x^2}{2} + \frac{x^3}{3} - \frac{x^4}{4} \ldots$. Thus $M = 2\ln(2) = 1.386$.

16.19 Use the Born-Haber cycle to calculate the crystal energy for KCl.

$$\Delta_c U = -\Delta_f H(KCl,s) + \Delta_{sub} H(K) + \frac{D_0(Cl_2)}{2} + IP(K) - EA(Cl) \ .$$ Using the following data: $\Delta_f H^\theta(KCl,s) = -435.9 \text{ kJ mol}^{-1}$, $\Delta_{sub} H(K) = 90.0 \text{ kJ mol}^{-1}$, $D_0(Cl_2) = 238.8 \text{ kJ mol}^{-1}$, $IP(K) = 418.8 \text{ kJ mol}^{-1}$ and $EA(Cl) = 348.8 \text{ kJ mol}^{-1}$, we find:

$$\Delta_c U = 715.3 \text{ kJ mol}^{-1} \ .$$

16.20 Calculate the theoretical crystal energy of KCl assuming $\kappa_T = 1.08 \times 10^{-11}$ cm^2/dyne.

The crystal energy is: $$\Delta_c U = \frac{Q_1 Q_2 ML\left(1 - \frac{1}{n}\right)}{R_e}$$ with

$Q_1 = Q_2 = 4.803 \times 10^{-10}$ esu , $M = 1.74756$,

$R_e = \left(\frac{133 + 181}{100}\right)\text{Å} = 3.14 \times 10^{-8}$ cm , $\kappa_T = 1.08 \times 10^{-11} \text{ cm}^2 \text{ dyne}^{-1}$

and $n = 1 + \frac{9cR_e^4}{\kappa_T Q_1 Q_2 M} = 5.02$. Plug in the numbers to find:

$$\Delta_c U = 618 \text{ kJ mol}^{-1} \ .$$

16.21 Assuming the repulsive energy of the atoms in the crystal is exponential:

$$E(R) = \frac{-q^2 \mathcal{M} L}{R} + A\, e^{-R/\rho}$$

show that

$$A = \frac{\rho q^2 \mathcal{M} L}{R_e^2 e^{-R_e/\rho}}$$

and the crystal energy is:

$$\Delta U_c = \frac{L \mathcal{M} q^2 (1 - \rho/R_e)}{R_e}$$

(ρ is a constant that can be determined from the compressibility of the crystal).

$E(R) = -q^2 \frac{ML}{R} + A\exp\left(\frac{R}{\rho}\right)$. Now $\frac{\partial E(R)}{\partial R} = 0$ at $R = R_e$, so that:

$\frac{\partial E(R)}{\partial R} = \frac{q^2 ML}{R^2} + \frac{A}{\rho}\left(\exp\left(\frac{R}{\rho}\right)\right) = 0$ (at $R = R_e$) . Thus

$A = -\frac{\rho q^2 ML}{R_e^2} \exp\left(-\frac{R_e}{\rho}\right)$, $\Delta_c U = -E(R_e) = q^2 \frac{ML}{R_e} - \frac{\rho q^2 ML}{R_e^2}$ and

$$\Delta_c U = \frac{LMq^2}{R_e}\left(1 - \frac{\rho}{R_e}\right) .$$

16.22 Calculate the efficiency of packing for bcc cells.

For the bcc arrangement, the spacing between atoms is $L = \frac{2}{\sqrt{3}} d$, where d is the atomic diameter. The volume of a unit cell is thus $V = \left(\frac{2}{\sqrt{3}} d\right)^3$. The volume occupied by atoms within the cell is: $V' = 2\left[\frac{4}{3} \pi \left(\frac{d}{2}\right)^3\right] = \frac{1}{3} \pi d^3$ corresponding to the volume of two atoms. The efficiency of packing is:

$$E = \frac{V'}{V} = \frac{\frac{\pi}{3}}{\left(\frac{2}{\sqrt{3}}\right)^3} = \frac{\pi\sqrt{3}}{8} .$$

16.23 Barium has a bcc cell with a = 5.025 Å. Calculate its density.

The body-centered cubic barium unit cell contains 2 barium atoms in a volume: $V = (5.025\ \text{Å})^3 \times 10^{-24}\ \text{cm}^3\ \text{Å}^{-3} = 1.269 \times 10^{-22}\ \text{cm}^3$. The mass of the 2 barium atoms is:

$$M = \frac{2(137.33\ \text{g mol}^{-1})}{6.022 \times 10^{23}\ \text{mol}^{-1}} = 4.561 \times 10^{-22}\ \text{g} .$$

Thus: $\rho = \frac{M}{V} = 3.595\ \text{g cm}^{-3}$.

16.24 Cadmium has a hcp cell with a = 2.979 Å, c = 5.618 Å. Calculate its density.

The hcp cell has a volume

$$V = abc[1 - \cos^2\alpha - \cos^2\beta - \cos^2\gamma + 2\cos\alpha\cos\beta\cos\gamma]^{1/2} .$$

With $a = b = 2.979$ Å , $c = 5.618$ Å , $\alpha = \beta = 90°$ and $\gamma = 120°$, we find $V = 4.317 \times 10^{-23}\ \text{cm}^3$. The cell contains 2 Cd atoms with mass $M = \frac{2(112.41\ \text{g mol}^{-1})}{6.022 \times 10^{23}\ \text{mol}^{-1}} = 3.733 \times 10^{-22}\ \text{g}$. Hence

$$\rho = \frac{M}{V} = 8.65\ \text{g cm}^{-3} .$$

16.25 Show that the Fermi energy for a metal containing N free (conduction) electrons per unit volume is:

$$E_F = \left(\frac{h^2}{8m_e}\right)\left(\frac{3N}{\pi}\right)^{2/3}$$

Estimate this quantity for sodium (density: 0.97 g/cm³).

For a particle in a 3-dimensional box: $E = \dfrac{(n_x^2 + n_y^2 + n_z^2)h^2}{8ma^2}$.

Let $n = (n_x^2 + n_y^2 + n_z^2)^{1/2}$ and $a^2 = V^{2/3}$ so that: $E = \dfrac{n^2h^2}{8mV^{2/3}}$.

Now $n = n_F$ at $E = E_F$ with N electrons in a volume V. The "volume" in "n" space will be $\left(\dfrac{4\pi n_F^3}{3}\right)\dfrac{1}{8} = \dfrac{NV}{2}$ ($\frac{1}{8}$ due to positive octant only, $\frac{N}{2}$ because of electron spin + or -). Thus:

$n_F^3 = \dfrac{3NV}{\pi}$ and $E_F = \dfrac{h^2}{8m}\left[\dfrac{3N}{\pi}\right]^{2/3}$. For sodium, with one valence electron per atom: $\dfrac{N}{L} = \dfrac{\rho}{MW} = (0.97 \text{ g cm}^{-3})\left(\dfrac{1}{22.99 \text{ g mol}^{-1}}\right)$.

$N = 2.54 \times 10^{22}$ e- cm^{-3} . Thus

$$E_F = \frac{h^2}{8m}\left[\frac{3N}{\pi}\right]^{2/3} = 5.049 \times 10^{-12} \text{ erg} = 3.15 \text{ eV} .$$

16.26 Estimate the lowest energy absorption for an F-center electron in a KCl lattice by using a particle-in-a-box model and assuming a cube size into which a Cl^- could be inscribed. The transition is observed around 2.6 eV = 21000 cm^{-1}.

For the particle in a box: $E = (n_x^2 + n_y^2 + n_z^2)\dfrac{h^2}{8ma^2}$. The lowest energy transition will thus correspond to:

$$\Delta E = \frac{3h^2}{8ma^2} = \frac{3(6.626 \times 10^{-27} \text{ erg s})^2}{8(9.109 \times 10^{-28} \text{ g})(3.62 \times 10^{-8} \text{ cm})^2}$$

$$\Delta E = 1.379 \times 10^{-11} \text{ erg s} = 1.379 \times 10^{-21} \text{ J} = 830.4 \text{ kJ mol}^{-1}$$

$$\Delta E = 8.60 \text{ eV} .$$

16.27 Draw a stress-strain diagram to illustrate the following characteristics of a material: initial modulus, yield stress, tensile strength, and ultimate strain.

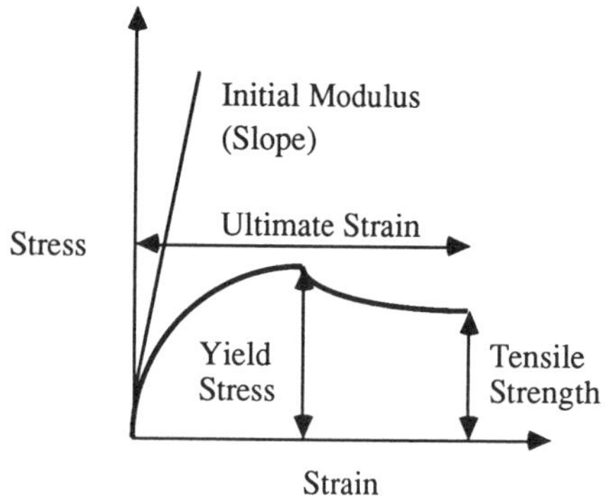

16.28 Which panel of Figure 16.39 would most nearly represent the behavior of household glass?

Panel (b); glass is rigid and brittle.

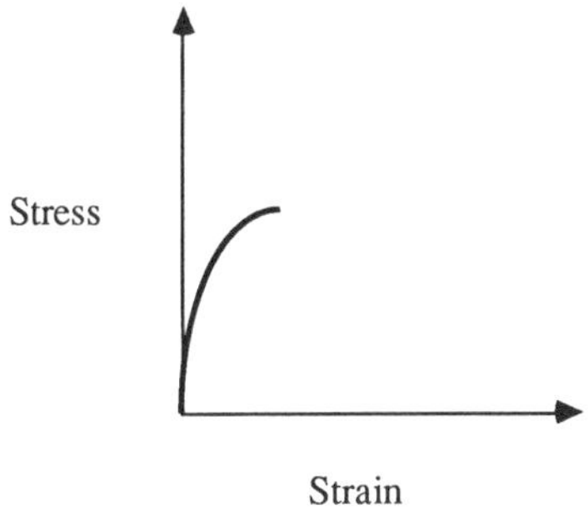

16.29 Use data in Table 16.6 to estimate the carbon chemical shifts to methyl groups on branches on polyethylene assuming branch lengths of 1, 2, 3, 4. What will happen for longer chains?

a)

```
                    CH3
                    |
... CH2 - CH2 - CH - CH2 - CH2 ...
```

$\delta = 8.85 + 2(9.51) + 2(-2.34) + 2(0.28) + 2(0.03) + (-0.96) - 2.35$

$\delta = 20.5$ ppm .

b)

```
                    CH3
                    |
                    CH2
                    |
... CH2 - CH2 - CH - CH2 - CH2 ...
```

$\delta = 8.85 + 9.51 + 2(-2.34) + 2(0.28) + 2(0.03) - 2.35$

$\delta = 11.8$ ppm .

c)

$$
\begin{array}{c}
CH_3 \\
| \\
CH_2 \\
| \\
CH_2 \\
| \\
\ldots\ CH_2 - CH - CH_2\ \ldots
\end{array}
$$

$\delta = 8.85 + 9.51 - 2.34 + 2(0.28) + 2(0.03) - 2.35 = 14.3$ ppm .

d)

$$
\begin{array}{c}
CH_3 \\
| \\
CH_2 \\
| \\
CH_2 \\
| \\
\ldots\ CH_2 - CH_2 - CH - CH_2 - CH_2\ \ldots
\end{array}
$$

$\delta = 8.85 + 9.51 - 2.34 + 0.28 + 2(0.03) - 2.35 = 14.0$ ppm .

16.30 Use data in Table 16.6 to estimate the chemical shifts of the three distinct carbons of polypropylene (ignoring tacticity effects).

```
... CH2 - CH - CH2 - CH - CH2 - CH - CH2 ...
          |         |         |
          CH3       CH3       CH3
```

methine:

$$\delta = 3(8.85) + 2(9.51) + 4(-2.34) + 2(0.28) + 4(0.03) + 2(-3.04) - 2.35$$

$$\delta = 28.5 \text{ ppm} .$$

methylene:

$$\delta = 2(8.85) + 4(9.51) + 2(-2.34) + 4(0.28) + 2(0.03) + 2(-2.11) - 2.35$$

$$\delta = 45.7 \text{ ppm} .$$

methyl:

$$\delta = 8.85 + 2(9.51) + 2(-2.34) + 4(0.28) + 2(0.03) + (-0.96) - 2.35$$

$$\delta = 21.1 \text{ ppm} .$$

16.31 In a carbon NMR spectrum of a branched polyethylene, the area of the methine peak was 15 and the area of the peak at 30 ppm was 747 (arbitrary units). Calculate the percent branching and the average run length.

The % branching is:

$$100\left(\frac{I_{38}}{I_{30} + 7I_{38}}\right) = 100\left(\frac{15}{747 + 7(15)}\right) = 1.76\% .$$

The average run length is: $\left(\frac{I_{30} + 6I_{38}}{I_{38}}\right) = \frac{747 + 6(15)}{15} = 56$.

16.32 In an isotactic polypropylene, a change in stereochemistry occurs every 100 units (i.e., the average run length is 100):

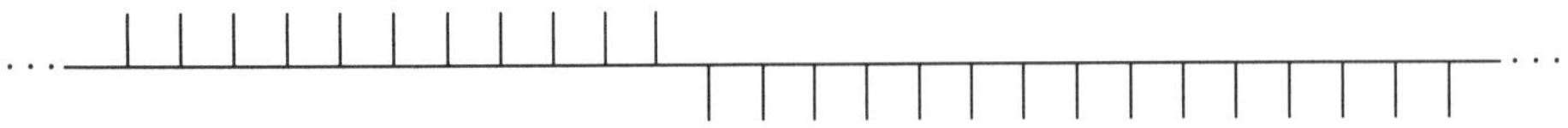

(Such an error suggests that the catalyst is sensitive only to the relative stereochemistry of the unit being added—see next problem.) List the tetrad sequences that would be observed, and their relative probabilities. For which carbon would these sequences be measurable from carbon NMR?

There are 99 m's followed by 1 r: etc. ← mmrmm → etc. Per 100 units, we would count 1 mrm, 2 mmr and 97 mmm groups. Relative stereochemistry is "visible" through NMR. Methylene carbon would "see" two possible environments:

Meso:

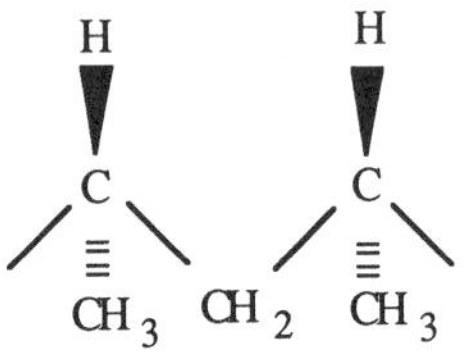

or

Racemic:

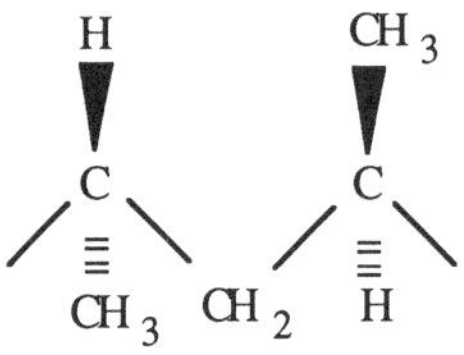

16.33 Repeat the previous problem assuming the error is:

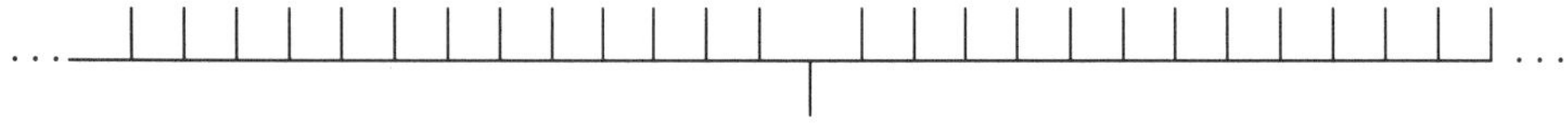

(Such an error suggests that the catalyst is sensitive to the absolute stereochemistry of the monomer units.)

In this case, there are 98 m's followed by 2 r's: etc. ← mmmrrmmm → etc. Per 100 units, we would count 2 mrr, 2 mmr, and 96 mmm groups.

16.34 Calculate the pentad sequences expected for the propylene chain of the previous two problems. Which carbon would show such features in its NMR spectrum?

```
For the sequence:   ← mmmmrmmmm →  we would count 2 mmmr,

2 mmrm, and 96 mmmm groups per 100 units.  For the sequence:

← mmmrrmmm →  we would count 2 mmmr, 2 mmrr, 1 mrrm, and

95 mmmm groups per 100 units.
```

16.35 Consider a random copolymer of 1-butene (B) and ethylene (E). (a) Use data in Table 16.6 to estimate the methine chemical shift for the center unit of the sequences: BBB, EBB, EBE. (Ignore the ε correction, for which you'd have to know the next unit in sequence.) (b) What would be the expected relative intensities of these resonances in a 50:50 random copolymer? (c) What would be the expected relative intensities of these resonances in a 50:50 copolymer assuming a block copolymer sequence length of 10 (only)?

```
CH2 = CH - CH2 - CH3     (1-butene)

CH2 = CH2                (ethylene)
```

a) BBB:

```
        CH3          CH3          CH3
         |            |            |
        CH2          CH2          CH2
         |            |            |
 ... CH2 - CH - CH2 - CH - CH2 - CH - ...
```

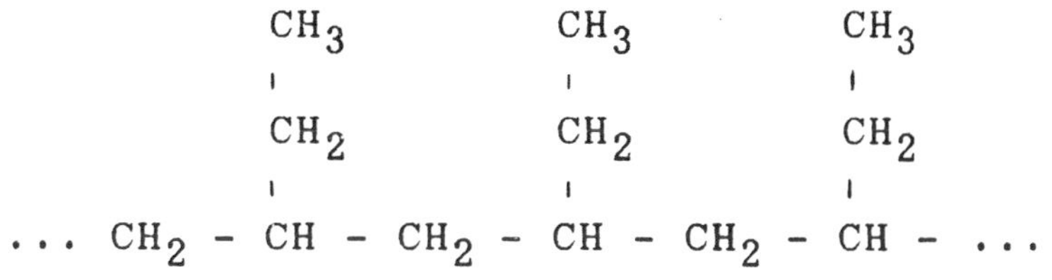

```
The methine resonance is:

   δ(BBB) = 3(8.85) + 3(9.51) + 4(-2.34) + 4(0.28) - 3(3.04) -
            2.35

   δ(BBB) = 35.4 ppm .
```

EBB:

```
                    CH3          CH3
                     |            |
                    CH2          CH2
                     |            |
 ... CH2 - CH2 - CH2 - CH - CH2 - CH - ...
```

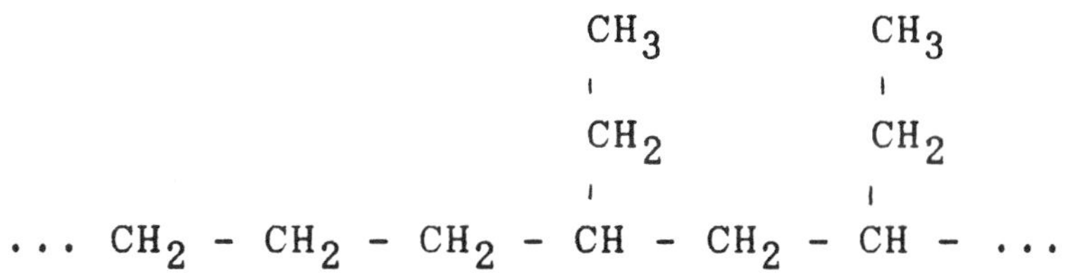

$\delta(EBB) = 3(8.85) + 3(9.51) + 3(-2.34) + 3(0.28) - 3(3.04) - 2.35$

$\delta(BBB) = 37.4$ ppm .

EBE:

$$
\begin{array}{c}
CH_3 \\
| \\
CH_2 \\
| \\
\cdots CH_2 - CH_2 - CH_2 - CH - CH_2 - CH_2 \cdots
\end{array}
$$

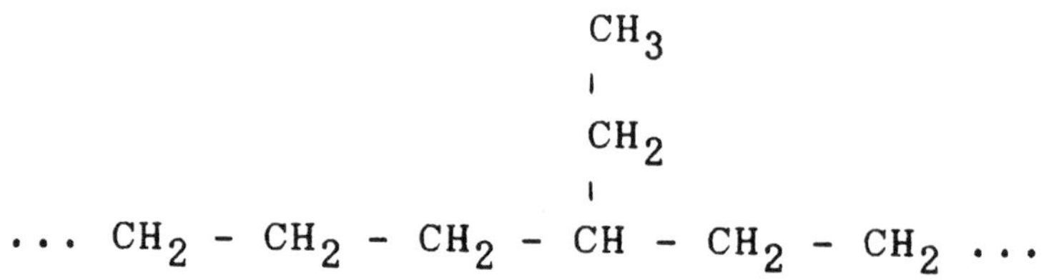

$\delta(EBE) = 3(8.85) + 3(9.51) + 2(-2.34) + 2(0.28) - 3(3.04) - 2.35$

$\delta(BBB) = 39.5$ ppm .

b)   Probability of B = 0.5 .   Probability of E = 0.5 .

Occurrences are random, so that relative intensities are:

$f = \sum n_i P_i$ where n_i = degeneracy of ith permutation .

$f(BBB) = (0.5)^3 = 0.125$ (1)

$f(EBB) = 2(0.5)^3 = 0.25$ (2)

$f(EBE) = (0.5)^3 = 0.125$ (1)

Thus we expect 1:2:1 relative intensities.

c)   Block copolymer: (10 B's) ... BBBEEE ... (10 E's) .

$f(BBB) = 8$ (4)

$f(EBB) = f(BEE) = 2$ (1)

$f(EBE) = 0$ (0)

Relative intensities are 4:1:0 .

16.36 Draw the chain structure for a polyester made from *p*-hydroxybenzoic acid. What type of properties would you expect for this material if it is drawn into a fiber? (Compare to the materials illustrated on Figure 16.52.)

Water is removed in polymerization.

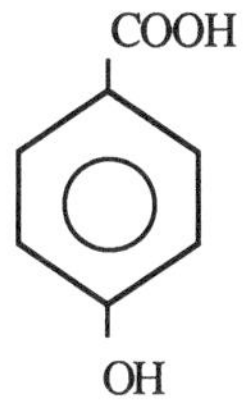

p-hydroxybenzoic acid

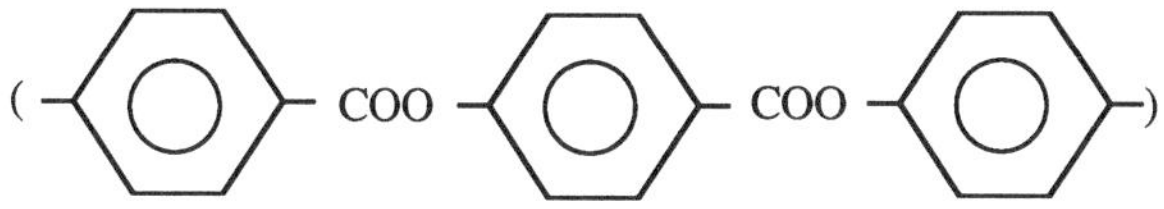

16.37 What is the SI unit for *compliance?*

The compliance is the reciprocal of the modulus. The modulus has units of $\left(\frac{\text{force}}{\text{area}}\right)$ so that SI units of the compliance are thus: $\frac{\text{area}}{\text{force}} = \frac{m^2}{N} = \frac{m^2}{kg\ m\ s^{-2}} = \frac{m\ s^2}{kg}$.